MANAGEMENT OF THE
Hypertensive
Patient

MANAGEMENT OF THE
Hypertensive Patient

LAWRENCE R. KRAKOFF, M.D.

Professor
Department of Medicine
Mount Sinai School of Medicine
of the City University of New York
New York, New York
Chief
Department of Medicine
Englewood Hospital
Englewood, New Jersey

Churchill Livingstone

New York, Edinburgh, London, Madrid, Melbourne, Milan, Tokyo

Library of Congress Cataloging-in-Publication Data

Krakoff, Lawrence R. (Lawrence Richard), date
    Management of the hypertensive patient / Lawrence R. Krakoff
        p.   cm.
    Includes bibliographical references and index.
    ISBN 0–443–08769–5
    1. Hypertension. I. Title.
    [DNLM: 1. Hypertension—prevention and control. 2. Hypertension—
diagnosis.   WG 340 K89m 1994]
    RC685.H8K73 1995
    616.1′32—dc20
    DNLM/DLC
    for Library of Congress   94–31119
                                              CIP

Distributed in the United Kingdom by Churchill Livingstone, Robert Stevenson House, 1–3 Baxter's Place, Leith Walk, Edinburgh EH1 3AF, and by associated companies, branches, and representatives throughout the world.

Accurate indications, adverse reactions, and dosage schedules for drugs are provided in this book, but it is possible that they may change. The reader is urged to review the package information data of the manufacturers of the medications mentioned.

The Publishers have made every effort to trace the copyright holders for borrowed material. If they have inadvertently overlooked any, they will be pleased to make the necessary arrangements at the first opportunity.

Acquisitions Editor: *Jennifer Mitchell*
Copy Editor: *Bridgett L. Dickinson*
Production Supervisor: *Christina Hippeli*
Desktop Coordinator: *Robb Quattro*
Cover Design: *Paul Moran*

Printed in the United States of America

First published in 1995   7 6 5 4 3 2 1

PREFACE

Systemic arterial hypertension (high blood pressure) is the most prevalent reversible cause of cardiovascular morbidity and mortality in adult populations of Western societies. This conclusion is supported by extensive epidemiologic surveys and by the results of a variety of randomized clinical trials. In the past 40 years, rapid progress has been made in understanding the pathophysiology, natural history, and treatment of high blood pressure. Development of many new and effective diagnostic and therapeutic methods has paralleled or followed the advances in basic science.

Applying the science and epidemiology of hypertension to the diagnosis and treatment of any one patient has become complex, yet it is the day-to-day activity of most internists and primary care physicians, cardiologists, nephrologists and endocrinologists. As new diagnostic modalities and therapies (invasive and pharmacologic) have proliferated, so has the need for careful reasoning and rational decisions in patient management.

Management of the Hypertensive Patient is addressed to the thinking physician as a guide for sorting out the decisions and strategy necessary for optimal treatment of each patient. It is based on the hypothesis that diseases and risk factors are abstractions, based in recent years on statistical simplifications that are valid but that fail to convey important differences between one patient and another. By contrast, the clinician often recognizes differences and heterogeneity. Through discerning the patient's individual characteristics, recalling past experience from training onward, and searching the separate knowledge bases of current literature, physicians can merge the requirements of science with the skill of the expert and compassionate craftsman for the patient's best interest.

When so very much has been written on hypertension, is another book needed? I believe it is because of the many and varied questions raised by clinicians whenever I lecture or talk shop with working doctors. Despite the more than 70,000 journal articles, 100 or more existing texts, innumerable reviews, chapters, audiovisual sets, videotapes, televised sessions, and postgraduate programs devoted to hypertension, the same questions tend to be asked. They are good questions, reflecting both curiosity and concern, that are not entirely satisfied by the enormous body of literature available to the physician, who has far too little time and energy to grapple with it.

Management of the Hypertensive Patient is devoted to those doctors who treat hypertensive patients. It is intended as a guide and will, I hope, be a companion. The current literature is referred to, but as a basis for strategy not as a set of lists to be memorized. The approach is based on science, while recognizing that science is abstract and faceless; patients are here, now and individual. No one literature source can be sufficient. Familiarity with a recent textbook of medicine, the journals of the previous month, and a good reference librarian or computer search system[1] are always necessary. Finally, our learning resources must include each patient. They (still) trust us to provide our best judgment on their behalf.

The management of hypertensive patients is part of preventive cardiology. Those patients who benefit from not suffering a stroke or experiencing a myocardial infarct rely on our confidence and security in the choices made for them. Frankly, I admire the many patients who do comply with our advice. Their trust and recognition of our effort should be a source of satisfaction equal to the diagnostic coup or surgical tour-de-force our colleagues sometimes achieve.

A few words about figures and diagrams. Several figures have been chosen because they clearly add important information or present crucial concepts better than a table or text could. In addition, I have provided line drawings and flow diagrams of my own as semiquantitative decision trees. Most of these I have found useful in my lectures in teaching medical students or postgraduate physicians.

Finally, what about references? There are simply too many to include in a book of this size and purpose. Where possible, I have chosen to list either the original publication or the most pertinent recent series published in widely respected, peer-reviewed journals. Little emphasis has been given to the 16th report that the wheel is indeed round. Reviews that add something have been included; reviews of reviews have been avoided. Meta-analyses are a recent development and are useful for furnishing a quantified summary of several trials.[2] They have their own pitfalls, however, and must not be considered as free from bias or invariably settling an issue.[3] There are those who would resolve a controversy by simply comparing the number of publications pro and con (the bean counting technique), avoiding the intellectual effort of grappling with the issues. This is not good medicine and is only a means of avoiding our contract with our patients to use the best of our abilities to address their health.

Where controversy exists and reference sources can be found for both sides of an important issue, I have tried to be fair, but give a rationale for my own conclusions. You, the reader, may well disagree and seek your own interpretation in relationship to the problem at hand. I congratulate you for the effort and hope my views are worthy of consideration as a basis for development of an alternate conclusion.

The goal of *Management of the Hypertensive Patient* is to provide the framework, using pertinent medical research as the guiding rationale, for management of hypertensive patients. In many areas, it agrees with current consensus reports and guidelines. In other areas, I provide my approach and the basis for that direction. Whether or not the reader agrees with my views, the time taken to consider the matter and reach a balanced conclusion will, without doubt, serve well the patient whose physician seeks a better answer.

Lawrence R. Krakoff, M.D.

REFERENCES

1. Wyatt J: Use and sources of medical knowledge. Lancet 338:1368, 1991

2. Lau J, Antman EM, Jimenez-Silva J et al: Cumulative meta-analysis of therapeutic trials for myocardial infarction. N Engl J Med 327:248, 1992

3. Thompson SG, Pocock SJ: Can meta-analyses be trusted? Lancet 338:1127, 1991

CONTENTS

Section IV   Special Problems

Section I

CLINICAL SCIENCE OF HYPERTENSION

Schema for Analysis of Clinical Hypertension

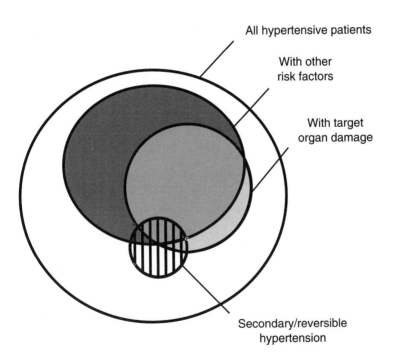

All hypertensive patients

With other
risk factors

With target
organ damage

Secondary/reversible
hypertension

1

DEFINITIONS

The term *hypertension* has become widely used, not only in medicine, but also in the health-related publications of the newspapers, popular press, and media. The public may interpret *hypertension* as something to do with stress or tension as ordinarily meant. In clinical medicine, however, a clear and consistent definition is necessary.

In this book, *hypertension* refers to high systemic arterial pressure. By *high,* I mean elevated enough for the physician to be concerned with the diagnosis of an underlying cause and to consider treatment because of the level of arterial pressure itself. Many other terms used to subdivide hypertension into more meaningful categories have found their way into the medical literature. They are defined, as ordinarily used by clinicians, in this chapter.

A broad range of systolic and diastolic arterial pressures is found in large surveys of adult populations. While these two pressures are generally correlated, there are instances when one or the other is sufficiently elevated for the term *systolic hypertension* or *diastolic hypertension* to be used. In the United States commonly accepted upper limits of normal are 140 mmHg for systolic pressure and 90 mmHg for diastolic pressure.[1] As of this writing, other countries and international advisory groups are increasingly accepting these limits.

The risks of cerebrovascular disease and coronary heart disease increase directly with the level of arterial pressure.[2] No clearly demarcated dividing line is yet established or generally accepted that marks the point at which increased risk of future cardiovascular disease begins so that a diagnosis of *hypertension* remains, to some extent, arbitrary. However, epidemiologic evidence suggests that adult systolic pressures below 130 mmHg and diastolic pressures below 85 mmHg convey minimal risk. The recognized range of *borderline* or *high normal* pressures is 130 to 140 mmHg for systolic pressure and 85 to 95 mmHg for diastolic pressure.

Elderly patients often have disproportionately increased systolic pressures (greater than 160 mmHg) when diastolic pressure is near or below 90 mmHg; this is called *isolated systolic hypertension* of the elderly. This condition is clearly related to increased cardiovascular mortality and morbidity; a clinical trial (Systolic Hypertension in the Elderly Program[3]) to establish whether antihypertensive therapy may reduce the risk of this disorder has recently been completed. Some elderly patients have apparent excessive elevation of their systolic pressure that, due to calcification of the arteries, is falsely high when determined by the occlusive cuff and auscultation (i.e., *pseudohypertension*).[4]

In younger subjects, a predominantly elevated systolic pressure with a normal diastolic pressure (e.g., 150/70 mmHg) may indicate a cardiovascular disorder with high cardiac output such as hyperthyroidism, anemia, or arteriovenous shunting. Aortic insufficiency may also cause a wide pulse pressure with elevated systolic pressure and normal or low diastolic pressure.

In children normal, borderline or high normal pressures, and hypertension are largely based on population-based norms for blood pressure distribution, defining those above the 90th and 95th percentiles as hypertensive.[5]

The likelihood of future cardiovascular morbidity is directly related to the height of the arterial pressure. It is useful to divide hypertension into several categories based on the level of pressure before treatment. All such classifications are somewhat arbitrary and use dividing lines that are convenient and easy to remember rather than precise (e.g., 90 rather than 91). The most recent scheme, advised in *The Fifth Report of the Joint National Committee on Detection, Evaluation and Treatment of High Blood Pressure*,[1] is shown in Table 1-1. Both systolic and diastolic pressures are included in determining the level of severity.

Morbid events due to cardiovascular, renal, and neurologic diseases are not invariably observed in those with hypertension. The term *uncomplicated* or *benign* hypertension refers to a stage before any such morbidity. Hypertension complicated by a cerebrovascular accident, CHD, renal insufficiency, or congestive heart failure conveys a greater risk to survival and the need for a more complex therapeutic strategy.

Malignant or *accelerated* hypertension refers to the combination of markedly elevated arterial pressure (usually diastolic pressure of 130 mmHg or higher), history of a recent increase in pressure, and retinal hemorrhage, exudate, and papilledema. Neurologic dysfunction or *hypertensive encephalopathy* may be present. Often there is evidence of left ventricular hypertrophy and strain (seen on the electrocardiogram) with pulmonary congestion due to left ventricular

Table 1-1. Classification of Blood Pressure for Adults 18 Years of Age or Older

	Systolic Range (mmHg)	Diastolic Range (mmHg)
Normal	<130	<85
High normal	130–139	85–89
Hypertensive		
Mild (stage 1)	140–159	90–99
Moderate (stage 2)	160–179	100–109
Severe (stage 3)	180–209	110–119
Very severe (stage 4)	>210	>120

The recommendation of the Joint National Committee on Detection and Treatment of Hypertension is that if systolic and diastolic pressures fall into different categories the *higher* category be used (e.g., 161/92 is considered stage 2 or moderate hypertension). Caution is needed, since the systolic pressure is likely to be more variable and less stable over time. Many patients will have a fall in either systolic or diastolic pressure over several months without treatment and thus "re-stage" themselves. Furthermore, *stage* is best used for an overall assessment of risk and concurrent morbidity, rather than for the level of pressure alone.

(From Joint National Committee on Detection and Treatment of Hypertension.[1])

decompensation. Proteinuria, microscopic or gross hematuria on urinalysis, and renal insufficiency (increased serum urea nitrogen and creatinine concentrations) may also be present. Malignant hypertension may occur in the course of inadequately treated essential hypertension or as a complication of chronic renal disease. It is characteristic of scleroderma renal crisis and may also occur in the course of secondary hypertension due to renal artery stenosis or pheochromocytoma. Strictly speaking, then, malignant hypertension is a phase or complicating event of severe hypertension.

Hypertension is, per se, a nonspecific finding. It may be the result of a specific detectable and reversible disorder and is, thus, *secondary* or may occur without any evident cause, termed *essential, primary,* or *idiopathic.* For the rest of this chapter and those that follow the term *essential hypertension* refers to those who have high blood pressure without obvious or detectable cause.

A recent entry in the vocabulary of hypertension is *white coat hypertension,* referring to the elevated pressure some persons experience only in the clinic or office, precipitated by the physician's presence but absent outside the medical setting.[6,7] In general, it is the average or usual arterial pressures that are best related to long-term risk.[2] However, the independent effects associated with episodic elevations in pressure or highly variable pressure can now be assessed by ambulatory blood pressure monitoring and may also contribute to cardiovascular risk.[8] Because of the trend toward a higher incidence of fatal and nonfatal myocardial infarctions in the morning hours, there is recent interest in diurnal variation in pressure and heart rate. In particular, the rapid increase in arterial pressure and heart rate that occur during the early phase of awakening (usually in the morning) is a subject of active research.[9–11]

The preceding terms form the nomenclature used in the discussions of the epidemiology, natural history, pathophysiology, diagnosis, and management of both essential and secondary hypertension presented in the following sections (Table 1-2).

Table 1-2. Summary of Terms

Hypertension
Systolic hypertension
Diastolic hypertension
Isolated systolic hypertension (ISH)
Pseudohypertension
Borderline blood pressure
Secondary hypertension
Essential or primary hypertension
Mild, moderate, or severe hypertension
High blood pressure
Systemic arterial hypertension
White coat hypertension
Malignant or accelerated hypertension
Hypertensive encephalopathy
Benign or complicated hypertension

REFERENCES

1. Joint National Committee on Detection and Treatment of Hypertension: The Fifth Report of the Joint National Committee on Detection, Evaluation and Treatment of High Blood Pressure (JNC V). Arch Intern Med 153:154, 1993

2. MacMahon S, Peto R, Cutler J et al: Blood pressure, stroke, and coronary heart disease. Part 1. Prolonged differences in blood pressure: prospective observational studies corrected for the regression dilution bias. Lancet 335:765, 1990

3. Systolic Hypertension in the Elderly Program Cooperative Research Group: Prevention of stroke by antihypertensive drug treatment in older persons with isolated systolic hypertension: final results of the Systolic Hypertension in the Elderly Program (SHEP). JAMA 265:3255, 1991

4. Messerli FH, Ventura HO, Amodeo C: Osler's maneuver and pseudohypertension. N Engl J Med 312:1548, 1985

5. Kaplan NM: Clinical Hypertension. 4th Ed. Williams & Wilkins, Baltimore, 1986

6. Mancia G, Bertinieri G, Grassi G et al: Effects of blood pressure measurement by the doctor on patient's blood pressure and heart rate. Lancet 2:695, 1983

7. Pickering TG, James GD, Boddie C et al: How common is white coat hypertension? JAMA 259:225, 1988

8. Parati G, Pomidossi G, Albini F et al: Relationship of 24-hour blood pressure mean and variability to severity of target-organ damage in hypertension. J Hypertens 5:93, 1987

9. Mitler MM, Hajdukovic RM, Shafor R et al: When people die. Cause of death versus time of death. Am J Med 82:266, 1987

10. Tofler GH, Brezinski D, Schafer AI et al: Concurrent morning increase in platelet aggregability and the risk of myocardial infarction and sudden cardiac death. N Engl J Med 316:1514, 1987

11. Muller JE, Toffler GH: Circadian variation and cardiovascular disease. N Engl J Med 325:1038, 1991

2

EPIDEMIOLOGY

This is a short chapter, despite the enormous number of publications dealing with the epidemiology of hypertension. The rationale for this brevity lies in the very simple notion that clinicians treat individual patients for whom the statistical trends evident in the epidemiology of hypertension convey a small number of fairly straightforward and well-characterized concepts. First, the blood pressures of populations vary over a wide range and are roughly normally distributed (i.e., a bell-shaped curve) if the frequency of a given pressure range is plotted against the level of pressure, as shown in Figure 2-1 (middle panel).[1]

From country to country, the position and width of the bell curve or population distribution may be different, especially at the higher (hypertensive) end; for adults, the prevalence of hypertension in China may be nearly 4 percent and in the United States it may be nearly 20 percent. Nonetheless, given the usual criteria for high blood pressure, there are plenty of hypertensive patients to evaluate and treat. This book does not address the concerns of the health care planner who must confront a population-wide problem and then be concerned about whether one population has a few or many more hypertensive people than another.

Next, it is evident that in Western societies arterial pressure tends to increase with age, more so for systolic than for diastolic pressure. This was identified nearly 50 years ago and has been amply confirmed[2] (Fig. 2-2).

The basis for the age-related disproportionate increase in systolic arterial pressure noted in Western societies is both well and poorly understood. The increased stiffness, or reduced large artery compliance, that occurs with the decades of adult life has been recognized since the 1930s[2] and is accompanied by progressive structural changes, fibrosis, and varying degrees of calcification. Weight gain, coupled with a high normal blood pressure, clearly indicates the likelihood of an increase in blood pressure with age.[3] Diet salt intake may play some small, but detectable role in the age-related increase in pressure.[4]

For the most part, however, the basic mechanisms accounting for progressive stiffness of the large arteries remain uncertain. No doubt obesity, diet, lack of exercise, alcohol use, smoking, diabetes, serum lipid or lipoprotein patterns, and behavioral factors participate to some extent.[5] Genetic predispositions must be considered as well.[6–8] Nonetheless, all these are merely imprecise correlates of arterial pressure in large statistical surveys. There is, however, little doubt that the elevation of systolic pressure in older patients is well correlated with cardiovascular risk, whether or not the diastolic pressure is elevated.[9]

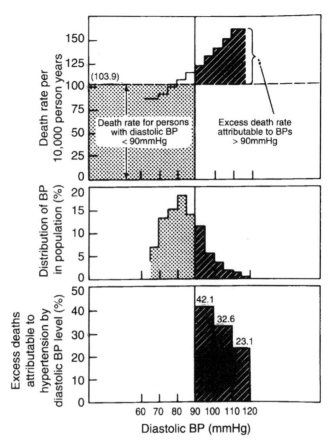

Fig. 2-1. Relationship between the frequency distribution of diastolic blood pressure from an "at home" screen of 158,906 subjects (center panel) and the predicted risk of mortality as death rate (upper panel) or fraction of excess deaths due to untreated hypertension. BP, blood pressure. (From Hypertension Detection and Follow-Up Program Cooperative Group,[1] with permission.)

Another well-recognized facet of the epidemiology of hypertension is that definable causes (i.e., secondary hypertension) affect a very small fraction of persons with elevated blood pressure. No more than 5 percent of those considered hypertensive have either chronic renal disease or one of the rare or reversible forms of hypertension.

What is most important about the epidemiology of arterial pressure to the clinician is the relationship between the height of either systolic or diastolic pressure and the risk of future cardiovascular disease. It is now readily apparent that the higher the pressure the greater the risk of stroke or coronary heart disease (CHD). This is readily apparent in Figure 2-2.

Figure 2-3 portrays the relationship between diastolic pressure and the risk of either stroke or CHD as derived from a meta-analysis of several large prospective surveys, mostly performed before the widespread application of antihypertensive drug treatment.[10] To me, it is the last word on this subject.

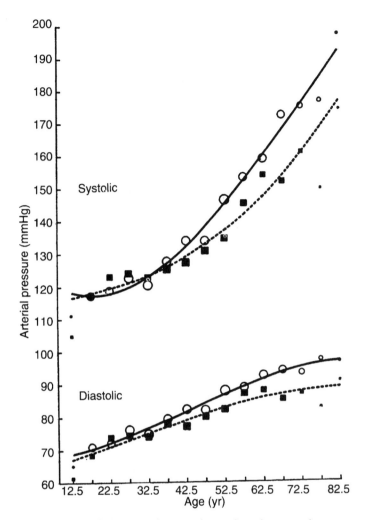

Fig. 2-2. Relationship between either systolic or diastolic arterial pressure and age in an untreated population from studies conducted in the United Kingdom. Open circles, females; closed squares, males. (From Pickering,[2] with permission.)

The importance of Figure 2-3 lies in three major points. First, the *slope* of the curves is different. The relationship between pressure and stroke is steeper than for CHD. In other words, for any given increase or decrease in pressure, it is expected that there will be a greater or smaller likelihood of stroke than of CHD. The expected benefit of blood pressure reduction will be different for these two different kinds of morbidity. Next, the margin of error (shaded boxes) in the relationship between pressure and stroke is smaller than for CHD. This agrees with many studies reporting that CHD is far more multifactorial than is stroke. This again predicts that a reduction in pressure alone might have different effects on either stroke or CHD. Finally, the legend includes the phrase, *usual diastolic pressure,* which comes from the use of several years of data from the Framingham study. Analysis of the data in the

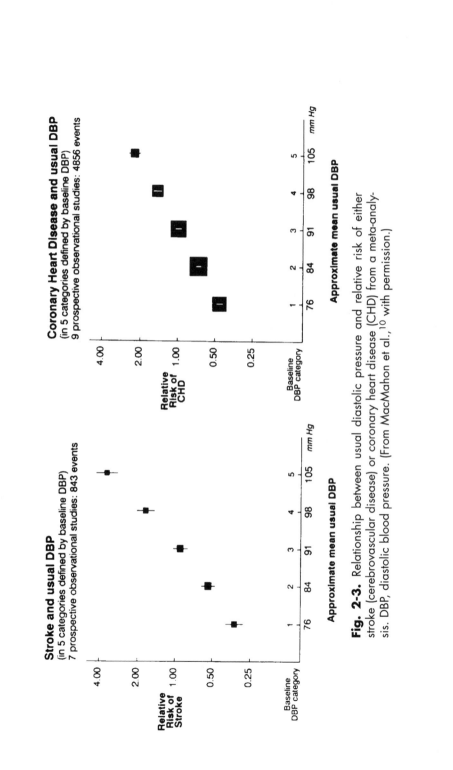

Fig. 2-3. Relationship between usual diastolic pressure and relative risk of either stroke (cerebrovascular disease) or coronary heart disease (CHD) from a meta-analysis. DBP, diastolic blood pressure. (From MacMahon et al.,[10] with permission.)

study indicates that "regression dilution" can decrease by not basing predictions on only a few measurements at baseline or entry. The *usual pressure* concept clearly implies that it is the long-term average level of pressure that is most tightly correlated with risk; it is less precise if only one or two clinical measurements are considered. This concept requires physicians to determine the *usual* pressure, through various methods, particularly for patients with high normal pressure or mild hypertension. The various methods are (1) longer observation periods, 3 to 6 months, before starting treatment[11]; (2) greater use of home and work-site pressure measurements, which are then averaged[12]; and (3) increased exploration of noninvasive ambulatory blood pressure monitoring. The latter is the best justified method or gold standard for the estimate of usual pressure.[13]

While the relationship between blood pressure and risk of either stroke or CHD is well quantified due to the large number of studies and the frequency of these forms of cardiovascular morbidity, hypertension is also an established risk factor for other, less common, morbidities. Severe hypertension leads to congestive heart failure, aortic dissection or abdominal aneurysm, and, to some extent, progression of chronic renal disease (particularly in diabetic patients). Together with other risk factors, hypertension may also contribute to the development of peripheral arterial occlusive disease.[14]

Often, chapters on the epidemiology of hypertension digress into the epidemiology of the other known risk factors, such as smoking, elevated serum low-density lipoprotein cholesterol, low high-density lipoprotein cholesterol, diabetes, and more recently described disorders. These can be summarized as nonhypertensive risk factors since their presence confers a greater likelihood of cardiovascular disease, whether or not the blood pressure is elevated. In general, these factors do not themselves elevate arterial pressure and are found in many normotensive people. For any one patient, cardiovascular risk correlates best to the number of risk factors present and to their quantitative effect, as is well defined in the many publications from the Framingham Study.[3] For groups of subjects, these quantitative effects are predictive and provide the rationale for management of individual patients. Nonetheless, individual patients do not always follow group trends. Some patients with high pressure and other risk factors develop little or no cardiovascular disease despite poor control. Others develop cardiovascular disease with few risk factors or with minimal deviation from normal. Most CHD still occurs in those with mild hypertension and serum cholesterol concentrations slightly above average. Thus, we have much to learn before *precise* predictions can be made for many individuals considered at risk because of elevated blood pressure with or without the presence of the nonhypertensive risk factors now identified.

These are then the most important concepts the epidemiology of hypertension has for the physician who will screen, evaluate, and manage individual patients with varying levels of arterial pressure, degrees of target organ pathology, an array of other risk factors, and, in some instances, a specific cause of the elevated pressure.

REFERENCES

1. Hypertension Detection and Follow-Up Program Cooperative Group: The Hypertension Detection and Follow-Up Program: a progress report. Circ Res, suppl. 1. 40:106, 1977

2. Pickering G: The Nature of Essential Hypertension. Grune & Stratton, New York, 1961

3. Leitschuh M, Cupples LA, Kannel W et al: High-normal blood pressure progression to hypertension in the Framingham Heart Study. Hypertension 17:22, 1991

4. Intersalt Cooperative Research Group: Intersalt: an international study of electrolyte excretion and blood pressure. Results for 24 hour urinary sodium and potassium excretion. BMJ 297:319, 1988

5. Beilin LJ: The fifth Sir George Pickering memorial lecture: epitaph to essential hypertension—a preventable disorder of known aetiology? J Hypertens 6:85, 1988

6. Watt GCM, Harrap SB, Foy CJW et al: Abnormalities of glucocorticoid metabolism and the renin-angiotensin system: a four-corners approach to the identification of genetic determinants of blood pressure. J Hypertens 10:473, 1992

7. Morris BJ: Identification of essential hypertension genes. J Hypertens 11:115, 1993

8. Lifton RP, Jeunemaitre X: Finding genes that cause human hypertension. J Hypertens 11:231, 1993

9. Lichtenstein MJ, Shipley MJ, Rose G: Systolic and diastolic blood pressure as predictors of coronary heart mortality in the Whitehall study. BMJ 291:243, 1985

10. MacMahon S, Peto R, Cutler J et al: Blood pressure, stroke, and coronary heart disease. Part 1. Prolonged differences in blood pressure: prospective observational studies corrected for the regression dilution bias. Lancet 335:765, 1990

11. Pearce KA, Grimm RH, Rao S et al: Population-derived comparisons of ambulatory and office blood pressures: implications for the determination of usual blood pressure and the concept of white coat hypertension. Arch Intern Med 152:750, 1992

12. Rademaker M, Lindsay A, McLaren JA, Padfield PL: Home monitoring of blood pressure: usefulness as a predictor of persistent hypertension. Scott Med J 32:16, 1987

13. Coats AJS, Radaelli R, Clark SJ et al: The influence of ambulatory blood pressure monitoring on the design and interpretation of trials in hypertension. J Hypertens 10:385, 1992

14. Goldhaber SZ, Manson JE, Stampfer MJ et al: Low-dose aspirin and subsequent peripheral arterial surgery in the Physicians' Health Study. Lancet 340:143, 1992

3

NATURAL HISTORY

Epidemiology tells us the likelihood or association between a risk factor such as hypertension and a future disease such as stroke. Prolonged observation of a group of untreated individuals with various levels of elevated pressure indicates, in greater detail, not only what, but when, future disease can be anticipated and how reversible it may be should treatment be successful. Thus, the concept of a "natural history" for hypertension is an old and an important one to be familiar with before evaluating the benefit or risk of treatment. However, recent studies have informed us that the natural history of a group with raised arterial pressure is complex, a set of histories that differ in their time course, appearance or lack of appearance of morbid events, and disease.

The natural history of untreated high blood pressure, particularly for moderate and severe hypertension, is based on observations made before 1970. Since then such a large fraction of those with moderate or severe hypertension have been treated that it is difficult to find descriptions of the course of those without therapy, except for reports of medically underserved groups such as are still found in our inner cities.[1,2] More recently, the patterns observed in the untreated or placebo groups of clinical trials have provided valuable information about the course of mild-to-moderate hypertension.[3–10] The sequence of events that occur in those with elevated systemic arterial pressure can be divided into three phases. However, it must be emphasized that the *rate of progression* from one phase to another is highly variable and should not be considered inevitable or highly predictable.

PHASES OF HYPERTENSION

Phase 1

Phase 1 hypertension is defined as increased pressure without evidence of target organ abnormality. Although symptoms (i.e., headache, epistaxes, or dizziness) may occur in phase 1 patients, they are nonspecific and are most often the basis for detection of hypertension rather than due to it. Other cardiovascular risk factors may be present that also require management for optimal prevention. Some studies suggest a tendency for risk factors to cluster in those with essential hypertension[11]; many of those with hypertension should be considered as "multi-risk" in this phase. The first phase of hypertension usually occurs in those younger than 50 years of age, with levels of pressure in the minimally elevated range (i.e., 135 to 150 mmHg systolic and

85 to 100 mmHg diastolic pressure). However, a few young individuals, despite having only slightly elevated pressure, will have an elevated left ventricular mass index by echocardiography and thus have already advanced to the next phase.[12]

Phase 2

Phase 2 hypertension is raised pressure with detectable abnormal cardiac, renal, neurologic, or vascular function, but *without symptoms* of cardiovascular, renal, or neurologic disease. The most frequently detected abnormalities in this stage are retinal artery irregularities, electrocardiographic signs of left atrial enlargement or left ventricular hypertrophy (or both) or left ventricular diastolic filling abnormalities,[12] microalbuminuria or mild proteinuria, and mild renal insufficiency. Asymptomatic vascular pathology (carotid or femoral artery bruit or aortic aneurysms) should be included in this category. Most phase 2 subjects are 50 years old or older, and many have other cardiovascular risk factors. With increasing age the likelihood of left ventricular enlargement and reduced renal function is greater. Nonetheless, many patients who are 60 to 80 years of age have little or no evidence of target organ abnormality. Risk of cardiovascular disease is dependent on age, level of pressure, other risk factors, and burden of target organ abnormality.

Phase 3

The third phase results in mortality or morbidity due to pathologic processes in organs that are the "targets" of the hypertensive process. Those diseases most related to the hypertensive process are cerebrovascular accidents or stroke, congestive heart failure, aortic aneurysm, and progressive renal failure. Atherosclerotic manifestations involving the carotid, coronary, peripheral, and renal arteries may be due to the combination of elevated arterial pressure with nonhypertensive risk factors: diabetes mellitus, smoking, and the hyperlipidemias. Two specific syndromes, the malignant phase of hypertension and hypertensive encephalopathy, are uniquely related to both the level of pressure and its rate of rise.

The likelihood that cardiac, neurologic, renal, and peripheral vascular disease will occur in hypertensive patients depends on several factors. These include age, duration and height of the pressure, presence of other risk factors, race, gender, and response to treatment. The state of the renin-angiotensin system may also predict future morbidity[13] (Fig. 3-1).

Although the rate of transition from the initial phase to a more advanced one is not well defined, eventually elevated arterial pressure may lead to overt disease in a substantial fraction of those with hypertension. This is particularly likely to occur in mild-to-moderate hypertension once the age of 50 is past. Stroke, cardiac disease, renal failure, or peripheral arterial insufficiency are the most common morbid or fatal events attributable to untreated hypertension. Table 3-1 indicates the accumulated prevalence of several of these events in a group of hypertensive men followed for 10 years.

Very high levels of arterial pressure (moderate and severe hypertension) are associated with specific morbidity caused by cerebral and subarachnoid

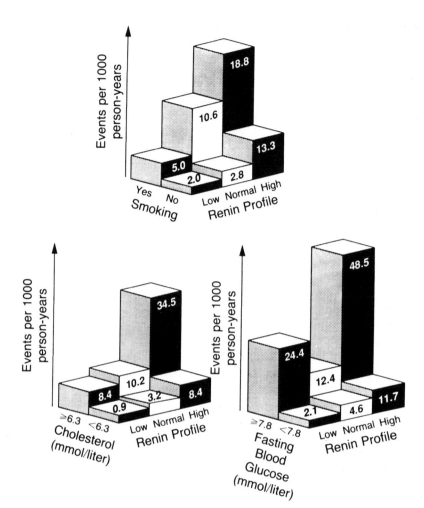

Fig. 3-1. Relationship between renin profile status (high, normal, or low) and occurrence of myocardial infarction at follow-up evaluation. Low renin status appears to be a protective trait, except in those with elevated blood glucose. (From Alderman et al.,[13] with permission.)

hemorrhage, thrombotic stroke, heart failure, aortic aneurysm, and progression of renal insufficiency due to nephrosclerosis.[7,8] Thus, these disorders are truly "hypertensive" in origin.

   In mild hypertension, coronary heart disease and extracranial, cerebrovascular, and peripheral thromboembolic and vascular occlusive disease may be more frequent when hyperlipidemia, diabetes, and smoking are present as additional risk factors. These diseases are due to atherosclerosis and thus are multifactorial in origin. This distinction indicates the expected benefit to be derived from reduction of arterial pressure, per se, compared with other measures targeted at overall reduction in cardiovascular risk.[14,15]

Table 3-1. Natural History of the Complications of Hypertension in a Cohort of Swedish Men Aged 47 to 54 Years at Baseline and Followed for 10 Years

Complication	Baseline Prevalence[a] (%)	10-Year Prevalence[b] (%)
Stroke	1.5	2.7
Myocardial infarction	1.5	4.0
Angina	3.9	12.6
Claudication	1.7	6.1
Congestive heart failure	1.0	5.9
None	93.7	78.3

[a]N = 686.
[b]N = 525.
(From Samuelsson et al.,[23] with permission.)

MALIGNANT HYPERTENSION

The malignant phase of hypertension is a unique and life-threatening clinical syndrome characterized by a rapid increase in arterial pressure, usually exceeding a diastolic pressure of 130 mmHg. The very high pressures are accompanied by advanced retinal pathology, flame-shaped or streak hemorrhages, and fluffy "cotton wool" exudates of retinal infarction (grade III) with or without papilledema (grade IV). Hypertensive encephalopathy marked by confusion, seizures, or focal neurologic deficits may be present in varying degree. In addition, left ventricular failure and renal dysfunction marked by proteinuria and hematuria, with progressive increases in serum urea nitrogen and creatinine levels, is often found. The degree of increase in pressure associated with the retinal findings, in the absence of other causes, defines the syndrome. Fibrinoid necrosis of renal arterioles is the pathologic counterpart of this syndrome; the resultant focal renal ischemia may lead to marked activation of the renin-angiotensin system. This in turn further elevates arterial pressure, resulting in a positive feedback cycle.

Malignant hypertension may occur in untreated essential hypertension, more often in black men than in other ethnic groups or in women, and has been associated with cigarette smoking.[16,17]

Any disease producing an abrupt and substantial increase in systemic arterial pressure may cause the malignant phase; it has been observed in renovascular hypertension, pheochromocytoma, acute and chronic glomerulonephritis, and the collagen vascular diseases, particularly scleroderma (scleroderma renal crisis).[18,19]

Before the advent of modern antihypertensive drug therapy and renal dialysis, more than one-half of those developing the malignant phase of hypertension died within 6 months of its appearance. At present, death from malignant hypertension can be eliminated due to the efficacy of current antihypertensive medication both for lowering arterial pressure and for preventing or reversing the vascular and renal pathology of this syndrome.[20]

Drug treatment of malignant hypertension with the earliest effective agents, the ganglionic blockers, was found to delay or avert death and irreversible renal failure. It was subsequently shown that treatment of severe essential hypertension by conventional agents (reserpine, hydrochlorothiazide, and hydralazine) could prevent development of the malignant phase.[7] Now that antihypertensive therapy is often started in mild and moderate hypertension, the malignant phase of essential hypertension has become infrequent (i.e., it is an entirely preventable complication of untreated hypertension).[21] However, in medically underserved urban areas, malignant hypertension still occurs far too often. This is best explained by the lack of adequate primary medical care delivery systems.[1]

HYPERTENSIVE ENCEPHALOPATHY

Hypertensive encephalopathy is an abrupt and sustained increase in arterial pressure to very high levels and may be associated with cerebral dysfunction, as revealed by convulsions and obtundation with or without focal neurologic abnormalities. Other possible causes of encephalopathy should be excluded. With modern diagnostic methods, particularly computed tomography, hypertensive encephalopathy is distinguishable from intracranial hemorrhage (subdural or subarachnoid bleeding), cerebral infarction, brain tumor, or other disorders.

The pathogenesis of hypertensive encephalopathy has been clearly delineated by clinical and experimental studies. Cerebral blood flow is normally kept constant over a wide range of arterial pressures (autoregulation), maintaining the constancy of capillary filtration pressure. The autoregulatory range is somewhat related to the usual pressure for any individual; it is higher in those with chronic hypertension than in normal subjects.[22] Substantial reductions in arterial pressure can diminish blood flow below the autoregulatory range, resulting in syncope—decreased cerebral perfusion and loss of consciousness. Large, sudden increases in arterial pressure, such as by experimental infusion of angiotensin II, may be sufficient to increase cerebral blood flow (breakthrough of autoregulation). The increased capillary flow at high pressure drives hyperfiltration, causing cerebral edema with its consequences—encephalopathy. Reduction of arterial pressure to within the autoregulatory range reverses the process and is the appropriate therapy for hypertensive encephalopathy.

The normal range of blood pressure for children and pregnant women is lower than that of adults. It is likely that the encephalopathy associated with nephritis in children or with toxemia in pregnancy may be due to cerebral edema. In these situations, the level of arterial pressure may be only moderately elevated but high enough to break through the autoregulatory range for that subject and cause hypertensive encephalopathy. Reduction of arterial pressure is then necessary to restore autoregulation of cerebral blood flow and reverse the hydraulic forces causing cerebral edema formation.

REFERENCES

1. Shea S, Misra D, Ehrlich MH et al: Predisposing factors for severe, uncontrolled hypertension in an inner city population. N Engl J Med 327:776, 1992

2. McCord C, Freeman HP: Excess mortality in Harlem. N Engl J Med 322:173, 1990

3. Amery A, Birkenhager W, Brixko P et al: Mortality and morbidity results from the European Working Party on High Blood Pressure in the Elderly Trial. Lancet 1:1349, 1985

4. The Management Committee: The Australian Therapeutic Trial in Mild Hypertension. Lancet 1:1261, 1980

5. Medical Research Council Working Party: MRC trial of treatment of mild hypertension: principal results. BMJ 291:97, 1985

6. The Management Committee: The Australian Therapeutic Trial in Mild Hypertension: untreated mild hypertension. Lancet 1:185, 1982

7. Veterans Administration Cooperative Study Group on Antihypertensive Agents: Effects of treatment on morbidity in hypertension: results in patients with diastolic blood pressures averaging 115 through 129 mmHg. JAMA 202:1028, 1967

8. Veterans Administration Cooperative Study Group on Antihypertensive Agents: Effects of treatment on morbidity in hypertension. II. Results in patients with diastolic blood pressure averaging 90 through 114 mmHg. JAMA 213:1143, 1970

9. Veterans Administration Cooperative Study Group on Antihypertensive Agents: Effects of treatment on morbidity in hypertension. III. Influence of age, diastolic pressure, and prior cardiovascular disease; further analysis of side effects. JAMA 45:991, 1972

10. Hypertension Detection and Follow-up Program Cooperative Group: Five-year findings of the Hypertension Detection and Follow-Up Program. I. Reduction in mortality of persons with high blood pressure, including mild hypertension. JAMA 242:2562, 1979

11. Julius S, Jamerson K, Mejia A et al: The association of borderline hypertension with target organ changes and higher coronary risk: the Tecumseh Study. JAMA 264:354, 1990

12. Phillips RA, Goldman ME, Ardeljan M et al: Determinants of abnormal left ventricular filling in early hypertension. J Am Coll Cardiol 14:979, 1989

13. Alderman MH, Madhavan S, Ooi WL et al: Association of the renin-sodium profile with the risk of myocardial infarction in patients with hypertension. N Engl J Med 324:1098, 1991

14. Rosenberg L, Kaufman DW, Helmrich SP, Shapiro S: The risk of myocardial infarction after quitting smoking in men under 55 years of age. N Engl J Med 313:1511, 1985

15. Samuelsson O, Wilhelmsen L, Andersson OK et al: Cardiovascular morbidity in relation to change in blood pressure and serum cholesterol levels in treated hypertension: results from the primary prevention in Goteborg, Sweden. JAMA 258:1768, 1987

16. Isles C, Brown JJ, Cumming AMM et al: Excess smoking in malignant-phase hypertension. BMJ 1:579, 1979

17. Bloxham CA, Beevers DG, Walker JM: Malignant hypertension and cigarette smoking. BMJ 1:581, 1979

18. Steen VD, Medsger TA Jr, Osial TA Jr et al: Factors predicting development of renal involvement in progressive systemic sclerosis. Am J Med 76:779, 1984

19. Traub YM, Shapiro AP, Rodnan GP et al: Hypertension and renal failure (scleroderma renal crisis) in progressive systemic sclerosis. Review of a 25-year experience with 68 cases. Medicine 62:335, 1983

20. Woods JW, Blythe WB, Huffines WD: Management of malignant hypertension complicated by renal insufficiency. N Engl J Med 291:10, 1974

21. Lee TH, Alderman MH: Malignant hypertension: declining mortality rate in New York City, 1958 to 1974. NY State J Med 1389, 1978

22. Strandgaard S: Autoregulation of cerebral blood flow in hypertensive patients. Circulation 53:720, 1976

23. Samuelsson O, Wilhelmsen L, Pennert K, Berglund G: Angina pectoris, intermittent claudication and congestive heart failure in middle-aged male hypertensives. Development and predictive factors during long-term antihypertensive care. The Primary Preventive Trial, Goteborg, Sweden. J Intern Med 221:23, 1987

4

PATHOPHYSIOLOGY

From the enormous literature of the past half century dealing with elevated systemic arterial pressure, several mechanisms have emerged that unequivocally account for brief or sustained periods of hypertension in humans. These mechanisms can be characterized by their general hemodynamic patterns or by the specific cardiovascular mechanisms that account for these patterns.

HEMODYNAMIC PATTERNS

In the most simplified view, systemic arterial pressure is usually considered the result of two components: cardiac output and systemic vascular resistance. This is expressed by a familiar equation in which the pressure term is mean arterial pressure:

Mean arterial pressure = cardiac output × systemic vascular resistance

From this point of view, increased arterial pressure could be due to elevation of either cardiac output or systemic vascular resistance, each of these components having many determinants. At one time, there was considerable interest in the view that, in its earliest phases, elevated arterial pressure was largely a result of increased cardiac output, alone, with a normal systemic vascular resistance. Some patients with this hemodynamic pattern are found during measurements made at rest. Usually, these are younger subjects and women to a greater extent than men.[1] When hemodynamic measurements are made during exercise, it is the sustained increase in systemic vascular resistance in those with higher pressures than normal that is more consistently observed.[2] Hypertension, then, is most often characterized by an elevated arterial systemic vascular resistance and a normal cardiac output.

REGULATION

Brief, minute to minute fluctuations in arterial pressure or heart rate are almost entirely a result of changes in activity of the autonomic nervous system, particularly neurosecretion of norepinephrine and adrenomedullary secretion of epinephrine[3,4] (Fig. 4-1).

During a 24-hour period, blood pressure in normal people and most hypertensive patients is higher during waking hours than during sleep, as established by many studies. Changes in autonomic function largely account for this pattern (Fig. 4-2).

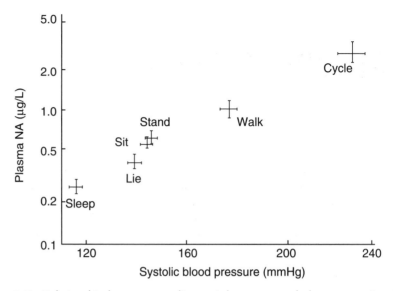

Fig. 4-1. Relationship between systolic arterial pressure and plasma norepinephrine (NA) in a group of mild-to-moderate hypertensive patients. Throughout a range of activities, pressure was measured by intra-arterial monitoring and blood samples for assay of norepinephrine were concurrently obtained. The very high correlation between physical or behavioral state and function of the sympathetic nervous system, as reflected by the plasma norepinephrine concentration, is evident. (Modified from Watson et al.,[3] with permission.)

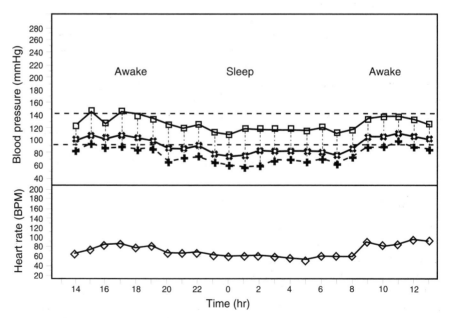

Fig. 4-2. Pattern of circadian systolic and diastolic pressure is shown from a subject with high normal blood pressure. During waking hours, both pressures are consistently higher than during sleep. This pattern is consistently observed in normal subjects and most hypertensive patients.

The trends in pressure that occur over long intervals, hours to days, are less well correlated with specific mechanisms. However, the action of the renin-angiotensin system, mineralocorticoid secretion (mainly aldosterone), tonic activity of the sympathetic nervous system, renal filtration, and tubular reabsorption of fluid, controlling extracellular and intravascular volume, all participate. Guyton has developed a complex model that centers long-term regulation of arterial pressure on the hydraulics of renal perfusion.[5,6]

MECHANISMS OF SYSTEMIC VASCULAR RESISTANCE

The causes of *clinical* hypertension are those mechanisms that raise systemic resistance; the best examples are based on research in secondary hypertension. My criteria for this rigorous selection are strict and depend on the following. For a mechanism to be identified as a *cause of hypertension* it must raise systemic vascular resistance, be measurable, and be present in excess when pressure is elevated. Furthermore, blockade or reversal by specific interventions should significantly reduce the elevated pressure. The role of norepinephrine in pheochromocytoma provides a simple example. In this disorder, plasma norepinephrine is markedly increased and administration of an α-receptor blocker (phentolamine in this paradigm) normalizes arterial pressure. Thus, we accept the sympathoadrenal system as a defined pathogenetic mechanism in some, albeit rare, forms of hypertension. Another example is the renin-secreting tumor in which hypertension can be explained entirely by increased secretion of active renin with ensuing generation of angiotensin II as the vasoconstrictor.

Table 4-1 lists those mechanisms that can at this point be accepted for their causative role. I have included only four basic categories: (1) the sympathoadrenal or adrenergic system, (2) the renin-angiotensin vasoconstrictor system, (3) salt/volume excess as due either to supranormal production of salt-retaining steroids or to impaired renal function, and (4) a vascular abnor-

Table 4-1. Causative Mechanisms for Human Hypertension

Mechanism	Disease/Example	Reversal by
Sympathoadrenal excess	Pheochromocytoma	α-Adrenergic receptors
Renin excess	Renin-secreting tumors	Angiotensin converting enzyme inhibitors
Renin excess	Unilateral renal artery stenosis	Angiotensin converting enzyme inhibitors
Salt/volume excess	Primary aldosteronism	Spironolactone
Salt/volume excess	Advanced or end-stage renal disease	Diuretic administration or dialysis
Primary vascular abnormalities, functional and/or structural	Essential hypertension	Calcium channel entry blockers
Secondary vascular abnormalities, functional and/or structural	Cushing syndrome, steroid excess, cyclosporine, others	RU 486, α-receptor blockers, calcium channel entry blockers

mality that can be reversed by widely employed and highly specific pharmacologic agents. Essential hypertension is considered a disorder in which the vascular disorder *may in some patients* be the only abnormality evident or is, in other words, a primary disorder.[7] By contrast, there are some forms of hypertension in which changes in properties of the vasculature may be secondary to other reversible processes or to the raised pressure itself.

The reader may be dismayed that I have limited the *known* causes of elevated arterial pressure to so few mechanisms when the experimental literature teems with potential causative agents, as represented in Table 4-2. However, but one must be skeptical of such claims until the proposed mechanism is clearly shown to account for hypertension in at least one, preferably several or many, patients. For another example, vasopressin—the antidiuretic hormone—is a well-characterized vasoconstrictor in some systems and briefly increases arterial pressure in animals. However, increased vasopressin in humans accounts only for the syndrome of hyponatremia, inappropriate antidiuretic hormone excess, which occurs without elevated blood pressure. Similarly, endothelin, a very potent peptide vasoconstrictor, remains unattached to any syndrome of human hypertension.

As of this writing, I await definitive reports that deficiencies of atrial natriuretic peptide, the potent vasodilator kinins, or the several prostaglandins account for *naturally* occurring high blood pressure in humans. By contrast, the occasional increase in pressure accompanying the use of nonsteroidal anti-inflammatory drugs may relate to drug-induced reduction of vasodilator prostaglandins. A recent report suggests that inhibition of endogenous synthesis of nitric oxide (the endothelial cell-derived vasodilator) by abnormal metabolites of arginine accumulating in chronic renal disease may participate in elevated pressure of those with renal failure.[8] Thus, there is some, if limited, evidence that loss of endogenous vasodilator function may participate in human hypertension.

CAUSES OF ESSENTIAL HYPERTENSION

Since I have drawn on the known causes of secondary or reversible hypertension for several mechanisms described above, one could conclude that these individually or together might account for the large fraction of cases of elevated pressure now classified as *essential hypertension*. After all, many patients have reductions in pressure when given adrenergic blockade, salt depletion (diuretics), or angiotensin converting enzyme inhibitors. Why not consider these patients as having raised arterial pressure secondary to increased participation of such systems as the sympathoadrenal or renin-angiotensin system or to salt/volume excess?

The problem that arises in trying to work backward from a therapeutic effect to a cause for essential hypertension is that often little correlation exists between the measured activity of the system and the therapeutic effect of the intervention. A fall in pressure due to diuretic administration is not necessarily strictly related to the degree of salt/volume loss. Plasma catecholamine

Table 4-2. Factors That May Control or Modify Systemic or Local Vascular Resistance[a]

Circulating hormones
    Plasma catecholamines: norepinephrine, epinephrine, dopamine
    Angiotensin II from the circulating renin system
    Plasma vasopressin
    Plasma insulin
    Parathyroid-hormone-like substances
    Plasma calcitonin-gene-related peptide
    Plasma atrial natriuretic peptide
Neurotransmitters
    Norepinephrine
    Acetylcholine
    Neuropeptide Y
    Substance P
Local paracrine or autocrine systems
    Arachidonic acid metabolites, prostaglandins, and leukotrienes
    Adenosine
    Nitric oxide
    Endothelin
    Kallikrein-generated peptides
    Tissue angiotensin converting enzyme
Cell receptors
    Adrenergic receptors: β_2, α_1, α_2, dopamine
    Angiotensin type 1
    Vasopressin type 1
    Endothelial acetylcholine receptors
Modulators of response or vascular reactivity
    Plasma steroids, aldosterone and cortisol
    Plasma Na/K-ATPase inhibitors, ouabain-like substances
    Salt intake
Structural changes in resistance vessels—growth, atrophy, remodeling
    Smooth muscle cell growth: hypertrophy and/or hyperplasia
    Fibrous tissue and matrix
    Rarification: loss of capillary density
Growth factors that may alter vascular structure

[a]This is a partial list.

concentrations are only slightly elevated in most hypertensive people, yet the response to α_1-receptor blockade is highly variable—large in some, small in others. Some correlation exists between the level of plasma renin activity and short-term reduction in pressure by the angiotensin converting enzyme inhibitors, but variability is high even in this response. In brief, once one departs from the known causes of secondary hypertension, close coupling between increased activation of a hypertensive mechanism and the effect of a specific therapeutic intervention falls apart.

Most of those with essential hypertension do not have evidence of markedly increased activity of the sympathoadrenal system, the renin-angiotensin system, or salt or volume excess. One might argue (some have) that raised arterial pressure by an unknown mechanism should be compensated by downward setting of the baroreflexes, and therefore the arterial baroreflexes must have adapted or become accustomed to maintaining high pressure, a mal-adaptation.[9] A similar position has been outlined for the renin system; its appropriate response to increased arterial pressure is to become hypoac-tive.[10] Perhaps this accounts for the 15 to 20 percent low renin fraction of the hypertensive population. If the renin system fails to become suppressed due to hypertension, this might reflect subtle intrarenal vascular narrowing, which would provide a stimulus for inappropriate renin release and also tend to retain salt and water/volume, as in a model of experimental hyperten-sion.[11] Finally, the systems analysis of Guyton[6] suggests that the appropriate response of the kidney to raised systemic pressure is a pressure-induced diure-sis and natriuresis that lower blood volume in compensation and thereby decreases cardiac output, with pressure returning to normal. From this per-spective, a normal blood volume in the presence of elevated arterial pressure is also a maladaptation.

What then accounts for the persistently raised systemic vascular resistance when no obvious pressor systems are clearly hyperactive? The obvious answer is that some of those with essential hypertension have primary disorder(s) of the resistance arteries and arterioles (including or even exclusively those of the kidney) that do not require hyperactivity of one of the neurocirculatory pressor systems or abnormal retention of salt and water/volume.

The concept that high arterial pressure might be substantially or primarily due to an altered vasculature is hardly new. In prior investigations, some patients with essential hypertension were found to have (1) increased pressor or vascular responsiveness to catecholamines or angiotensin II, suggesting increased vascular hyperreactivity; (2) impaired maximal dilation to ischemia or vasodilator substances, implying structural abnormalities limiting maximal vasorelaxation or vasodilation; and (3) increased resistance vessel wall/lumen ratios consistent with altered structural characteristics of the vascular wall. The latter may occur as a result of (1) increased absolute wall thickness (cross-sectional area) at the extraluminal or adventitial surface, giving a mechanical advantage to outer layers of smooth muscle for vasoconstric-tion[12]; (2) increased growth of the wall at the luminal surface; or (3) a per-manent reduction in luminal diameter, resulting from remodeling of the wall without an increase in its cross-sectional area.[7] Which of these alterations are truly primary and which occur as a result of elevated pressure is not yet fully determined. Nonetheless, these mechanisms imply that altered growth and the microanatomy of resistance arteries and arterioles, as determined by the genetic and molecular mechanisms now being explored for vascular tissues, may provide an excellent basis for understanding essential hypertension in the future (Fig. 4-3).

To conclude this section, several well-defined mechanisms may account for increased arterial pressure in patients with secondary hypertension. In addi-tion, some of those with the diagnosis of essential hypertension may have evi-dence of increased activity of these systems. There are well-defined subgroups (i.e., high-renin, hyperadrenergic, or salt-sensitive hypertensive patients). In addition, there is a substantial fraction of those with "normal in everything currently measurable" essential hypertension in whom a set of primary vas-

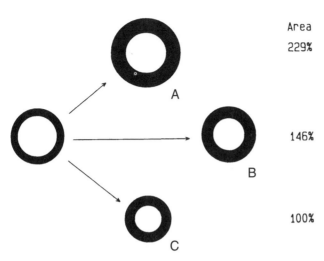

Area

229%

A

146%

B

100%

C

Fig. 4-3. Schema depicting the potential effects of vascular growth in relationship to lumen and wall thickness (cross-sectional area). In each figure, the wall/lumen ratio has been doubled. **(A)** Outer wall is increased without a change in lumenal diameter. **(B)** Growth at the inner wall, reducing lumenal diameter. In Figs. A and B, growth has occurred and the cross-sectional area of the vascular wall increased. **(C)** Alternatively, the lumen is reduced without increased cross-sectional area of the wall, the concept of "remodelling." (Adapted from Heagerty et al.,[7] with permission.)

cular abnormalities may be operative. There is no reason not to consider the group of subjects labeled as having essential hypertension by current clinical criteria as substantially heterogeneous regarding the mechanisms that raise systemic vascular resistance, perhaps the only other trait these individuals have in common.

TRAITS ASSOCIATED WITH ESSENTIAL HYPERTENSION

Practicing physicians and other health care professionals know what essential hypertension is, but hardly any agree on the definition, a situation that has been compared with the story of the blind men and the elephant. In that fable each observer, touching a small different part of the whole animal, gave a description based on his limited perspective (whether he touched a tail, trunk, leg, and so forth). However, the story is an oversimplified analogy for hypertension because, in fact, many clinicians view hypertensive patients in a variety of ways and are quite familiar with many pertinent issues. Yet that apparent familiarity may generate different opinions about what constitutes essential hypertension (i.e., those with elevated arterial pressure, unexplained by the rare diagnosable and reversible disorders).

Confusion regarding essential hypertension arises because of the many (almost too numerous to count) studies in which various traits are associated with a group having higher blood pressure than a comparison group, variably called *control, normal,* or *normotensive.* I have chosen one example to illustrate this point. Figure 4-4 displays results from such a study.[13]

The individual measurements for red cell sodium-lithium countertransport are shown for both groups, and usual statistical comparisons are given. It is evident from the data that several conclusions might be drawn, but only some will be accurate; others would be misleading. Some examples follow:

1. Most, but not all, hypertensive individuals have higher sodium-lithium countertransport than most normotensive individuals.
2. The average sodium-lithium countertransport for hypertensive patients is higher than the average for normotensive patients. The odds are less than 1 in 20 ($P < 0.05$) that this is due to chance, should other groups be compared.
3. Hypertensive patients have higher sodium-lithium countertransport than normal patients.
4. Essential hypertension is characterized by a high sodium-lithium countertransport.

Inspection of statements 1 and 2 reveals that they accurately describe the data shown in Figure 4-1 and violate no logical principles or those of reasonable inference. Statement 3, however, is either false (if it is meant to say that all hypertensive individuals have higher sodium-lithium countertransport than normal persons) or misleading since some hypertensive patients do not have higher sodium-lithium countertransport than normal persons. Statement 4, quite typical of medical literature, creates an entity (essential

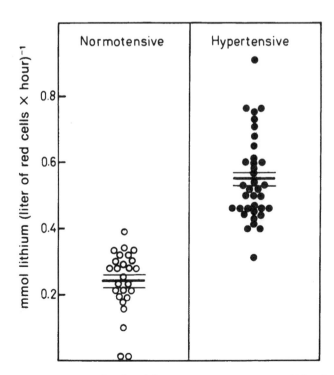

Fig. 4-4. Measurements of sodium-lithium countertransport in red blood cells from normotensive or hypertensive subjects. (Adapted from Canessa et al.,[13] with permission.)

hypertension) that somehow magically exists apart from any individual and endows that entity with a high sodium-lithium countertransport. However, there is no such thing, there are only patients with high arterial pressure. The intellectual concept of essential hypertension has no separate existence. For convenience, we use the term hypertension but sometimes forget that it has no meaning other than the implication that a patient or group in which we are interested have high blood pressure. If we find a patient with high blood pressure (e.g., 160/110 mmHg) who does not have secondary hypertension, but without a high sodium-lithium countertransport, what should we call the disorder, if not essential hypertension? There will certainly be many individuals to consider as either having or not having this trait. Of course, we could recognize the trait as an option and refer to patients as having essential hypertension with or without the trait of increased sodium-lithium countertransport. However, since so many traits have a vague but statistically significant association with elevated blood pressure, diagnostic terms would quickly become cumbersome. Even worse, often no evidence exists that such a trait might raise pressure or that reducing the trait would lower the pressure.

Previous writers on this problem have important lessons for the present. In a small book, full of important insights, Pickering,[14] having recognized this dilemma, gave a set of definitions that have not been surpassed. In brief, essential hypertension is nothing other than a quantitative upward deviation of arterial pressure. The *significance* of the deviation lies in its relationship to future risk. Those with high pressure without obvious causes (renal or endocrine disease, and so forth) are defined as having essential hypertension by default. Some, but not all, of those with high blood pressure share certain traits or characteristics. In the past 30 years, this list of characteristics has expanded, as indicated in Table 4-3. As new causes of secondary hypertension have become recognized, essential hypertension will inevitably become a more restricted or slightly smaller fraction of all those with elevated pressure.

Table 4-3. Examples of Traits Found in Some Hypertensive Patients

Type of Trait	Correlation With Level of Pressure	Cause of Increased Pressure
Retinal artery sclerosis	Fair	No
Nephrosclerosis	Fair	Uncertain
Blood cell transport abnormalities	Poor	Unknown
Insulin resistance	Fair to poor	Unknown
Increased plasma norepinephrine	Poor	Unknown
Increased plasma renin activity	Fair	In some patients
Salt sensitivity	Poor	Perhaps in some groups
Circulating Na/K-ATPase inhibitors	Poor	Unknown
Platelet intracellular $[Ca^{2+}]$	Good	Unknown
Increased cardiac output	Poor	Uncertain
Overweight	Fair	Likely in many, but not all patients

While essential hypertension is nothing other than high blood pressure, important insights may be gained from recognizing that some hypertensive persons have one or more other traits and some do not. Three important aspects come immediately to mind: (1) prognosis, (2) pathogenesis, and (3) treatment.

For the same level of pressure, group outcomes differ in part because of presence or absence of nonhypertensive risk factors or the activity of the renin system.[15] Other traits, such as insulin resistance or those exposed by measurements of red cell transport characteristics, have yet to be explored for their independent effects on long-term rates of cardiovascular disease.

Several traits seem related to salt sensitivity in hypertensive patients. It is tempting to consider that the transport characteristics of an accessible cell (red cell or leukocyte) might predict the effect of a change in dietary salt intake. Few such attempts have been made. Salt sensitivity has been linked to insulin resistance in reports limited by small numbers.[16–18]

The causal relationship between increased plasma renin activity and elevated blood pressure in some patients is well known. Where there is a pathogenetic link between a trait and the level of arterial pressure, a therapeutic strategy is implied. Ideally, one would like to be able to predict the response of a given hypertensive patient to the spectrum of agents now available (or to be developed) on the basis of these traits. At present, however, age, ethnic status, and the renin system offer a minimum basis for variation and response, leaving large gaps between the ability to find hypertension-related traits and specific and/or selective therapeutic choices.

MULTIFACTORIAL NATURE OF ESSENTIAL HYPERTENSION

What determines the usual level of a patient's arterial pressure? Many factors operating to a varying degree at any time determine pressure. This heterogeneity has been recognized as the concept of a "multifactorial nature" as employed by Pickering[14] or by using the analogy of a mosaic, a concept conceived by Page.[19] Elevated pressure is primarily a disorder of increased systemic vascular resistance. Therefore, the various factors capable of affecting systemic vascular resistance are now seen as participating, to a greater or lesser extent, in the multifactorial nature of essential hypertension. In other words, individual patients differ from each other in the spectrum of causal mechanisms accounting for their raised pressure.

Since the original descriptions of the multifactorial nature of essential hypertension, many new mechanisms have emerged that may play a role in the determination of increased blood pressure. Some of these mechanisms may be under strict genetic control for their expression; some may be activated by specific environmental or acquired conditions (e.g., high salt intake or weight gain). Others may be adaptive or maladaptive responses to the hemodynamic or structural consequences of vasoconstriction or increased systemic vascular resistance. Those changes that represent adaptive effects occurring over months to years represent age-related phenomena. For any individual patient with high blood pressure, mechanisms may vary in a time-dependent manner from childhood or adolescence to middle and late age.

Presently, most studies characterizing mechanisms related to age in hypertensive persons rely on cross-sectional studies comparing different age groups. For the older groups, this represents the survivors, a selection bias. Thus, that elderly hypertensive patients are considered a "low-renin" group could be because middle- or high-renin patients have a higher mortality rate at a younger age.

The previous considerations lead to several conclusions regarding most subjects with high blood pressure (i.e., those given the label of essential hypertension). First, patients differ from each other with regard to their average or usual level of pressure, nonhypertensive risk, pathophysiologic mechanisms, and target organ damage (i.e., they are a very heterogeneous group). Second, the mechanisms accounting for elevated pressure in most patients are poorly characterized, that is, the specific cause(s) of their upward deviation in pressure is not well defined. Third, adaptive changes and aging may alter these mechanisms so that the characteristics of the patient with high blood pressure when seen early in life may be altered as that individual gets older. Conceptually, their hypertension is a moving target. Fourth, antihypertensive interventions, whether they are life-style changes or drug treatment, are beneficial in the statistical sense that applies to group trends. However, the effects of such approaches also remain largely uncharacterized, especially with regard to recently defined vasoactive systems and traits.

Thus, each patient with high blood pressure represents a complex problem to be carefully appraised during the initial and subsequent management. It is all too easy to evade some of these complexities by oversimplification and to consider most or all of those with high blood pressure as similar to each other. I find that few physicians will easily accept this monolithic approach. Most recognize the pertinent differences between one hypertensive patient and another. In general, these physicians wish to address the need for efficient and pertinent strategies to give optimal care to each of their hypertensive patients, without unduly minimizing the sophistication that current medical science now offers.

REFERENCES

1. Messerli FH, Garavaglia GE, Schmieder RE et al: Disparate cardiovascular findings in men and women with essential hypertension. Ann Intern Med 101:158, 1987

2. Amery A, Julius S, Whitlock LS, Conway J: Influence of hypertension on the hemodynamic response to exercise. Circulation 36:231, 1967

3. Watson RDS, Stallard TJ, Flinn RM: Factors determining direct arterial pressure and its variability in hypertensive man. Hypertension 2:303, 1980

4. Krakoff LR, Dziedzic S, Mann SJ et al: Plasma epinephrine concentration in healthy men: correlation with systolic pressure and rate-pressure product. J Am Coll Cardiol 5:352, 1985

5. Guyton AC, Coleman TG, Cowley AW et al: Arterial pressure regulation: overriding dominance of the kidneys in long-term regulation and in hypertension. Am J Med 52:584, 1972

6. Guyton AC: Blood pressure control—special role of the kidneys and body fluids. Science 252:1813, 1991

7. Heagerty AM, Aalkjaer C, Bund SJ et al: Small artery structure in hypertension. Hypertension 21:391, 1993

8. Vallance P, Leone A, Calver A et al: Accumulation of an endogenous inhibitor of nitric oxide synthesis in chronic renal failure. Lancet 339:572, 1992

9. Julius S: The blood pressure seeking properties of the central nervous system. J Hypertens 6:177, 1988

10. Sealey JE, Blumenfeld JD, Bell GM et al: On the renal basis for essential hypertension: nephron heterogeneity with discordant renin secretion and sodium excretion causing a hypertensive vasoconstriction-volume relationship. J Hypertens 6:763, 1988

11. Gavras H, Brunner HR, Vaughan ED, Laragh JH: Angiotensin-sodium interaction in blood pressure maintainence of renal hypertensive rats and normotensive rats. Science 180:1369, 1973

12. Folkow B, Grimby G, Thulesius O: Adaptive structural changes of the vascular walls in hypertension and their relation to the control of the peripheral resistance. Acta Physiol Scand 44:255, 1958

13. Canessa M, Adragna N, Solomon HS et al: Increased sodium-lithium countertransport in red cells of patients with essential hypertension. N Engl J Med 302:772, 1980

14. Pickering G: The Nature of Essential Hypertension. Grune & Stratton, Orlando, FL, 1961

15. Brunner HR, Laragh JH, Baer L et al: Essential hypertension: renin, and aldosterone, heart attack and stroke. N Engl J Med 286:441, 1972

16. Sharma AM, Ruland K, Spies K-P, Distler A: Salt sensitivity in young normotensive subjects is associated with a hyperinsulinemic response to oral glucose. J Hypertens 9:329, 1991

17. Sharma AM, Schorr U, Distler A: Insulin resistance in young salt sensitive normotensive subjects. Hypertension 21:273, 1993

18. Rocchini AP, Key J, Bondie D et al: The effect of weight loss on the sensitivity of blood pressure to sodium in obese adolescents. N Engl J Med 321:580, 1989

19. Page IH: A unifying view of renal hypertension. p. 391. In Page IH, McCubbin JW (eds): Renal Hypertension. Year Book, Chicago, 1968

5

CLINICAL TRIALS

CLINICAL TRIALS

Is the treatment of hypertension beneficial? For any one clinic or physician, this question is difficult to answer, since the experience would include too few patients for a definitive conclusion. By the mid-1960s, however, it became both necessary and feasible to proceed with formal trials of therapy because (1) hypertension was a highly prevalent disorder, (2) the risk of elevated blood pressure had been well defined by a variety of epidemiologic studies, and (3) effective and relatively safe drugs for lowering blood pressure had become available. The treatment of hypertension has since become one of the most well-studied subjects through the conduct of prospective clinical trials.

Over the past 25 years, a succession of multicenter randomized therapeutic clinical trials have provided a robust body of evidence for the conclusion that drug treatment of hypertension is both effective (i.e., blood pressure can be decreased for long periods) and beneficial in preventing cardiovascular disease. In perhaps no other area of medicine have randomized clinical trials played such a major role in providing physicians with a rationale for their therapeutic decisions on a day-to-day basis.

Despite the number and variety of therapeutic clinical trials for hypertension that have already been published, many issues physicians must deal with in choosing therapeutic strategies for their patients are unsettled or controversial. Clinical trials are large-scale, expensive experiments that require simplified and orderly methods to achieve their goal (i.e., "Is one form of treatment better or worse than another?"). The treatments might be placebo versus active drug, one drug versus another, or one system of care versus another. To study enough patients to obtain definitive answers and to be certain that unrelated factors do not obscure endpoints, clinical trials recruit large numbers of patients, but have inclusion and exclusion criteria that account for the kinds of patients to be studied. Simplified, easily standardized methods are necessary to be able to compare rates of disease (e.g., stroke or myocardial infarction) in large numbers of patients. More subtle differences between patients or patients who require expensive technology are generally not included. In other words, clinical trials have their own limits, and conclusions from them should not be substituted for careful thought in the management of any one patient.

Any one clinical trial, even if well planned, may fail to reveal the expected result, of either establishing or eliminating the hypothesis that a treatment is beneficial. Pooling separate studies has become formally recognized as *meta-*

analysis. Meta-analysis can be used to summarize previously performed trials as a group. However, a recent report describes methods for this type of analysis in sequence, adding each new trial in a given area to those that preceded it.[1] It is suggested that this approach may well detect statistically significant effects of treatment long before they would otherwise be recognized. The reader is advised, however, that even meta-analysis has its limitations and controversies.[2]

This chapter summarizes the randomized therapeutic clinical trials that are the basis for drug treatment of hypertension. Both the value and the limitations of these trials, as pertinent to the treatment of individual hypertensive patients, are emphasized.

SEVERE AND MODERATE HYPERTENSION

In 1967, publication of the results of the Veterans Administration (VA) Cooperative Trial[3] for those with severe hypertension (defined as entering diastolic pressures of 115 mmHg or higher on placebo) established, beyond reasonable doubt, the need to treat this group with effective blood pressure lowering medication. The study included only men and the size of the trial was small, but the differences in outcome between those treated with active drugs (reserpine, chlorthiazide, and hydralazine) and the placebo group were unequivocally significant by clinical and statistical appraisal. Subsequent publications from an extension of this study, including those with less severe hypertension, demonstrated that antihypertensive therapy was clearly beneficial in men with moderate hypertension, defined as pretreatment diastolic pressures of at least 105 to 114 mmHg.[4,5]

Since 1970, several studies with different designs and goals have been conducted to establish the benefit of antihypertensive therapy in mild-to-moderate hypertension, pretreatment diastolic pressures defined as 90 to 110 mmHg. The individual trials have been reviewed and analyzed in several meta-analyses.[6–9] The summary figure from one of the best known of these analyses is shown in Figure 5-1.

Randomized clinical trials for the treatment of mild-to-moderate hypertension have differed from each other in several important features, including (1) age and sex of those recruited; (2) inclusion or exclusion of those with nonhypertensive risk factors; (3) duration of follow up; (4) open, single, or double blind methodology; 5) placebo, untreated, or community-treated "control" groups for comparison with those given antihypertensive therapy by protocol; and (6) nature of the ancillary services provided to keep patients in treatment or in the study. Several trials have focused specifically on older patients, recruiting only those above 60 years of age.

DRUGS USED IN THE CLINICAL TRIALS

The drugs chosen for therapy in the trials have varied. Many of the early trials employed diuretics plus a variety of antiadrenergic agents for control of

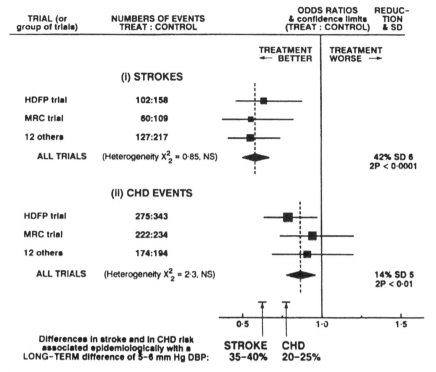

TRIAL (or group of trials)	NUMBERS OF EVENTS TREAT : CONTROL	ODDS RATIOS & confidence limits (TREAT : CONTROL)	REDUC-TION & SD

TREATMENT ← BETTER   TREATMENT WORSE →

(i) STROKES

HDFP trial	102:158		
MRC trial	60:109		
12 others	127:217		
ALL TRIALS	(Heterogeneity x^2_2 = 0·85, NS)		42% SD 6 2P < 0·0001

(ii) CHD EVENTS

HDFP trial	275:343		
MRC trial	222:234		
12 others	174:194		
ALL TRIALS	(Heterogeneity x^2_2 = 2·3, NS)		14% SD 5 2P < 0·01

0·5   1·0   1·5

Differences in stroke and in CHD risk associated epidemiologically with a LONG-TERM difference of 5–6 mm Hg DBP:

STROKE   CHD
35–40%   20–25%

Fig. 5-1. Composite figure from an often quoted meta-analysis of the clinical trials of drug treatment for hypertension. Reductions (odds ratios) are compared for stroke (fatal and nonfatal) with nonfatal and fatal coronary heart disease (CHD). The *actual benefit* from pooled estimates for stroke and CHD are 42 and 14 percent, respectively. The *predicted benefit* from epidemiologic surveys for stroke and CHD are 35 to 40 and 20 to 25 percent, respectively. This analysis clearly shows the greater and more consistent value of antihypertensive drug treatment for prevention of stroke compared with the inconsistent and less effective prevention of CHD. MRC, Medical Research Council; HDFP, Hypertension Detection Follow-Up Program; NS, not significant; SD, standard deviation; DBP, diastolic blood pressure. (From Collins et al.,[7] with permission.)

pressure in comparison to a placebo or untreated group (Table 5-1). The initial VA studies combined a diuretic with reserpine and hydralazine. Before β-receptor blockers were widely employed, methyldopa was often combined with a diuretic.[10–12] The Medical Research Council[13] (MRC) trial compared a thiazide and propranolol as active treatment against placebo in a single blind, three-limb, design. Only the most recent study (Trial of Mild Hypertension Study[14] [TOMHS]) of antihypertensive drug therapy included an angiotensin converting enzyme (ACE) inhibitor and a calcium channel blocker. Some have concluded that only diuretics and β-blockers are effective antihypertensive drug therapy for mild hypertension. As seen from the preceding discussion, this is not so. Many drugs have been used in the successful trials.

COMPARISON GROUP

Six of the eight trials referred to in Table 5-1 compared drug-treated subjects with placebo-treated or untreated controls. These were both VA trials, Goteborg, Oslo, MRC, Australian and TOMHS. The two exceptions were the Hypertension Detection and Follow-up Program (HDFP) study and the Multiple Risk Factor Intervention Trial (MRFIT), in which special clinics treated one-half the patients; the other half were referred back to their community-based sources of treatment (offices or clinics). The special clinics provided free medication and used various strategies to achieve high compliance. These differences in design have often been discussed; skeptics emphasize that the lack of placebo-controlled groups for comparison in the HDFP and MRFIT studies limits interpretation.

INITIAL CONCLUSIONS

Overall conclusions to be drawn from summarizing the available clinical trials of therapy for mild hypertension are as follows:

1. Antihypertensive therapy reduces morbidity and mortality from cerebrovascular disease in a consistent and highly significant manner; the reduction in morbidity (approximately 40 percent) is almost exactly that predicted by epidemiologic forecasts.
2. Overall and cardiovascular mortality are reduced by antihypertensive therapy by 10 to 15 percent (i.e., to a lesser extent than that of cerebrovascular disease and below that predicted by epidemiologic surveys).
3. The effect of antihypertensive drug treatment on ischemic or coronary heart disease is definitely less than predicted from epidemiologic forecasts and varies greatly from study to study. Even meta-analyses do not agree on the effect, reporting 6 to 14 percent reductions in risk.[6,7]
4. Age is a determinant of results, especially in mild hypertension. No trial has shown a significant reduction in events in those less than 50 years of age. Most trials have focused on the middle aged (50 to 65 years), for whom benefit of treatment is well documented.

Some of the controversial issues arising from this overview of the conservative conclusions of the trials are explored in the following sections of this chapter.

TREATMENT AND CORONARY HEART DISEASE

Since coronary heart disease is such a frequent outcome in those with mild hypertension, two to four times more common than stroke, several explanations have been offered for the difference in observable effect of antihypertensive therapy in relationship to the benefit predicted by epidemiologic surveys: (1) time and duration of therapy, (2) differences in nonhypertensive risk as altered by treatment, (3) expectations for the β-blockers, and (4) the J-curve effect of excessive reduction in arterial pressure on treatment. Each of these is briefly discussed.

Table 5-1. The Important Clinical Trials of Therapy for Hypertension for Middle-Aged Patients[a]

Name	Year Published	Drugs Used
Veterans Administration, severe hypertension[3] (VA-1)	1967	Reserpine, thiazide, hydralazine
Veterans Administration, mild/moderate hypertension[4] (VA-2)	1970	Reserpine, thiazide, hydralazine
Australian[10]	1980	Thiazide, methyldopa, propranolol, pindolol
Oslo[46]	1980	Thiazide, methyldopa, propranolol
Hypertension Detection and Follow-Up Program[12] (HDFP)	1979	Thiazide, reserpine, methyldopa, propranolol
Multiple Risk Factor Intervention Trial[16,47] (MRFIT)	1985, 1990	Thiazide, chlorthalidone, reserpine, propranolol, others
Medical Research Council[13] (MRC)	1985	Thiazide, propranolol
Goteborg (Sweden)[48]	1978	Various β-blockers, diuretics, hydralazine
Trial of Mild Hypertension Study[14] (TOMHS)	1993	Acebutolol, amlodipine, chlorthalidone, enalapril, doxazosin

[a]Active treatment compared to placebo, no treatment or community control (HDFP).

Duration of Treatment

Most clinical trials have lasted 4 to 5 years. By contrast, the atherosclerotic lesions causing coronary heart disease evolve (and possibly regress) over decades. This discrepancy may account for the result in one meta-analysis[7] that antihypertensive drug treatment in the trials reduced coronary heart disease morbidity by 14 percent, whereas a 22 percent reduction was predicted by epidemiologic studies.

Risk Trade-Off During Treatment

Coronary atherosclerosis is multifactorial in origin, with hyperlipidemia and diabetes participating in addition to hypertension. Effects of the various antihypertensive drugs on nonhypertensive risk factors may be significant. Thiazide diuretics have been shown to impair glucose tolerance, increase total and high-density lipoprotein cholesterol and reduce serum potassium, all of which might lead to an increase in nonhypertensive risk, offsetting the benefit of decreased arterial pressure.[15] It has been suggested that reliance on diuretic treatment accounts for the negative results of the initial report of the MRFIT.[16] In that study, those hypertensive patients with abnormal electrocardiograms at entry had a worse outcome despite attending special intervention clinics than did those randomized to care by their community physicians.

Role of β-Blockers

In the 1970s, the consensus was that β-receptor blockers, as antihypertensive agents, should be effective in reducing ischemic or coronary heart disease. Several studies were designed to address this hypothesis in various ways. These are summarized in Table 5-2.

Results of the MRC trial suggested that the β-blocker propranolol conferred better protection in nonsmoking men against ischemic heart disease than did a diuretic. This was less clear in the other subgroups. A slight trend in the same direction was found in the International Prospective Primary Prevention Study in Hypertension (IPPPSH) and in the Metoprolol Atherosclerosis Prevention in Hypertension (MAPHY) study. However, the Heart Attack Primary Prevention in Hypertension (HAPPHY) trial, which included patients in MAPHY but on atenolol as well, failed to demonstrate that the β-blocker group benefitted significantly, compared with those on the diuretic. The differences between the HAPPHY and MAPHY studies have never been entirely explained.[17] Summary by meta-analysis failed to confirm that β-blockers had a unique benefit for primary prevention of coronary heart disease compared with other antihypertensive treatments.[18]

In contrast to the treatment of hypertension as a *primary* intervention, use of β blockers as *secondary* prevention after an initial myocardial infarction has been successful for hypertensive and nonhypertensive patients.[8,19] This conclusion cannot be overlooked in a comprehensive assessment of current drug therapy. Perhaps the design of trials of antihypertensive treatment have underestimated the value of β-blockade for pertinent subgroups.

J-Curve

Does excessive reduction of arterial pressure lead to an increase in cardiovascular morbidity on treatment, a "J-curve" effect? Cruikshank et al.[20] reviewed the course of 902 patients treated with atenolol plus other drugs over a 10-year follow-up period. Of those with previous ischemic disease, the group with diastolic pressures of 85 to 90 mmHg *during* treatment had a lower occurrence of myocardial infarction than groups with pressures either higher or lower. In a 12-year follow-up study of 686 men treated for moderate hypertension in Goteborg, Sweden, as part of a multiple risk reduction pro-

Table 5-2. Clinical Trials Comparing a β-Blocker Versus Thiazide or Other Treatment

Name	Year Published	Drugs Used
IPPPSH[49]	1985	Oxprenolol versus placebo, other drugs
HAPPHY[50]	1987	Metoprolol or atenolol versus thiazide
MAPHY[51]	1988	Metoprolol versus thiazide
MRC[13]	1985	Thiazide or propranolol versus placebo

gram,[21] reduction of systolic pressure to below 143 mmHg (lowest quartile on treatment) was associated with a slightly higher incidence of coronary heart disease compared with those with systolic pressures of 143 to 159 mmHg. However, those with pressures above 159 mmHg had the highest incidence of coronary disease. The occurrence of coronary disease decreased in those with on-treatment diastolic pressures of greater than 97 to 86 mmHg, but increased slightly in the 86 mmHg or less group. It was concluded that there may be a level of blood pressure during treatment (140 to 150 mmHg systolic/85 to 90 mmHg diastolic) below which no further benefit would be gained by antihypertensive medication. A recent meta-analysis supports the J-curve hypothesis that the optimal on-treatment level of diastolic pressure for prevention of coronary heart disease is about 85 mmHg[22] (Fig. 5-2).

Mechanisms accounting for increased coronary heart disease in those with the lowest diastolic pressure on treatment are not fully established. It has been suggested that the J-curve is due to presence of ischemic heart disease before treatment. If this effect is limited to those with pretreatment atherosclerosis of the coronary arteries, a reduced ability of stiffened coronary arteries to permit flow at lower diastolic pressures (an upward shift of the autoregulatory range for coronary flow) might occur.[23] However, reanalysis of the Goteborg study indicates that the J-curve pattern is observed both in those with and in those without evidence of ischemic heart disease before treatment.[24] A recent report suggests that it is the excessive reduction from pretreatment pressure rather than the level of arterial pressure achieved on treatment that is related to increased morbidity.[25] This observation is not confirmed in the reanalysis of the Goteborg study.[24]

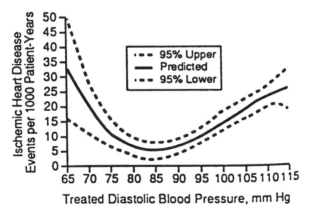

Fig. 5-2. J-curve (summary curve model) from a meta-analysis of the clinical trials of hypertension. This composite suggests that the optimal on-treatment diastolic pressure is nearly 85 mmHg. Confidence limits are shown and increase as pressure falls below the "optimal pressure." (From Farnett et al.,[22] with permission.)

TREATMENT IN THE ELDERLY

Before 1980, there was considerable skepticism that drug treatment of older or elderly hypertensive patients (above 60 to 65 years, then perceived as elderly) would be beneficial. In part this may have been due to the limited availability of antihypertensive drugs without adverse effects on central nervous function. Such agents as reserpine, methyldopa, clonidine, and the then available β-blocker propranolol were well known for causing depressive symptoms, fatigue, disturbing dreams, and impaired mental function. In older patients, these adverse effects were often intolerable. Furthermore, no studies were specifically designed to evaluate whether drug treatment would prevent cardiovascular disease, as had been shown for middle-aged patients, 50 to 65 years old. In addition, the pathophysiology of hypertension in the elderly was thought to be a result of reduced compliance of larger arteries and the aorta rather than vasoconstriction of resistance vessels, characteristic of younger hypertensive patients. Theoretically, older patients would be less likely to respond to drug treatment primarily designed to diminish vasoconstriction. Nonetheless, the well-established risk of either systolic or diastolic pressure elevations in older populations provided the basis for randomized trials of drug therapy.

Five randomized clinical trials have now been conducted in elderly hypertensive patients,[10–12,26–30] and the older subgroups from additional trials have been reanalyzed (Table 5-3). All but one included those with diastolic hypertension. The European Working Party on Hypertension in the Elderly (EWPHE) trial[26] first demonstrated that drug treatment significantly reduced cardiovascular disease in older patients. The benefit of treatment was greater for prevention of cardiac events than for cerebrovascular disease. A similar, but less impressive trend was found in the study by Coope and Warrender.[27] Neither of these trials demonstrated that treatment could achieve a reduction in overall mortality.

Two recently published studies[29,30] add support to the conclusion that antihypertensive drug treatment is beneficial for elderly patients with diastolic hypertension. In the MRC trial,[30] atenolol (a β-blocker) was compared with diuretic therapy. Stroke was reduced by both drugs compared with placebo. However, coronary events were decreased by the diuretic drug but not by the

Table 5-3. Clinical Trials of Hypertension in the Elderly

Name of Trial	Year Published	Drugs Used
EWPHE[26]	1985	Thiazide-triamterene, methyldopa
Coope and Warrender[27]	1986	Thiazide, atenolol, methyldopa
SHEP[28]	1991	Chlorthalidone, atenolol
STOP-Hypertension, Sweden[29]	1991	Thiazide/amiloride, β-blockers
MRC Trial[30]	1992	Thiazide or propranolol versus placebo

β-blocker. Cardiovascular mortality was significantly reduced by treatment compared with placebo. All cause mortality was, however, not affected by drug therapy. The Swedish Trial in Old Patients with Hypertension[29] compared several β-blockers and a diuretic combination designed to minimize hypokalemia (thiazide and amiloride) with a placebo. This study was discontinued by the monitoring committee because of a clear, significant trend toward reduction in stroke and cardiovascular deaths in the treated subjects. Of note, however, was a pattern suggesting that antihypertensive drug treatment conferred no benefit in those over 84 years of age.

The Systolic Hypertension in the Elderly Program study[28] evaluated antihypertensive drug treatment (low-dose diuretic medication with the β-blocker atenolol as the second step) in relatively healthy elderly patients with isolated systolic pressures of 160 mmHg or higher and diastolic pressures of less than 90 mmHg at baseline. Compared with the placebo group, the treated patients had significant reductions in cerebrovascular disease (stroke), myocardial infarction, left ventricular failure, and death due to coronary heart disease. Adverse effects possibly related to drug treatment were somewhat more frequent in those on active drugs compared with the placebo group.

These studies indicate that antihypertensive drug treatment is surprisingly beneficial in elderly populations. The more recent studies emphasize that this benefit may be achieved with relatively low doses of the antihypertensive agents. Table 5-4 summarizes the impact of antihypertensive drug therapy in elderly patients.

OTHER ISSUES

Left Ventricular Hypertrophy

Many clinically relevant issues are not yet fully addressed in randomized clinical trials of antihypertensive therapy. For example, the presence of left ventricular hypertrophy with hypertension confers a worse prognosis.[31,32] Antihypertensive drugs (antiadrenergic agents, calcium channel entry blockers, and ACE inhibitors) may reduce left ventricular hypertrophy through reduction in wall thickness. Diuretics may also reduce left ventricular mass, but primarily by a decrease in diastolic chamber dimension rather than a

Table 5-4. Effect of Antihypertensive Drug Treatment for Elderly Patients[a]

Event	Risk Reduction (%)
Stroke	34
Coronary heart disease	19
Congestive heart failure	48
All cardiovascular disease	25

[a]Pooled results of seven studies; weighted average based on number of subjects in each study. (From the Joint National Committee on Detection and Treatment of Hypertension.[52])

change in wall thickness.[33] However, no trial yet confirms that reduction of left ventricular mass (regression of left ventricular hypertrophy) has an independent benefit distinct from reduction in arterial pressure itself. However, it may be quite difficult to design a study in which blood pressure is lowered *without* some reduction in left ventricular mass, no matter how the subjects were to be treated. Furthermore, I am not certain it would be ethically suitable, given our present knowledge, to embark on such an effort if it were likely that one group would be treated with an agent (e.g., minoxidil) that would achieve this effect.

Progression of Renal Insufficiency

Retrospective surveys suggest that antihypertensive drug therapy delays progression of renal insufficiency in those with chronic renal disease, particularly diabetic nephropathy.[34-36] On theoretical grounds and some clinical experience, ACE inhibitors have been thought to be particularly suited to delay progression in this disorder.[34] A recent randomized trial comparing an ACE inhibitor, captopril, with placebo was conducted in insulin-dependent diabetics with proteinuria nephropathy. The results clearly demonstrate a beneficial effect for those receiving the ACE inhibitor. They had a significantly reduced rate of progression of renal insufficiency as assessed by reduction in glomerular filtration rate or requirement for dialysis or renal transplantation.[37] The benefit of ACE inhibitor therapy in this study was most marked in those who entered with a serum creatinine level of 1.5 mg/dl or more. Not all patients in this study were hypertensive; the value of ACE inhibition could not be related to any change in blood pressure. ACE inhibitors can reduce microalbuminuria over a 5-year period in normotensive persons with noninsulin-dependent diabetes.[38] It is not yet known, however, whether this strategy will prevent progression to renal insufficiency requiring renal replacement therapy (dialysis or transplantation) in adults with noninsulin-dependent diabetes.

End-stage renal disease requiring renal replacement therapy occurs far more often in black (African-American) than in nonblack hypertensive persons. It has been suggested that this is the result of inadequate blood pressure reduction in those with increased sensitivity to the nephrosclerotic effect of hypertension or to factors, not yet characterized, independent of arterial pressure level. The value of aggressive antihypertensive therapy with either calcium channel blockers or ACE inhibitors for preventing progression of renal insufficiency in nondiabetic hypertensive groups, especially black patients, is now being studied actively. Some studies will compare pressure reduction with the usually accepted therapeutic range (diastolic pressures 80 to 90 mmHg) with attempts to achieve much lower pressures (in the diastolic range of 70 to 80 mmHg).

Newer Drugs

Are the newer antihypertensive drug classes, the ACE inhibitors, α-receptor blockers, and calcium entry blockers, equal or superior to the older agents (thiazide-type diuretics, β-blockers, methyldopa, and hydralazine) in preventing cardiovascular mortality or morbidity for those with the usual form of mild-to-moderate hypertension? A pilot study (TOMHS) has been conducted to assess the feasibility of such an approach.[14,39] In this trial, approximately 900 middle-aged mild hypertensive individuals were recruited for evaluation. All received training in diet and exercise (nutritional-hygienic) intervention and were randomized to receive either placebo or one of the following drugs given once per day: amlodipine (5 mg), acebutolol (400 mg), chlorthalidone (15 mg), doxazosin (2 mg), or enalapril (5 mg). During the first year of the study, pressure fell in *all* groups, but to a greater (and similar) extent in the five drug-treated groups compared with the placebo-treated group. Side effect profiles were remarkably similar among the various treatment groups.[39] After completion of the trial, with an average of 4.4 years of follow up, major events (death from any cause, nonfatal myocardial infarction or stroke, congestive heart failure, surgery for aneurysm, coronary bypass surgery, angioplasty, thrombolytic therapy or hospitalization for unstable angina) were found to be 7.1 percent for the placebo group and 5.1 percent for all drug-treated groups combined. The 31-percent reduction for events in those treated with antihypertensive drugs was not statistically significant ($P = 0.21$).[14] When major events were combined with minor events (transient ischemic attacks, angina, or claudication as determined by questionnaire), the rates were 16.2 percent in the placebo group and 11.1 percent in the combined drug-treated groups, a significant difference ($P = 0.03$). The TOMHS trial was too small to compare the different drugs used. Nonetheless, all five drugs were well tolerated at low doses and were effective for blood pressure reduction; they can now all be considered as appropriate for monotherapy of mild hypertension.

Of the newer antihypertensive agents, only the ACE inhibitors have found a secure role in the treatment of those with impaired left ventricular systolic function reflected as either overt congestive failure or reduced left ventricular ejection fraction without symptoms. Several studies indicate that use of ACE inhibitors improves the outcome for such subjects.[40–43]

INTERPRETATION OF CLINICAL TRIALS

Before concluding this chapter, a few words of caution are in order for the physician who would rely on available results of randomized clinical trials as the sole basis for therapeutic decisions in the treatment of hypertension. At issue are the problems of (1) generalization and (2) extrapolation. It is expected that the outcome of a clinical trial will best predict the future results of a group of patients most nearly like those enrolled in the trial and who are treated in a similar way to those treated in the study. If an individual patient is unlike those in the trial, the same results may not be as likely to occur; more or less benefit may accrue. For example, diabetic hypertensive persons were excluded from several of the randomized trials of antihypertensive therapy. Can we expect that, as a group, diabetic hypertensive persons will derive the same benefit from reduction in arterial pressure as do nondiabetic hypertensive persons? We may hope so, but there is no certainty that this will happen. When we extrapolate the results of the clinical trials well beyond the entry criteria or the treatment protocol employed, our ability to determine the expected outcome becomes more and more imprecise. As a result, therapeutic decisions become more of an informed guess than a statistical likelihood. However, when patients do resemble those of the trial, the guesswork is reduced. Evidence shows that reports of such studies influence physicians' therapeutic choices.[44]

Even if many of our patients are similar to those whose experiences are reported in one or more randomized clinical trials, what results should we expect? The results of clinical trials can be reported in various ways. Most often, the benefit of a treatment is presented as the reduction in risk ratio or in relative risk (e.g., a decrease in stroke of 40 percent). However, if displayed as the change in absolute rate of stroke, from 1 percent to 0.6 percent (0.4 percent absolute reduction), the perspective changes. It then becomes apparent that many will be treated to benefit a single patient through prevention of a single event. Calculation of the number needed to treat can be made. This is illustrated in Figure 5-3. Other methods for putting the results of a clinical trial into perspective may be interesting or useful from time to time, such as calculation of the cost/benefit ratio (total dollar amount needed to prevent one event) or, more recently, the tons of drug needed to prevent an event.[45]

Other pitfalls may be overlooked if one fails to examine the fine print of the methods and results sections of clinical trials: (1) Were there large dropout rates? Perhaps many could not tolerate the treatment. Do the results take this into account by reporting *intention to treat* outcomes, as well as out-

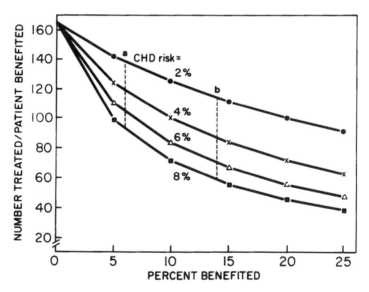

Fig. 5-3. Efficiency of treatment: relationship to incidence of coronary heart disease (CHD). Calculation of number of patients treated over 5 years to benefit one patient by reduction of either stroke or CHD. Rates for stroke are based on the British MRC trial.[13] Calculations were made for added benefit by varying incidence rates of CHD from 2 to 8 percent and for reduction in risk by treatment from 0 to 25 percent. Meta-analyses suggest, however, that the achieved benefit for reducing CHD is from 6 to 14 percent (lines a and b), implying that, at best, 60 are treated for every 1 patient who benefits by prevention of serious disease. (Courtesy of Dr. L.R. Krakoff.)

comes for subjects completing the trial? Were adverse effects presented fairly? (2) Was the study stable, or were there changes along the way because of unforeseen events? (3) Were differences between two or more treatments present for a main effect (i.e., comparing all subjects), or were they limited to selected subgroups? If limited to subgroups, were they identified at the start of the study or only by retrospective analysis? (4) As a last consideration, do the results make sense if viewed from the known pathophysiology of the disease and the pharmacology of the drugs used?

Randomized clinical trials, in spite of their limitations, provide useful information and are the backbone of sound clinical decision making when they are applicable. Nonetheless, despite the abundance of clinical trials for therapy of hypertension, many patients do not match entry criteria of trials already conducted. Furthermore, new developments in the drug treatment of hypertension have not been fully tested through the mechanism of randomized controlled trials of outcome, yet appear valuable for the therapy of many patients. Physicians considering the therapeutic options for each patient they encounter will still have to employ sound clinical judgment by balancing the conclusions of randomized clinical trials with several other pertinent factors to arrive at optimal strategy.

REFERENCES

1. Lau J, Antman EM, Jimenez-Silva J et al: Cumulative meta-analysis of therapeutic trials for myocardial infarction. N Engl J Med 327:248, 1992
2. Thompson SG, Pocock SJ: Can meta-analyses be trusted? Lancet 338:1127, 1991
3. Veterans Administration Cooperative Study Group on Antihypertensive Agents: Effects of treatment on morbidity in hypertension: results in patients with diastolic blood pressures averaging 115 through 129 mmHg. JAMA 202:1028, 1967
4. Veterans Administration Cooperative Study Group on Antihypertensive Agents: Effects of treatment on morbidity in hypertension. II. Results in patients with diastolic blood pressure averaging 90 through 114 mmHg. JAMA 213:1143, 1970
5. Veterans Administration Cooperative Study Group on Antihypertensive Agents: Effects of treatment on morbidity in hypertension. III. Influence of age, diastolic pressure, and prior cardiovascular disease: further analysis of side effects. JAMA 45:991, 1972
6. MacMahon SW, Cutler JA, Furberg CD, Payne GH: The effects of drug treatment for hypertension on morbidity and mortality from cardiovascular disease: a review of randomized clinical trials. Prog Cardiovasc Dis 24:99, 1986
7. Collins R, Peto R, MacMahon S et al: Blood pressure, stroke, and coronary heart disease. Part 2. Short-term reductions in blood pressure: overview of randomized drug trials in their epidemiological context. Lancet 335:827, 1990
8. Yusuf S, Wittes J, Friedman L: Overview of results of randomized clinical trials in heart disease. 1. Treatments following myocardial infarction. JAMA 260:2088, 1988
9. Yusuf S, Wittes J, Friedman L: Overview of results of randomized clinical trials in heart disease. II. Unstable angina, heart failure, primary prevention with aspirin, and risk factor modification. JAMA 260:2259, 1988

10. Report by the Management Committee: The Australian Therapeutic Trial in Mild Hypertension. Lancet 1:1261, 1980

11. Hypertension Detection and Follow-up Program Cooperative Group: Five-year findings of the Hypertension Detection and Follow-Up Program. II. Mortality by race, sex and age. JAMA 242:2572, 1979

12. Hypertension Detection and Follow-Up Program Cooperative Group: Five-year findings of the Hypertension Detection and Follow-Up Program. I. Reduction in mortality of persons with high blood pressure, including mild hypertension. JAMA 242:2562, 1979

13. Medical Research Council Working Party: MRC trial of treatment of mild hypertension: principal results. BMJ 291:97, 1985

14. Neaton JD, Grimm RH Jr, Prineas RJ et al: Treatment of Mild Hypertension Study: final results. JAMA 207:713, 1993

15. Grimm RH, Leon AS, Hunninghake DB et al: Effects of thiazide diuretics on plasma lipids and lipoproteins in mildly hypertensive patients: a double blind controlled trial. Ann Intern Med 94:7, 1981

16. Multiple Risk Factor Intervention Trial Research Group: Multiple risk factor intervention trial: risk factor changes and mortality results. JAMA 248:1465, 1982

17. Moser M, Sheps S: Confusing messages from the newest of the beta-blocker/diuretic hypertension trials. Arch Intern Med 149:2174, 1989

18. Fletcher AE, Bulpitt CJ, Chase DM et al: Quality of life with three antihypertensive treatments: cilazapril, atenolol, nifedipine. Hypertension 19:499, 1992

19. Goldman L, Sia STB, Cook EF et al: Costs and effectiveness of routine therapy with long-term beta-adrenergic antagonists after acute myocardial infarction. N Engl J Med 319:152, 1988

20. Cruickshank JM, Thorp JM, Zacharias FJ: Benefits and potential harm of lowering high blood pressure. Lancet 1:581, 1987

21. Samuelsson O, Wilhelmsen L, Andersson OK et al: Cardiovascular morbidity in relation to change in blood pressure and serum cholesterol levels in treated hypertension: results from the primary prevention in Goteborg, Sweden. JAMA 258:1768, 1987

22. Farnett L, Mulrow CD, Linn WD et al: The J-curve phenomenon and the treatment of hypertension. Is there a point beyond which pressure reduction is dangerous? JAMA 265:489, 1991

23. Polese A, De Cesare N, Montorsi P et al: Upward shift of the lower range of coronary flow autoregulation in hypertensive patients with hypertrophy of the left ventricle. Circulation 83:845, 1991

24. Samuelsson OG, Wilhemsen LW, Pennert KM et al: The J-shaped relationship between coronary heart disease and achieved blood pressure level in treated hypertension: further analyses of 12 years of follow-up of treated hypertensives in the Primary Prevention Trial in Gothenburg, Sweden. J Hypertens 8:547, 1990

25. Alderman MH, Ooi WL, Madhavan S, Cohen H: Treatment-induced blood pressure reduction and the risk of myocardial infarction. JAMA 262:920, 1989

26. Amery A, Birkenhager W, Brixko P et al: Mortality and morbidity results from the European Working Party on High Blood Pressure in the Elderly Trial. Lancet 1:1349, 1985

27. Coope J, Warrender TS: Randomized trial of treatment of hypertension in elderly patients in primary care. BMJ 293:1145, 1986

28. SHEP Cooperative Research Group: Prevention of stroke by antihypertensive drug treatment in older persons with isolated systolic hypertension: final results of the Systolic Hypertension in the Elderly Program (SHEP). JAMA 265:3255, 1991

29. Dahlof B, Lindholm LH, Hansson L et al: Morbidity and mortality in the Swedish Trial in Old Patients with hypertension (STOP-hypertension). Lancet 338:1281, 1991

30. MRC Working Party: Medical Research Council trial of treatment of hypertension in older adults: principal results. BMJ 304:405, 1992

31. Casale PN, Devereux RB, Milner M et al: Value of echocardiographic measurements of left ventricular mass in predicting cardiovascular morbid events in hypertensive men. Ann Intern Med 105:173, 1986

32. Levy D, Garrison RJ, Savage DD et al: Prognostic implications of echocardiographically determined left ventricular mass in the Framingham Heart Study. N Engl J Med 322:1561, 1990

33. Dahlof B, Pennert K, Hansson L: Reversal of left ventricular hypertrophy in hypertensive patients: a metaanalysis of 109 treatment studies. Am J Hypertens 5:95, 1992

34. Keane WF, Anderson S, Aurell M et al: Angiotensin converting enzyme inhibitors and progressive renal insufficiency. Ann Intern Med 111:503, 1990

35. Parving HH, Andersen AR, Smidt UM, Svendsen PA: Early aggressive antihypertensive treatment reduces rate of decline in kidney function in diabetic nephropathy. Lancet 1:1175, 1983

36. Klahr S: The modification of diet in renal disease study. N Engl J Med 320:864, 1989

37. Lewis EJ, Hunsicker LG, Bain RP, Rohde RD for the Collaborative Study Group: The effect of angiotensin-converting-enzyme inhibition on diabetic nephropathy. N Engl J Med 329:1456, 1993

38. Ravid M, Savin H, Jutrin I et al: Long-term stabilizing effect of angiotensin-converting enzyme inhibition on plasma creatinine and on proteinuria in normtensive type II diabetic patients. Ann Intern Med 118:577, 1993

39. Treatment of Mild Hypertension Research Group: The treatment of mild hypertension study: a randomized, placebo-controlled trial of a nutritional-hygienic regimen along with various drug monotherapies. Arch Intern Med 151:1413, 1991

40. The SOLVD Investigators: Effect of enalapril on survival in patients with reduced left ventricular ejection fractions and congestive heart failure. N Engl J Med 325:293, 1991

41. Cohn JN, Johnson G, Ziesche S, et al: A comparison of enalapril with hydralazine-isosorbide dinitrate in the treatment of chronic congestive heart failure. N Engl J Med 325:303, 1991

42. The CONSENSUS Trial Study Group: Effects of enalapril on mortality in severe congestive heart failure: results of the Cooperative North Scandinavian Enalapril Survival Study (CONSENSUS). N Engl J Med 316:1429, 1987

43. Pfeffer MA, Braunwald E, Moye LA et al: Effect of captopril on mortality and morbidity in patients with left ventricular dysfunction after myocardial infarction: results of the survival and ventricular enlargement trial. N Engl J Med 327:669, 1992

44. Lamas GA, Pfeffer MA, Hamm P et al: Do the results of randomized clinical trials of cardiovascular drugs influence medical practice? N Engl J Med 327:241, 1992

45. Naylor CD, Chen E, Strauss B: Measured enthusiasm: does the method of reporting trial results alter perceptions of therapeutic effectiveness? Ann Intern Med 117:916, 1992

46. Helgeland A: Treatment of mild hypertension: a five year controlled drug trial. Am J Med 69:725, 1980

47. The Multiple Risk Factor Intervention Trial Research Group: Mortality rates after 10.5 years for participants in the Multiple Risk Factor Intervention Trial. Findings related to a priori hypotheses of the trial. JAMA 263:1795, 1990

48. Berglund G, Sannerstedt R, Andersson O et al: Coronary heart-disease after treatment of hypertension. Lancet 8054:1, 1978

49. The IPPPSH Collaborative Group: Cardiovascular risk and risk factors in a randomized trial of treatment based on the beta-blocker oxprenolol: the International Prospective Primary Prevention Study in Hypertension (IPPPSH). J Hypertens 3:379, 1985

50. Wilhelmsen L, Berglund G, Elmfeldt D et al: Beta-blockers versus diuretics in hypertensive men: main results from the HAPPHY trial. J Hypertens 5:561, 1987

51. Wikstrand J, Warnold I, Olsson G et al: Primary prevention with metoprolol in patients with hypertension: mortality results from the MAPHY study. JAMA 259:1976, 1988

52. Joint National Committee on Detection and Treatment of Hypertension: The 5th Report of the Joint National Committee on Detection, Evaluation and Treatment of High Blood Pressure (JNC V). Arch Intern Med 153:154, 1993

Section II

DIAGNOSTIC ASSESSMENT

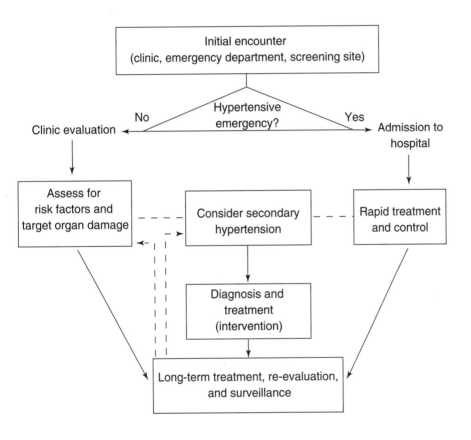

6

DIAGNOSIS: GENERAL CONSIDERATIONS

What do we need to know for the diagnosis of hypertensive patients before starting either treatment or a detailed search for reversible causes? Since patients are so different from each other, no single list of procedures or tests is appropriate. However, common categories of information can be delineated to organize our priorities before making decisions such as "antihypertensive drug treatment must begin," "this patient needs additional observation," or "this patient is normotensive, but other risk factors need correction."

The sections of this chapter focus on the diagnostic strategy applicable to most hypertensive patients, in particular those who will be evaluated and treated in the clinic or office. The areas to be evaluated are summarized in Table 6-1.

For most of the categories listed in Table 6-1, methods of measurement or detection include basic clinical skills, the medical history and physical examination, and widely available technologies and laboratory tests. Some patients, however, benefit from more complex and sophisticated assessments, such as 24-hour ambulatory blood pressure monitoring or magnetic resonance imaging. Each procedure or test has its own accuracy, potential for benefit or harm, and cost. In some cases, test accuracy is well known or characterized. For others, accuracy and other characteristics have not been well studied. Thus, the large menu of diagnostic evaluations at our disposal for the diagnosis of hypertension should be employed judiciously and with good sense.

MEASUREMENT OF ARTERIAL PRESSURE

When a patient is first seen, how high is the blood pressure? Ordinarily the pressure will be taken manually by auscultation, the method used for the past 100 years. Blood pressure should be taken in both arms (to exclude subclavian artery stenosis) and in the legs (if there is reason to suspect peripheral arterial occlusive disease or coarctation of the aorta). The size of the cuff should be appropriate for the size of the arm or leg. When possible, the patient should be seated for a few minutes before the pressure is taken, in the hope that the patient will relax (to the extent possible in a physician's presence). If performed correctly, the usual clinical method for measurement of arterial pressure is suitable for defining those with clearly normal (less than 130/85 mmHg systolic/diastolic pressure) and very high blood pressure

Table 6-1. Initial Diagnostic Evaluation for Hypertensive Patients

Accurate, unbiased determination of arterial pressure
Assessment of nonhypertensive risk status
Staging for complications or pathology due to cardiovascular disease
Investigation for reversible causes of hypertension
Overall medical status with regard to additional disorders, allergies,
    and other factors pertinent to individual management

(180/110 mmHg or higher) on the initial visit. For such patients, supplemental methods of measurement are not needed. If the pressure falls between these extremes, as it does in many patients, a strategy to determine the usual or average pressure becomes necessary. Figure 6-1 provides an approach to this problem.

When mild hypertension or a borderline blood pressure (diastolic pressure 90 to 100 mmHg) is initially detected, two or three blood pressure determinations in the clinic may not reflect the average daily blood pressure with enough accuracy.[1] The small sample size and limited standardization for determining blood pressure on a casual basis may be a source of error for noninvasive measurement of the average blood pressure. Dividing lines between normal pressure, high-normal pressure, and mild hypertension are all situated on the upper part or down-slope of the population distribution curve. Thus, small errors in measurement of blood pressure (e.g., 5 mmHg) are more likely to misclassify normal persons as hypertensive (false-positive diagnoses) than hypertensive patients as normal (false-negative diagnoses).[2] In addition to this statistical consideration, other sources of error include bias by the nurse or physician[3] and an excessive "stress" response by the subject to the physician or clinic setting.[4,5] The results of serial measurements of clinic blood pressure in therapeutic trials have shown that over a 6-month period a substantial fraction (nearly 20 percent) of the blood pressure of those initially thought to have mild hypertension will decrease to the normal range on placebo alone.[6,7] Hence, repeated clinic measurements, using an unbiased method for five to eight visits[1,2,8] may be needed to determine the diagnosis.

Greater precision in determining average pressure may be provided by noninvasive ambulatory blood pressure monitoring or by self-taken home blood pressure measurements. These methods are described in the following sections.

Ambulatory Blood Pressure Monitoring

Ambulatory blood pressure monitoring with automatic devices has been widely studied[9,10] and found to have clinical utility. This technique has received increasing scrutiny as an improved means for predicting future cardiovascular mortality and morbidity when compared with casual measurements made in the clinic.[11] Noninvasive ambulatory blood pressure monitoring has also been shown to give better correlation with left ventricular hypertrophy, as determined by echocardiography, than casual blood pressure mea-

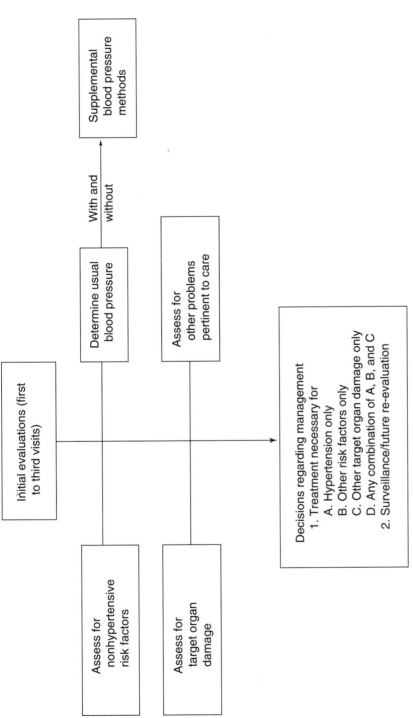

Fig. 6-1. Strategy for determining average or usual arterial pressures in those with high normal pressures or mild hypertension (i.e., initial clinic diastolic pressures of 85 to 100 mmHg).

surement.[12] This technique shows promise for the detection of those with elevated pressure only in the clinic—a form known as *white coat hypertension*[2,13–16]—or during brief episodes, as in the panic disorder syndrome.[17]

Figure 6-2 displays the pattern of white coat hypertension. Only the initial pressures, taken in a clinic at the time when the monitor was placed on the patient, are elevated. All other hourly average pressures are less than 140/90 mmHg. The white coat pattern is not limited to the first few visits, but may persist for long periods. We have observed a patient with white coat hypertension for more than 8 years, as shown in Figure 6-3.

Of untreated patients with clinic pressures in the mild hypertensive range, 20 to 40 percent will have average daytime pressures far lower when measured by ambulatory blood pressure monitoring. Usually, these patients are younger, have a recent diagnosis of hypertension, and are more likely to be women than men.[13,16,18] Studies to define the normal range for ambulatory blood pressure are in progress. Nonetheless, it is highly likely that those with average pressures below 130 to 135/85 mmHg have minimal or normal risk and clearly overlap the normal range.[13,19–21] The use of ambulatory blood pressure monitoring is cost-effective because of the improved accuracy in classifying those with mild hypertension, which then reduces the need to prescribe antihypertensive drugs for those with normal average pressures.[22]

Usual or average daily pressure may be *underestimated* by clinic or casual pressure measurements. Those with high job strain, defined as the combination of increased demand and low control over activity, tend to have higher daytime ambulatory pressures at work. This pattern of 24-hour blood pressure is shown in Figure 6-4. In addition, this group has an increased left ventricular mass index by echocardiography.[23] Cigarette smokers may also have higher pressures during usual activity compared with clinic measurements made during a brief escape from their habit.[24] Those with average daytime pressures disproportionately higher than their clinic or casual pressures should be considered at greater risk of future cardiovascular disease and thus targeted for more aggressive antihypertensive treatment and comprehensive risk intervention.

Noninvasive ambulatory blood pressure monitoring may also reveal abnormal patterns of diurnal variation, notably the lack of a sleep-related decrease in arterial pressure, as occur in autonomic neuropathy, chronic renal disease,[25] Cushing syndrome,[26] and after cardiac transplantation.[27] An example of such an abnormality is shown in Figure 6-5. A summary of conditions for which ambulatory blood pressure monitoring may be valuable is given in Table 6-2.

Home or Self-Determined Blood Pressure

The usefulness of home blood pressure measurement by the patient has been studied.[28–30] This approach is limited by the variable accuracy of the many devices available for home use,[31] the problems of "quality control" in teaching the patient and of a selection bias for choosing nonrepresentative pressures (those the patient may wish to have), and the lack of any correlation

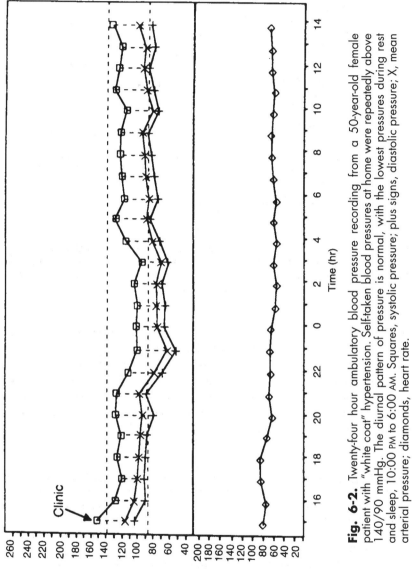

Fig. 6-2. Twenty-four hour ambulatory blood pressure recording from a 50-year-old female patient with "white coat" hypertension. Self-taken blood pressures at home were repeatedly above 140/90 mmHg. The diurnal pattern of pressure is normal, with the lowest pressures during rest and sleep, 10:00 PM to 6:00 AM. Squares, systolic pressure; plus signs, diastolic pressure; X, mean arterial pressure; diamonds, heart rate.

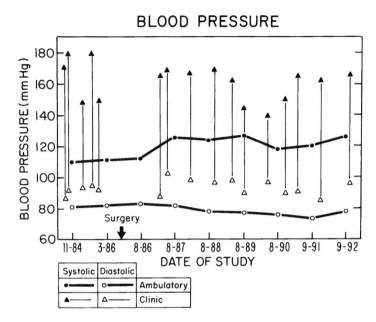

Fig. 6-3. White coat hypertension over several years.[97] While clinic pressures were always elevated, 24-hour ambulatory pressures were consistently less than 130/85 mmHg. A benign parathyroid adenoma was removed in 1986, as indicated by the arrow. (From Martin et al.,[97] with permission.)

with long-term outcome. Furthermore, the act of taking one's own pressure may increase it when compared with having it taken by someone else or by a device.[32] However, home blood pressure measurements are correlated with left ventricular mass,[33] left ventricular diastolic filling abnormalities, and reduced forearm vascular resistance in mild hypertension.[34] In addition, patients taught to take their own pressures may require fewer clinic visits, telephone calls to their doctor, and laboratory tests.[35]

Table 6-2. Situations for Which Ambulatory Blood Pressure Monitoring is Useful

Borderline blood pressure (seated pressures 135–150/85–100 mmHg after two to three office visits)

Apparent "refractory hypertension" (to determine true average pressure while on treatment)

Suspected white coat hypertension syndrome when clinic or casual pressures seem inappropriately high in relationship to patient's status

Suspected work-time hypertension due to occupation with high job strain

Panic disorder syndrome

Unexplained syncope, usually with concurrent Holter monitoring of electrocardiogram for rate and rhythm

Some forms of secondary hypertension (pheochromocytoma, Cushing syndrome, disorders of autonomic regulation, suspected disorders of diurnal blood pressure pattern)

Suspected disorders of diurnal rhythm in pressure

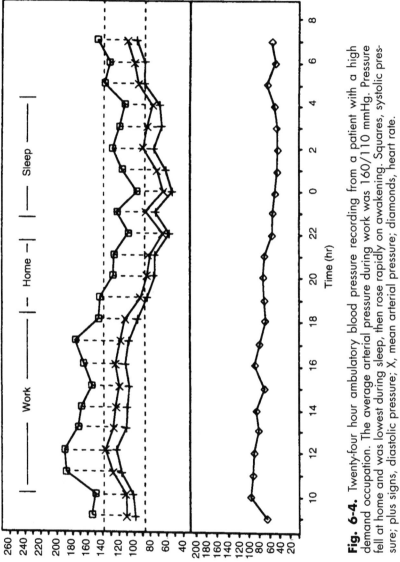

Fig. 6-4. Twenty-four hour ambulatory blood pressure recording from a patient with a high demand occupation. The average arterial pressure during work was 160/110 mmHg. Pressure fell at home and was lowest during sleep, then rose rapidly on awakening. Squares, systolic pressure; plus signs, diastolic pressure; X, mean arterial pressure; diamonds, heart rate.

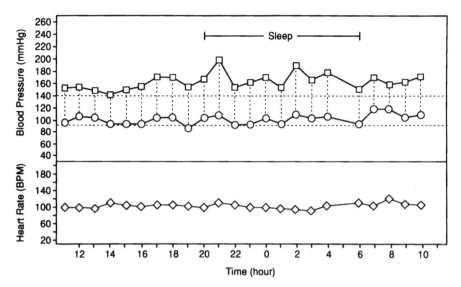

Fig. 6-5. Twenty-four hour ambulatory blood pressure recording from a patient with diabetic autonomic neuropathy and nephropathy. The diurnal pattern of pressure is distinctly abnormal. Throughout the day and night arterial pressure exceeds 140/90 mmHg. Highest pressures were recorded during sleep. Squares, systolic pressure; circles, diastolic pressure; diamonds, heart rate.

Exercise Blood Pressures

It has been suggested that blood pressures taken during programmed exercise, as in stress tests, may be helpful in deciding who is hypertensive. In one study, excessive elevation of systolic pressure (greater than 210 mmHg) correlated with the presence of left ventricular hypertrophy.[36] However, in other studies, changes in pressure during aerobic exercise or other challenges did not correlate well with ambulatory pressures.[14,37] This is not surprising, since the pattern of activity encountered during one's usual day need not have any relationship to hemodynamic changes for a short interval in unusual or artificial circumstances (i.e., stress or behavior testing).

Pseudohypertension

Older patients often have a disproportionate elevation of systolic pressure due in part to reduced compliance (stiffness) of large arteries. Noninvasive measurement of pressure may significantly overestimate the true intra-arterial pressure.[38] Patients with this pattern sometimes have palpable brachial and radial arteries despite cuff inflation to above their apparent systolic pressure, the Osler sign. A noninvasive method using infrasonic wave detection to detect pseudohypertension has been suggested.[39] Some elderly patients with pseudohypertension will have extensive calcification of the brachial artery and its major branches, which is easily seen on conventional radiographs of the arm. Rarely, the noninvasive blood pressure will be so much higher than expected by the clinical situation that direct intra-arterial measurement by catheterization of the radial or brachial artery will be necessary.

Postural Change

All patients, but especially the elderly, should have blood pressure measurements compared in the sitting and upright positions before and during treatment. The normal blood pressure response to standing is a small reduction (less than 10 mmHg) in systolic pressure, an increase in heart rate (2 to 10 BPM) and a small (2 to 5 mmHg) increase in diastolic pressure. Detection of a significant reduction, orthostatic hypotension (reduction greater than 20 mmHg in systolic pressure), may occur as a consequence of an underlying neuropathy (most often in patients with diabetes), disease of the central nervous system (multisystem atrophy, the Shy-Drager syndrome), drugs that reduce sympathetic reflex tone (α-receptor antagonists, peripheral neuron depletors, antidepressants), or excessive volume depletion due to diuretics. Some elderly patients have a tendency to orthostatic hypotension, which must be recognized before they are given antihypertensive medication.

Postprandial Hypotension

Elderly patients may have significant reductions in systolic pressure, averaging 25 mmHg, after large meals, presumably due to splanchnic pooling of blood and impaired baroreflexes.[40] This condition, *postprandial hypotension*, should be detectable by a trained observer or by a noninvasive ambulatory blood pressure monitor.

NONHYPERTENSIVE RISK FACTORS

What other reversible risk factors are present in the patient that may require treatment or management for optimal prevention? Some clarification is needed. Many factors are associated with cardiovascular disease. Some are predictors, but not causes (e.g., uric acid); others may be causative, but are not known to be reversible (familial or genetic tendencies). The term *risk factor* as used in cardiovascular disease means a predictor that is causative, treatable, and reversible (Table 6-3). Furthermore, reasonable evidence should be present that correcting the risk factor prevents future disease. The best evidence comes from well-conducted randomized clinical trials. However, other well-designed studies using a case-control method may be sufficient, as in the case of cigarette smoking.[41]

Weight, Health Behavior, or Life-Style Assessment

Some of the most important risk factors are those that patients control through their choices of ordinary activity. These include cigarette smoking, weight as determined by diet (calories) and exercise, exercise pattern itself, diet composition with regard to alcohol, salt, potassium, lipids, possibly calcium, and fish oil. The initial evaluation of all hypertensive patients must

Table 6-3. Test to Determine Metabolic or Additional Risk in Hypertensive Patients

Fasting plasma/serum glucose

Hemoglobin A1C
   Useful for integrating overall glucose level in patients whose fasting glucose is
      in the borderline range

Serum cholesterol profile
   Total cholesterol
   HDL cholesterol
   Total cholesterol/HDL ratio
   Triglycerides
   LDL_c cholesterol calculated as total cholesterol $- [HDL + \dfrac{triglycerides}{5}]$

Additional serum lipoprotein fractions[a]
   Lipoprotein (a)[b]
   Apolipoprotein levels

Plasma renin activity, renin profile when related to daily sodium excretion

---

[a]These tests have predictive value. It is not yet known whether they can be changed by treatment or whether such changes confer benefit.
[b]Not routinely available; primarily a research test.

---

include adequate assessment of these areas. Brief but well-designed questionnaires may be useful for this purpose.

Height and weight should be measured for all patients at the initial visit. Weight should be measured at all follow-up visits as well. The definition of overweight or obesity depends on relationships to height and body build, and can be quantified by various published tables or formulas. The body mass index (BMI) has achieved widespread use in epidemiologic studies and is easily calculated using the metric system for weight (kilograms) and height (meters). The formula is BMI = (kg/m^2). Since many health care providers in the United States still use the English system (pounds and inches), a simple corrected calculation can be made:

$$BMI = 705 \times \frac{weight\ (pounds)}{height\ (inches)^2}$$

For women, the desirable weight is based on a BMI of 24 or less; at 10 percent above this limit, the BMI is 26.4. For men the desirable weight is based on a BMI of 25 or less, with a 10 percent upper limit of 27.5. Table 6-4 lists desirable weights related to height for both genders and the 10 percent upper limits. These measurements may be helpful in counseling patients about the amount they are overweight and reasonable targets for weight reduction.

Serum Cholesterol and Fractions

The status of serum lipids or lipoproteins as risk factors is as important for hypertensive as for normotensive patients. Total serum cholesterol and its component fractions, low-density lipoprotein (LDL) and high-density lipoprotein (HDL) cholesterol, and their ratios serve as a the major guide to risk classification.[42] More recently described serum lipoproteins, such as

Table 6-4. Upper Limits of Desirable Weight Adjusted for Height in Women and Men[a]

Gender	Height (in.)	Height (cm)	Desirable Weight (lb)	10% Limit (lb)	Desirable Weight (kg)	10% Limit (kg)
Women						
	60	152	123	135	55.7	61.3
	61	155	127	139	57.6	63.3
	62	157	131	144	59.5	65.4
	63	160	135	149	61.4	67.6
	64	163	139	153	63.4	69.7
	65	165	144	158	65.4	71.9
	66	168	148	163	67.4	74.1
	67	170	153	168	69.5	76.4
	68	173	157	173	71.6	78.7
	69	175	162	178	73.7	81.0
	70	178	167	183	75.8	83.4
	71	180	172	189	78.0	85.8
	72	183	176	194	80.2	88.2
	73	185	181	200	82.5	90.7
	74	188	186	205	84.7	93.2
Men						
	62	157	136	150	62.0	68.2
	63	160	141	155	64.0	70.4
	64	163	145	160	66.0	72.6
	65	165	150	165	68.1	74.9
	66	168	154	170	70.2	77.2
	67	170	159	175	72.4	79.6
	68	173	164	180	74.5	82.0
	69	175	169	186	76.7	84.4
	70	178	174	191	79.0	86.9
	71	180	179	197	81.3	89.4
	72	183	184	202	83.6	91.9
	73	185	189	208	85.9	94.5
	74	188	194	214	88.3	97.1
	75	191	199	219	90.7	99.7
	76	193	205	225	93.1	102.4

[a]Upper limits for desirable weight based on body mass index of 24 for women and 25 for men. Values for 10% above desirable weight are shown also.

lipoprotein (a), may be predictive or even pathogenetically linked to atherogenesis due to its homology with thrombosis-related proteins, specifically plasminogen.[43] As yet, however, these serum proteins fail to qualify as risk factors, since it is not known whether they can be modified by specific therapy or whether such modification would reduce future cardiovascular disease in randomized clinical trials. One study suggests that neither β-blockers nor other antihypertensive agents alter lipoprotein (a) levels.

Low High-Density Lipoprotein, High Triglyceride Pattern

The role of serum triglyceride concentration as an independent risk factor remains uncertain. It is evident, however, that a fraction of the hypertensive population, considered at high risk of cardiovascular disease, has the combination of obesity, noninsulin-dependent diabetes mellitus (NIDDM), low serum HDL cholesterol, and high serum triglyceride concentrations. Often these hypertensive persons have demonstrable resistance to the action of insulin and are hyperinsulinemic with varying degrees of glucose intolerance. This risk cluster or syndrome X may be the result of a genetically linked condition or the common product of a single pathogenetic sequence.[44–46]

Diabetes Mellitus, Intermediate Glucose Tolerance, and Insulin Resistance

In many series, 6 to 7 percent of the hypertensive population is classified as diabetic.[47,48] Most adult hypertensive diabetics are non-insulin dependent (NIDDM) and are also overweight. A lesser fraction of the adult hypertensive diabetic group is insulin dependent (IDDM). Some of those with IDDM, as adults, were previously juvenile or early onset diabetics who developed diabetic nephropathy as the basis of their elevated pressure. It has been suggested that such patients had a predisposition to become hypertensive, on the basis of red cell sodium-lithium countertransport abnormalities, which in turn led to additional renal (glomerular) pathology.[49,50] Other hypertensive patients with IDDM represent those with prior NIDDM who may have exhausted their insulin production.

Measurement of postprandial glucose levels in hypertensive patients or performance of glucose tolerance tests will expose a sizable fraction (10 to 15 percent) who are not clearly diabetic (i.e., fasting glucose remains less than 140 mg/dl), but who are now labeled as having impaired glucose tolerance. In many instances, the impairment will be accompanied by persistently elevated insulin levels, implying that the metabolic derangement is due to *insulin resistance* (i.e., a diminished cellular response to the action of circulating insulin). Furthermore, several recent studies have demonstrated that insulin resistance and persisting hyperinsulinemia may be present in many hypertensive subjects, without abnormal glucose tolerance.[51–53] While often found in obese subjects, insulin resistance has been described in nonoverweight hypertensive persons also.[54,55]

Is insulin resistance in hypertensive patients itself a risk factor? At this time, the answer must remain in doubt. The association between either hyperinsulinemia or insulin resistance and elevated arterial pressure is evident in some but not all groups. For example, the relationship between insulin resistance and arterial pressure found in whites is absent in blacks, those of subcontinental Indian extraction, Pima native Americans, and women with the polycystic ovary syndrome.[41,51,52,54–60] Hyperinsulinemia has been suggested as a cause of raised pressure by an action on either the central nervous system and sympathoadrenal function or on renal excretion of salt and water.[61–64] Confirmatory studies are needed before elevated insulin can be viewed as a direct cause of hypertension. Drugs that selectively reduce insulin resistance (metformin) may cause vasodilation; but their effects on arterial pressure need additional study. Finally, no studies document that reduction of insulin resistance, per se, causes sustained reduction in blood pressure with concurrent diminution in cardiovascular disease.

Renin Level

Hypertensive patients have either low, normal, or high renin patterns. The renin pattern is determined by the relationship of the plasma renin level to urine sodium excretion, as shown in Figure 6-6. Whether the renin-angiotensin system is a risk factor for hypertensive patients has been a controversial matter since a report in 1972 linked increased cardiovascular complications in hypertensive patients to normal or high renin levels.[66] In those with normal blood pressure, plasma renin activity may be a less significant predictor of future risk.[67] However, a large recently published prospective study now strongly supports the view that plasma renin activity can accurately predict future ischemic heart disease, independent of smoking history, glucose level, or cholesterol status within a hypertensive population. In that study, the low renin patients had a lower risk of myocardial infarction than normal and high renin patients.[65]

These results imply that normal and high renin patients may gain extra benefit from therapy that specifically reduces the action of the renin-angiotensin system (i.e., β-receptor antagonists, which decrease renin secre-

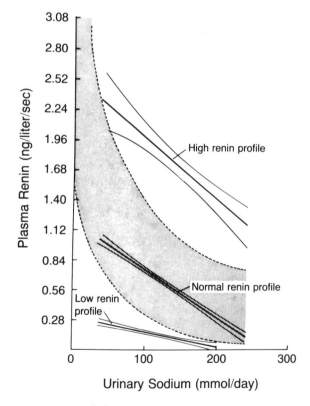

Fig. 6-6. Summary pattern of plasma renin in relationship to urine sodium excretion in a large cohort of untreated hypertensive patients. The normal relationship between renin and sodium excretion is indicated by the shaded area. Groups of low, normal, and high renin measurements within the hypertensive population are shown. (From Alderman et al.,[65] with permission.)

tion; ACE inhibitors, which inhibit formation of angiotensin II; direct angiotensin II antagonists, now in clinical trial; or direct renin inhibitors, currently being developed for clinical use). The above, together with the relatively low cost of performing plasma renin activity assays, suggest that renin profiling be added to the initial appraisal of many hypertensive patients. In addition, some forms of secondary hypertension (renal artery stenosis or primary aldosteronism) may be detected earlier when plasma renin levels are much higher or lower than the normal or expected range.

STAGE

Is the patient free of any cardiovascular disorder attributable to hypertension or nonhypertensive risk factors when first seen? Thorough evaluation of hypertensive patients may reveal the presence of cardiovascular disease in those organs affected by sustained elevations of pressure—the heart, retina, brain, kidneys, and peripheral arteries. A careful history, physical examination, selected laboratory tests, and the resting electrocardiogram were thought sufficient to answer this question. However, recent studies provide needed data regarding the value of this approach and also indicate when additional diagnostic assessment may be helpful.

Retinopathy

The retinae are the only sites where pathology of the hypertensive process can be seen directly by noninvasive means. Papilledema, hemorrhages, and/or exudates indicate the malignant or accelerated phase of hypertension, possibly due to uncontrolled essential hypertension, renal disease, scleroderma renal crisis, or renal artery stenosis.[68] Less severe retinal pathology, as reflected only in arteriolar abnormalities (focal constriction, arteriovenous crossing defects), is often present but fails to correlate well with the level of clinic or daytime ambulatory blood pressure, left ventricular mass (echocardiography), or microalbumin excretion.[69]

Cardiac Status

In the past, the electrocardiogram and the chest radiograph were used to detect left ventricular hypertrophy due to hypertension, a finding that confers a poorer prognosis. In recent years, a variety of new noninvasive approaches have become available that can, when used appropriately, add important data in determining the cardiac status of the hypertensive patient, as shown in Table 6-5.

Several studies indicate the superior sensitivity of echocardiography in detecting left ventricular hypertrophy compared with the electrocardiogram or chest radiograph. Furthermore, it is now established that the presence of echocardiographic left ventricular hypertrophy or higher left ventricular mass independently increases the likelihood of future cardiovascular morbidity.[70–72]

Antihypertensive drug treatment can reduce left ventricular mass,[73–75] and several drug classes have proved effective.[76] In obese patients, weight reduction may be useful.[77] It has yet to be shown, however, that regression of left ventricular hypertrophy or a decrease in left ventricular mass associated with

Table 6-5. Noninvasive Tests for Cardiac Disease in Hypertensive Patients

Chest radiograph
> Limited sensitivity and specificity; little use in most
> cases; helpful for pulmonary congestion; low cost

12-Lead electrocardiogram
> Limited sensitivity and specificity for left ventricular enlargement and ischemic
> heart disease; inexpensive, widely available, and can be well standardized

Echocardiogram
> The "gold standard" for left ventricular enlargement; useful for systolic and
> diastolic function (with Doppler measurement of flow velocity); can detect
> wall motion abnormalities of ischemic heart disease; high cost; subjective
> interpretation

Gated nuclear ventricular function (MUGA) scans
> The "gold standard" for noninvasive measurement of systolic function (ejection
> fraction) and useful for diastolic function; can be used with exercise; can
> detect wall motion abnormalities of ischemic heart disease; objective tech-
> nique; high cost

Stress thallium myocardial imaging
> For noninvasive detection of coronary artery disease; false-positive results often
> found in hypertensive patients without epicardial coronary stenosis

Adenosine or dipyrridamole thallium imaging
> Alternative to the exercise stress test; false-positive and -negative rates for hyper-
> tensive patients not well characterized

treatment of hypertension confers a better outlook, independent of the reduction in pressure, per se.

Left ventricular filling abnormalities (diastolic dysfunction) may occur in hypertensive patients, independent of left ventricular hypertrophy.[78–81] Severe left ventricular diastolic dysfunction may cause pulmonary congestion without diminished systolic or "pump" action.[82] It has been suggested that calcium channel entry blockers may be preferentially beneficial in reversing left ventricular diastolic dysfunction.[74]

Evidence of ischemic heart disease due to coronary artery atherosclerosis is often found in hypertensive patients, indicated by a history of angina pectoris or electrocardiographic signs of ischemia or previous myocardial infarction. Echocardiography or nuclear studies may reveal evidence of regional scars or ischemia reflected in wall motion abnormalities at rest or with exertion. Patients with left ventricular hypertrophy may have abnormal stress electrocardiogram results, which are then falsely positive for epicardial coronary artery lesions. Appropriate use of stress testing or adenosine thallium nuclear imaging may be helpful for noninvasive detection of coronary artery pathology when suspected by history. However, the rate of false-positive test results varies from study to study, implying that a positive stress thallium test does not guarantee a significant epicardial coronary lesion will be found in the hypertensive patient with an abnormal scan.[83,84]

How far should diagnostic testing go for assessment of the cardiac status of each hypertensive patient? Should all patients have echocardiography to determine left ventricular mass? Are noninvasive assessments for ischemic heart disease useful in asymptomatic patients? While these questions cannot be answered in an oversimplified way, most patients without either symptoms or abnormalities on physical examination of the heart can be effectively managed with nothing more than a resting electrocardiogram.

Nephropathy

Renal function in hypertensive patients is assessed by urinalysis and serum creatinine or urea nitrogen level. In selected situations, estimation of glomerular filtration rate by creatinine clearance and determination of total (24-hour or timed collection) protein excretion may be useful. Urinary excretion of albumin (microalbuminuria) is related to the presence of cardiac and vascular disease and the level of clinic or daytime ambulatory arterial pressure in hypertensive patients.[69,85] Tests useful for assessing renal function or defining the stage of chronic renal disease are shown in Table 6-6.

Cerebrovascular Disease

A brief, but pertinent neurologic examination should be part of each hypertensive patient's workup initially and at regular (every 1 to 2 years) intervals. In addition, the examiner should listen for carotid bruits in all patients with recent neurologic symptoms and periodically in those without obvious deficits. When abnormalities are found, additional studies may be needed. Noninvasive assessment of the extracranial cerebral vasculature by ultrasound may detect occlusive arterial disease. Computed tomography or magnetic resonance imaging may, on occasion, be pertinent. If reversible disease is highly suspected, arteriography is necessary. Detection of high-grade carotid artery stenosis in patients with compatible neurologic syndromes raises the possibility that vascular surgery may be beneficial.[86–89] Tests useful for establishing the neurologic status of hypertensive patients are shown in Table 6-7.

Peripheral Arterial Occlusive Disease

Diminished peripheral pulses or the symptom of intermittent claudication reflecting occlusive disease of the peripheral (leg) arteries is usually found in hypertensive patients with accompanying nonhypertensive risk factors (especially smoking, hyperlipidemia, and diabetes). Reduced pressure in the leg arteries is characteristic of coarctation of the aorta. As a minimum examination, the femoral, posterior tibial, and dorsalis pedis pulses should be palpated in all recently detected hypertensive persons. In addition, auscultation of the femoral areas is necessary to detect the bruit of iliac or femoral arterial stenosis.

Table 6-6. Tests of Renal Function and Progression of Renal Disease

"Dipstick" urinalysis for semiquantitative measurement of protein, glucose, red and white blood cells; microscopic evaluation of cells; casts may be helpful

Serum urea nitrogen and serum creatinine as markers of glomerular filtration

24-Hour urine or timed urine collection for total protein, creatinine excretion to calculate creatinine clearance

24-Hour urine or timed excretion of albumin (microalbuminuria)

Table 6-7. Neurologic Assessment of Hypertensive Patients

Comprehensive neurologic examination

Noninvasive evaluation of cerebral circulation (Doppler flow studies and B-scan of carotid and accessible arteries); ophthalmodynamometry

Noninvasive imaging for hemorrhage or infarction (computed tomographic scan or magnetic resonance imaging)

Cerebral arteriography

In the past, clinicians have tended to ignore asymptomatic peripheral vascular disease and wait for symptoms of claudication to develop before evaluating the arteries to the legs, unless they were searching for coarctation of the aorta. Recent studies, however, suggest that a more thorough assessment of these arteries is necessary in the initial evaluation even when coarctation is not likely to be present. This is especially so for those over 50 years of age or with a history of other risk factors that might hasten the appearance of atherosclerosis.

The systolic arterial pressure in the calf can be easily measured with a normal or large adult cuff and either palpation of the ankle or foot (dorsalis pedis or posterior tibial arteries) or use of inexpensive Doppler probes. Measurement of the ankle artery pressure can then be compared with that of the arm (brachial artery). Those with normal arteries to the legs will have equal or higher pressures in the lower leg arteries compared with the brachial artery, as reflected by an ankle/arm systolic pressure ratio of 1.0 or higher. Those with ankle/arm ratios of less than 0.9 have a two- to fourfold greater risk of cardiovascular pathology, especially carotid and coronary artery disease and death due to cardiovascular disease.[90–92] These observations suggest that such patients may benefit from aggressive control of their pressure and all pertinent risk factors to delay progression and perhaps even reverse their arterial pathology.

When peripheral arterial disease has advanced to the point of causing symptoms (i.e., intermittent claudication), noninvasive assessment by plethysmography and Doppler signal detection may be used to localize the site(s) of arterial obstruction. If claudication is mild and stable, a conservative, noninterventional approach is recommended.[93] For those with severe disabling manifestations of arterial occlusive disease, vascular surgery or angioplasty may be necessary. Digital vascular imaging of intravenously injected dye is a promising alternative to intra-arterial catheterization when the risk of complications during the latter procedure is high, before choosing an invasive approach to therapy.

Abdominal Aortic Aneurysms

The presence of abdominal aortic aneurysms in older patients, more than 55 years of age, especially those with hypertension, other risk factors, and chronic obstructive pulmonary disease (no doubt reflecting the effect of high levels of smoking), is a significant cause of morbidity and mortality. Rupture of undetected or untreated aneurysms causes either death or emergency surgery, often leading to a prolonged and complicated hospital course.[94] Many abdominal aneurysms can be detected by palpation, but sonography is far more sensitive and should be considered for asymptomatic patients,[95] for both initial detection and serial follow-up of small aneurysms. Recent surveys suggest that the rupture rate over 5 years for asymptomatic abdominal aortic aneurysms is less than 2 percent for those less than 4 cm in diameter, 3 to 12 percent for those 4 to 5 cm in diameter, and 25 to 40 percent for those 5 cm or above in diameter.[94] These considerations have led to the view that abdominal sonography may be a cost-effective screening strategy for detection and early surgical treatment in patients 55 to 60 years of age or older.[95,96]

SUMMARY OF THE INITIAL EVALUATION

After one or two visits to the clinic or office, the status of the patient with regard to level of pressure, nonhypertensive risk, staging (retinal, cardiac, renal, neurologic, and retinal status), likelihood of secondary hypertension, and other medical features can be summarized. Most often, the initial workup can be performed with the tests listed in Table 6-8. The important findings need to be organized so that a quick review can be made for efficient decisions concerning the need for additional evaluation or the initiation of treatment. The development of a problem list is often useful.

I have found that organizing this information into a micro-computer data base system is most helpful for a brief review before arriving at a therapeutic plan (Fig. 6-7). At this point, the sequence of decisions becomes more clear, and the following options alone or in combination can be initiated:

1. Begin antihypertensive therapy: pharmacologic and/or nonpharmacologic
2. Start treatment for nonhypertensive risk factors
3. Initiate additional tests for secondary hypertension
4. Administer additional tests for suspected target organ abnormalities or other medical disease
5. Limit management to surveillance, which may include ambulatory blood pressure monitoring or home blood pressure measurement

Table 6-8. Initial or Baseline Tests for Hypertensive Patients

Complete medical history and physical examination

Complete urinalysis

Serum electrolytes, blood count, urea nitrogen or creatinine (or both), uric acid, calcium, glucose[a]

Serum lipid profile (fasting cholesterol, HDL cholesterol, triglycerides)[a]

Standard 12-lead electrocardiogram

Chest radiograph optional, depending on presence of smoking, exposure to industrial irritants, symptoms of pulmonary disease, or other pertinent medical conditions

[a]These items are often combined in "chemical profiles," which also give results for general status, including hepatic function and other evaluations.

CARDIOVASCULAR RISK REPORT

M. Wellbeck, M.D.
Preventive Cardiology (PC) Associates
275 Osler Avenue
Englewood, NJ 07631

Thursday, April 21, 1994

Patient name: Risque, Hy (58-year-old white man)

Address: 300 Butterball Lane

Riverdale, NY 10463

Home phone: (212) 333-1111

Business phone: (212) 444-6666   Date first seen: 04/01/86

Date of birth: 04/15/36   Date last seen: 12/11/89

ID number: 222333355

Risk Profile

Hypertension status: Mild essential hypertension

Lipid status: Other

Diabetic status: Suspect

Smoking status: Used to - 60.0 pack years - stopped 06/86

Alcohol use: Moderate

Exercise: Never

Height: 1.73 m Weight: 85.0 kg (13.6% overweight) Body mass index: 28.4

Family history: Premature coronary diabetes

Stage Status

Retinal status: 2 (focal)

Cardiac: None

Neurologic: None

Renal: Hyperuricemia (06/84)

Vascular: None

Notes

Hypertension since 1979 associated with headaches, dizzyness.

Adverse reactions to many medications. Hypokalemia on thiazides.

Normal plasma renin (3.0). Echocardiograph: mild LVH. Last

LDL 150, HDL 35. High-stress job. Pressure well controlled.

Past year on ACE inhibitor. Still promises to lose weight

and exercise.

Fig. 6-7. Sample cardiovascular risk report for patient named "Hy Risque."

REFERENCES

1. Schechter CB, Adler RS: Bayesian analysis of diastolic blood pressure measurement. Med Decis Making 8:182, 1991

2. Perry HM Jr, Miller JP: Difficulties in diagnosing hypertension: implications and alternatives. J Hypertens 10:887, 1992

3. Bruce NG, Shaper AG, Walker M et al: Observer bias in blood pressure studies. J Hypertens 6:375, 1988

4. Mancia G, Bertinieri G, Grassi G et al: Effects of blood pressure measurement by the doctor on patient's blood pressure and heart rate. Lancet 2:695, 1983

5. Simons RJ, Baily RG, Zelis R, Zwillich CW: The physiologic and psychologic effects of the bedside presentation. N Engl J Med 321:1273, 1989

6. Management Committee of the Australian Therapeutic Trial in Mild Hypertension: untreated mild hypertension. Lancet 1:185, 1982

7. Medical Research Council Working Party: MRC trial of treatment of mild hypertension: principal results. BMJ 291:97, 1985

8. Pearce KA, Grimm RH, Rao S et al: Population-derived comparisons of ambulatory and office blood pressures: implications for the determination of usual blood pressure and the concept of white coat hypertension. Arch Intern Med 152:750, 1992

9. Pickering TG, Harshfield GA, Kleinert HD et al: Blood pressure during normal daily activities, sleep, and exercise. JAMA 247:992, 1982

10. Drayer JI, Weber MA, Nakamura DK: Automated ambulatory blood pressure monitoring: a study in age matched normotensive and hypertensive men. Am Heart J 109:1334, 1985

11. Perloff D, Sokolow M, Cowan R: The prognostic value of ambulatory blood pressures. JAMA 249:2792, 1983

12. Devereux RB, Pickering TG, Harshfield GA: Left ventricular hypertrophy in patients with hypertension: importance of blood pressure response to regular recurring stress. Circulation 68:470, 1983

13. Pickering TG, James GD, Boddie C et al: How common is white coat hypertension? JAMA 259:225, 1988

14. Siegel WC, Blumenthal JA, Divine GW: Physiological, psychological, and behavioral factors and white coat hypertension. Hypertension 16:140, 1990

15. Myers MG, Reeves RA: White coat phenomenon in patients receiving antihypertensive therapy. Am J Hypertens 4:844, 1991

16. Hoegholm A, Kristensen KS, Madsen NH, Svendsen TL: White coat hypertension diagnosed by 24-h ambulatory monitoring. Am J Hypertens 5:64, 1992

17. White WB, Baker LH: Ambulatory blood pressure monitoring in patients with panic disorder. Arch Intern Med 147:1973, 1987

18. Eison H, Phillips RA, Ardeljan M, Krakoff LR: Differences in ambulatory blood pressure between men and women with mild hypertension. J Hum Hypertens 4:400, 1990

19. Staessen J, Bulpitt CJ, Fagard R et al: Reference values for the ambulatory blood pressure and the blood pressure measured at home: a population study. J Hum Hypertens 5:355, 1991

20. O'Brien E, Murphy J, Tyndall A et al: Twenty-four-hour ambulatory blood pressure in men and women aged 17 to 80 years: the Allied Irish Bank Study. J Hypertens 9:355, 1991

21. Staessen J, Fagard RH, Ljinen PJ et al: Mean and range of the ambulatory pressure in normotensive subjects from a meta-analysis of 23 studies. Am J Cardiol 67:723, 1991

22. Krakoff LR, Schechter C, Fahs M, Andre M: Ambulatory blood pressure monitoring: is it cost-effective? J Hypertens 9:S28, 1991

23. Schnall PL, Pieper C, Schwartz JE et al: The relationship between "job strain," workplace diastolic pressure, and left venticular mass index: results of a case control study. JAMA 263:1929, 1990

24. Mann SJ, James GD, Wang RS, Pickering TG: Elevation of ambulatory systolic blood pressure in hypertensive smokers. JAMA 265:2226, 1991

25. Portulupp F, Montanari L, Massari M et al: Loss of nocturnal decline of blood pressure in hypertension due to chronic renal failure. Am J Hypertens 4:20, 1991

26. Imai Y, Abe K, Sasaki S, et al: Altered circadian blood pressure rhythm in patients with Cushing's syndrome. Hypertension 12:11, 1988

27. Reeves RA, Shapiro AP, Thompson ME, Johnsen AM: Loss of nocturnal decline in blood pressure after cardiac transplantation. Circulation 73:401, 1986

28. Julius S, Ellis CN, Pascual AV et al: Home blood pressure determination: value in borderline ("labile") hypertension. JAMA 229:663, 1974

29. Kleinert HD, Harshfield GA, Pickering TG et al: What is the value of home blood pressure measurement in mild hypertension? Hypertension 6:574, 1984

30. Rademaker M, Lindsay A, McLaren JA, Padfield PL: Home monitoring of blood pressure: usefulness as a predictor of persistent hypertension. Scot Med J 32:16, 1987

31. Evans CE, Haynes RB, Goldsmith CH, Hewson SA: Home blood pressure-measuring devices: a comparative study of accuracy. J Hypertens 7:133, 1989

32. Veerman DP, van Montfras GA, Wieling W: Effects of cuff inflation on self-recorded blood pressure. Lancet 335:451, 1990

33. Mejia AD, Egan BM, Schork NJ, Zweifler AJ: Artefacts in measurement of blood pressure and lack of target organ involvement in the assessment of patients with treatment-resistant hypertension. Ann Intern Med 112:270, 1990

34. Julius S, Jamerson K, Mejia A et al: The association of borderline hypertension with target organ changes and higher coronary risk: the Tecumseh Study. JAMA 264:354, 1990

35. Soghikian K, Casper SM, Fireman BH et al: Home blood pressure monitoring: effect on use of medical services and medical care costs. Med Care 30:855, 1992

36. Gottdiener JS, Brown J, Zoltick J et al: Left ventricular hypertrophy in men with normal blood pressure: relation to exaggerated blood pressure response to exercise. Ann Intern Med 112:161, 1990

37. Floras JS, Hassan MO, Jones JV, Sleight P: Pressor responses to laboratory stresses and daytime blood pressure variability. J Hypertens 5:715, 1987

38. Messerli FH, Ventura HO, Amodeo C: Osler's maneuver and pseudohypertension. N Engl J Med 312:1548, 1985

39. Hla KM, Feussner JR: Screening for pseudohypertension: a quantitative, noninvasive approach. Arch Intern Med 148:673, 1988

40. Lipsitz LA, Nyquist RP, Wei JY, Rowe JW: Postprandial reduction in blood pressure in the elderly. N Engl J Med 309:81, 1983

41. Rosenberg L, Kaufman DW, Helmrich SP, Shapiro S: The risk of myocardial infarction after quitting smoking in men under 55 years of age. N Engl J Med 313:1511, 1985

42. The Expert Panel: Report of the National Cholesterol Education Program Expert Panel on Detection, Evaluation and Treatment of High Blood Cholesterol in Adults. Arch Intern Med 148:36, 1988

43. Jenner JL, Ordovas JM, Lamon Fava S et al: Effects of age, sex, and menopausal status on plasma lipoprotein(a) levels. Circulation 87:1135, 1993

44. Reaven GM: Role of insulin resistance in human disease. Diabetes 37:1595, 1988

45. Zavaroni I, Dall'Aglio E, Bonaro E et al: Evidence that multiple risk factors for coronary artery disease exist in persons with normal glucose tolerance. Am J Med 83:609, 1987

46. Zavaroni I, Bonora E, Pagliara M et al: Risk factors for coronary artery disease in healthy persons with hyperinsulinemia and normal glucose intolerance. N Engl J Med 320:702, 1989

47. Hypertension Detection and Follow-up Program Cooperative Group: Five-year findings of the Hypertension Detection and Follow-up Program. I. Reduction in mortality of persons with high blood pressure, including mild hypertension. JAMA 242:2562, 1979

48. Krakoff LR, Bravo EL, Tuck ML, et al: Nifedipine gastrointestinal therapeutic system in the treatment of hypertension: results of a multicenter trial [Modern Approach to the Treatment of Hypertension (MATH) Study Group]. Am J Hypertens 3:318S, 1991

49. Krowlewski AS, Canessa M, Warram JH et al: Predisposition to hypertension and susceptibility to renal disease in insulin-dependent diabetes mellitus. N Engl J Med 318:140, 1988

50. Mangili R, Bending JJ, Scott G et al: Increased sodium-lithium countertransport activity in red cells of patients with insulin-dependent diabetes and nephropathy. N Engl J Med 318:146, 1988

51. Saad MF, Lillioja S, Nyomba BL et al: Racial differences in the relation between blood pressure and insulin resistance. N Engl J Med 324:733, 1991

52. Shen DC, Sheih SM, Chen YD, Reaven GM: Resistance to insulin-stimulated glucose uptake in patients with hypertension. J Clin Endocrinol Metab 66:580, 1988

53. Sheu WH-H, Jeng C-Y, Shieh S-M et al: Insulin resistance and abnormal electrocardiograms in patients with high blood pressure. Am J Hypertens 5:444, 1992

54. Ferrannini E, Buzzigoli G, Bonadonna R et al: Insulin resistance in essential hypertension. N Engl J Med 317:350, 1987

55. Natali A, Santoro D, Palombo C et al: Impaired insulin action on skeletal muscle metabolism in essential hypertension. Hypertension 17:170, 1991

56. Swislocki A, Hoffman B, Reaven G: Insulin resistance, glucose tolerance, and hyperinsulinemia in patients with hypertension. Am J Hypertens 2:419, 1989

57. Manicardi V, Camellini L, Belloidi G et al: Evidence for an association of high blood pressure and hyperinsulinemia in obese man. J Clin Endocrinol Metab 62:1302, 1986

58. Moller DE, Flier JS: Insulin resistance—mechanisms, syndromes, and implications. N Engl J Med 325:938, 1991

59. Cruickshank JK, Cooper J, Burnett J et al: Ethnic differences in fasting plasma C-peptide and insulin in relation to glucose tolerance and blood pressure. Lancet 338:842, 1991

60. Zimmerman S, Phillips RA, Dunaif A et al: Polycystic ovary syndrome: lack of hypertension despite profound insulin resistance. J Clin Endocrinol Metab 75:508, 1992

61. Rocchini AP, Key J, Bondie D et al: The effect of weight loss on the sensitivity of blood pressure to sodium in obese adolescents. N Engl J Med 321:580, 1989

62. Rowe JW, Young JB, Minaker KL et al: Effects of insulin and glucose infusions on sympathetic nervous system activity in normal man. Diabetes 30:219, 1981

63. Rocchini AP, Katch V, Kveselis D et al: Insulin and renal sodium retention in obese adolescents. Hypertension 14:367, 1989

64. Rocchini AP, Moorehead C, DeRemer S et al: Hyperinsulinemia and the aldosterone and pressor responses to angiotensin II. Hypertension 15:861, 1990

65. Alderman MH, Madhavan S, Ooi WL et al: Association of the renin-sodium profile with the risk of myocardial infarction in patients with hypertension. N Engl J Med 324:1098, 1991

66. Brunner HR, Laragh JH, Baer L et al: Essential hypertension: renin, and aldosterone, heart attack and stroke. N Engl J Med 286:441, 1972

67. Meade TW, Coope JA, et al: Plasma renin activity and ischemic heart disease. N Engl J Med 329:616, 1993

68. Davis BA, Crook JE, Vestal RE, Oates JA: Prevalence of renovascular hypertension in patients with grade III or IV hypertensive retinopathy. N Engl J Med 301:1273, 1979

69. Dimmitt SB, West JNW, Eames SM et al: Usefulness of ophthalmoscopy in mild to moderate hypertension. Lancet 1:1103, 1989

70. Casale PN, Devereux RB, Milner M et al: Value of echocardiographic measurements of left ventricular mass in predicting cardiovascular morbid events in hypertensive men. Ann Intern Med 105:173, 1986

71. Levy D, Garrison RJ, Savage DD et al: Prognostic implications of echocardiographically determined left ventricular mass in the Framingham Heart Study. N Engl J Med 322:1561, 1990

72. Koren MJ, Devereux RB, Casale PN et al: Relation of left ventricular mass and geometry to morbidity and mortality in uncomplicated essential hypertension. Ann Intern Med 114:345, 1991

73. Shahi M, Thom S, Poulter N et al: Regression of hypertensive left ventricular hypertrophy and left ventricular diastolic function. Lancet 336:458, 1990

74. Schulman SP, Weiss JL, Becher LC et al: The effects of antihypertensive therapy on left ventricular mass in elderly patients. N Engl J Med 322:1350, 1990

75. Geizhals M, Phillips RA, Ardeljan M, Krakoff LR: Sustained calcium channel blockade in the treatment of severe hypertension. Am J Hypertens 3(No. 10, Pt. 2):313S, 1990

76. Dahlof B, Pennert K, Hansson L: Reversal of left ventricular hypertrophy in hypertensive patients: a metaanalysis of 109 treatment studies. Am J Hypertens 5:95, 1992

77. MacMahon SW, Wilcken DEL, MacDonald GJ: The effect of weight reduction on left ventricular mass: a randomized controlled trial in young, overweight hypertensive patients. N Engl J Med 314:334, 1986

78. Phillips RA, Coplan NL, Krakoff LR et al: Doppler echocardiographic analysis of left ventricular filling in treated hypertensive patients. J Am Coll Cardiol 9:317, 1987

79. Smith VE, Schulman P, Karimeddini M et al: Rapid left ventricular filling in left ventricular hypertrophy II. Pathological hypertrophy. J Am Coll Cardiol 5:869, 1985

80. Fouad FM, Slominiski JM, Tarazi RC: Left ventricular diastolic function in hypertension: relation to left ventricular mass and systolic function. J Am Coll Cardiol 3:1500, 1984

81. Harizi RC, Bianco JA, Alpert JS: Diastolic function of the heart in clinical cardiology. Arch Intern Med 148:99, 1988

82. Topol EJ, Traill GV, Fortuin NJ: Hypertensive cardiomyopathy of the elderly. N Engl J Med 312:277, 1985

83. Houghton JL, Frank MJ, Carr AA et al: Relations among impaired coronary flow reserve, left ventricular hypertrophy and thallium perfusion defects in hypertensive patients without obstructive coronary disease. J Am Coll Cardiol 15:43, 1990

84. Chin WL, O'Kelly B, Tubau JF et al: Diagnostic accuracy of exercise thallium-201 scintigraphy in men with asymptomatic essential hypertension. Am J Hypertens 5:465, 1992

85. Yudkin JS, Forrest RD, Jackson CA: Microalbuminuria as predictor of vascular disease in non-diabetic subjects. Lancet 2:530, 1988

86. European Carotid Surgery Trialists' Collaborative Group: MRC European Carotid Surgery Trial: interim results for symptomatic patients with severe (70–99%) or mild (0–29%) carotid stenosis. Lancet 337:1235, 1991

87. Grotta JC: Current medical and surgical therapy for cerebrovascular disease. N Engl J Med 317:1505, 1987

88. North American Symptomatic Carotid Endarterectomy Trial Collaborators: Beneficial effect of carotid endarterectomy in symptomatic patients with high-grade carotid stenosis. N Engl J Med 325:445, 1991

89. Kistler JP, Buananno FS, Gress DR: Carotid endarterectomy- specific therapy based on pathophysiology. N Engl J Med 325:505, 1991

90. Ogren M, Isacsson S-O, Janzon L et al: Non-invasively detected carotid stenosis and ischaemic heart disease in men with leg arteriosclerosis. Lancet 342:1138, 1993

91. Vogt MT, Cauley JA, Newman AB et al: Decreased ankle/arm blood pressure index and mortality in elderly women. JAMA 270:465, 1993

92. Newman AB, Sutton-Tyrell K et al: Morbidity and mortality in hypertensive adults with a low ankle/arm index. JAMA 270:487, 1993

93. Coffman JD: Intermittent claudication—be conservative. N Engl J Med 325:577, 1991

94. Ernst CB: Abdominal aortic aneurysm. N Engl J Med 328:1167, 1993

95. Collin J, Araujo L, Walton J, Lindsell D: Oxford Screening Programme for abdominal aortic aneurysm in men aged 65 to 74 years. Lancet 2:613, 1988

96. Frame PS, Fryback DG, Patterson C: Screening for abdominal aortic aneurysm in men ages 60 to 80 years. Ann Intern Med 119:411, 1993

97. Martin K, Phillips RA, Krakoff LR: Persistent white coat hypertension. Am J Hypertens 7:368, 1994

7

SECONDARY OR CURABLE HYPERTENSION

A small fraction (1 to 5 percent) of those with hypertension have unique disorders that cause their elevated arterial pressure. In some instances (e.g., pheochromocytoma or renal artery stenosis), the cause is curable by invasive means or can be reversed without the need for prolonged antihypertensive drug treatment. Ideally, all those with curable hypertension should be detected and reversed long before the disease or hypertension, itself, causes morbidity or fatality. However, accurate diagnosis and curative treatment may require procedures with some risk (e.g., angiography, surgery) or excessive cost, which must be balanced against the benefit of invasive interventions for either diagnosis or treatment. In general, strategies for detection and treatment begin with noninvasive, simpler procedures with less risk and cost. If these initial tests are positive or suggestive of the suspected diagnosis, the more definitive, but more costly and risky, procedures are justified.

Within the spectrum of secondary hypertension, some disorders are highly dangerous and should be unmasked and cured with dispatch (pheochromocytoma), while others are less likely to cause immediate risk and can be treated with antihypertensive medication, even for long periods (e.g., primary aldosteronism, unilateral renal artery stenosis). A new category of reversible hypertension includes those disorders caused by drugs, drug interactions, and environmental substances. Often their diagnosis depends on careful history, since routine tests will be unrevealing.

Ordinarily we think of the need for accurate diagnosis of secondary hypertension only in terms of the individual patient. However, several forms of secondary hypertension have a familial or genetic distribution. Detection of the first such family member may and often should lead to strategies for survey of all relevant family members, as would be the case in familial endocrine neoplasia, polycystic kidney disease, or the genetic disorders of adrenocorticosteroid-related hypertension. Rather than wait for clinical manifestations of these disorders to occur in genetically related family members, molecular biologic techniques are being developed to detect affected individuals early in the disease course and perhaps even in utero.[1-3]

The best-known forms of naturally occurring reversible secondary hypertension are pheochromocytoma, primary aldosteronism, Cushing syndrome, renal artery stenosis, and coarctation of the aorta. Apart from elevated arterial pressure, these diseases are unequivocally distinct from each other. However, they tend to be grouped together when physicians wish to "rule out secondary hypertension." It has been my impression that secondary hypertension is often not considered for an undue length of time and that patients are treated as if they had essential hypertension or unrelated disorders until the eventual discovery (sometimes by accident) of the correct diagnosis. The tests developed for diagnosis of these disorders are well characterized. Often they only confirm an astute clinical suspicion. However, when and how should clinical suspicion begin? A few suggestions for initiating the hunt for reversible secondary hypertension are given in Table 7-1.

TEST STRATEGY AND CHARACTERISTICS

The detection of secondary hypertension has been a fruitful area for those interested in the probability and statistics, often called decision analysis,

Table 7-1. Initial Detection of Secondary Hypertension

Cause of Hypertension	How to Start the Process of Diagnosis
Pheochromocytoma	*Think of it:* the patient's symptoms and/or family history should suggest the possibility of pheochromocytoma
Cushing syndrome	*Look for it:* this disease will be missed unless it is suspected on the basis of the physical examination; perform the look test
Renal artery stenosis	*Listen for it:* not all those with renal artery stenosis will have bruits, but many do; patients with atherosclerotic renal artery stenosis often have narrowed carotid or peripheral arteries that also make noise detectable to the stethoscope
Primary aldosteronism	*Test for it:* unprovoked hypokalemia remains the most likely basis for initial detection of mineralocorticoid excess; all too often serum potassium levels of 3.0–3.5 are ignored
Coarctation of the aorta	*Feel for it:* without examination of the femoral and distal pulses, coarctation will not be considered; every year a few young adults with this disease turn up without prior detection
Oral contraceptive pill–induced hypertension, diet pill overdose, monoamine oxidase inhibitor/tyramine syndrome, clonidine withdrawal, cocaine administration	*Ask about them:* only the history, taken carefully, will unmask the pheochromocytoma-like disorders or use of birth control pills; consider a toxicology screening test for cocaine when warranted

applied to diagnosis of uncommon diseases. Hypertension is frequent; curable forms are rare. Many are screened, few are detected. By now there is an extensive literature on the use of Bayes theorem in conjunction with fairly well-established characteristics of the tests used to unmask curable hypertension. This section briefly reviews some of the important terms and concepts useful for applying decision analysis to the detection of secondary hypertension.

First, some definitions of the various terms as they are currently used in the literature of decision analysis are necessary. These are provided in Table 7-2.

When different tests are used to detect curable secondary hypertension, their *predictive value* is related both to their sensitivity and specificity and to the prevalence of the sought for disease in the population being tested. As quantified by Bayes theorem, the increase in likelihood of diagnosis, conferred by a positive test, is a function of the ratio of true positive results to false-positive results in the population. For a test with 90 percent sensitivity and specificity applied to a population with a 1-percent incidence of a disease, the increase in likelihood or conditional probability rises from 1 to 9.1 percent for a positive test. If the prevalence of the disease were 20 percent in the target population, a positive test would increase the predictive value to 69 percent. The effect of varying prevalence on the predictive value of such a test is shown in Figure 7-1.

Characteristics of many of (but not all) the diagnostic tests often used to detect reversible hypertension have been defined in large series or compiled

Table 7-2. Definition of Terms Used in Decision Analysis[a]

Term	Definition
T+	Number of positive tests
D+	Number with disease
T+/D+	True-positive rate or *sensitivity*
T−	Number of negative tests
D−	Number without disease
T−/D−	True-negative rate or *specificity*
T+/D−	False-positive rate = 1 − specificity
T−/D+	False-negative rate = 1 − sensitivity
Prevalence × (T+/D+)/ (prevalence × [T+/D+]) + (1 − prevalence) × (T+/D−)	Predictive value (conditional probability as defined by Bayesian analysis)
Test accuracy	Fraction of true-positive and true-negative results in total group studied, with and without the disease
Positive likelihood ratio	Sensitivity/false-positive rate (should be >1.0)
Negative likelihood ratio	False-negative rate/specificity (should be <1.0)

[a]More than one noninvasive test is often used to evaluate patients with suspected causes of secondary hypertension. The likelihood ratio of two or more tests is the product of their positive or negative likelihoods.

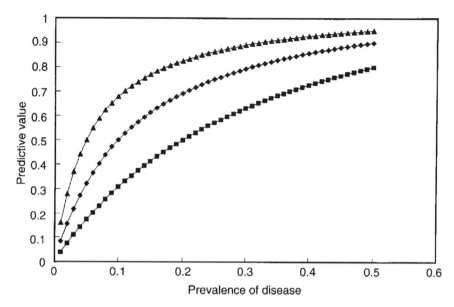

Fig. 7-1. Bayes calculations. Graphic representation of the predictive value for three levels of sensitivity/specificity using single screening tests at varying rates of disease (prevalence) in the population. Squares, 80 percent sensitivity/specificity; diamonds, 90 percent sensitivity/specificity; triangles, 95 percent sensitivity/specificity.

in reviews. Where there is a very large experience shared among several centers using similar and (one hopes) standardized methods, it seems reasonable that this represents a "community" standard that the clinician practicing outside a large referral center can rely on. For those tests performed on a smaller scale in a limited number of studies at a few sites or at only one center, there is little basis for assuming that another laboratory or facility will easily replicate a different facility's results. Tables 7-3 to 7-6 present characteristics of several available tests or procedures for the detection of reversible hypertension as provided by the current literature.

At one time, many studies devoted themselves to the search for the "single best screening test" for a given cause of secondary hypertension. In nearly every case, the test in question failed to meet expectations. How did anyone ever find these diseases? Most often, by using more than one test, not merely repeating the same one over and over. Since many of the more commonly used tests do not cost much, have little or no risk, and the use of a combination of tests results in increased precision, the likelihood ratios for combined tests and the resulting increased precision are given in Tables 7-3 to 7-6. For example, in an untreated hypertensive patient with hypokalemia and a below normal plasma renin activity, primary aldosteronism is highly expected to be present, yet the cost of these two tests is less than $100. Recent developments

Table 7-3. Test Characteristics for Pheochromocytoma

Test	Characteristics

Metanephrine excretion[4]	Sensitivity 83%
	Specificity 95%
	Likelihood ratio
	    Positive 16.6
	    Negative 0.18

Vanillylmandelic acid excretion[4]	Sensitivity 81%
	Specificity 95%
	Likelihood ratio
	    Positive 16.2
	    Negative 0.20

Catecholamine excretion[4]	Sensitivity 82%
	Specificity 95%
	Likelihood ratio
	    Positive 16.4
	    Negative 0.19

I^{131}-mono-iodo-benzylguanidine scan[5–7]	Sensitivity 90%
	Specificity 96%
	Likelihood ratio
	    Positive 22.5
	    Negative 0.10

Plasma catecholamines[8,9]	Sensitivity 75%
	Specificity 95%
	Likelihood ratio
	    Positive 15.0
	    Negative 0.26

Computed tomography scan[4]	Sensitivity 92%
	Specificity 80%
	Likelihood ratio
	    Positive 4.6
	    Negative 0.10

Combined tests
    Combination of urine metanephrine
        excretion and plasma catecholamine
        concentration
	Both positive
	    Likelihood ratio 240
	Both negative
	    Likelihood ratio 0.05

Table 7-4. Characteristics of Diagnostic Tests for Renovascular Hypertension

Test	Characteristics

Plasma renin activity	Sensitivity 65%
	 Specificity 84%
	 Likelihood ratio
	     Positive 4.1
	     Negative 0.42

Captopril test	Sensitivity 74%
	 Specificity 89%
	 Likelihood ratio
	     Positive 6.7
	     Negative 0.29

Intravenous urogram	Sensitivity 75%
	 Specificity 86%
	 Likelihood ratio
	     Positive 5.4
	     Negative 0.29

Captopril renal scan (postcaptopril scan)	Sensitivity 93%
	 Specificity 95%
	 Likelihood ratio
	     Positive 18.6
	     Negative 0.07

Renal vein renin study	Sensitivity 77%
	 Specificity 75%
	 Likelihood ratio
	     Positive 3.1
	     Negative 0.31

Combined tests
     Combination of plasma renin
       activity and captopril renal scan
	Both positive
	     Likelihood ratio 76
	 Both negative
	     Likelihood ratio 0.03

(Data from Mann and Pickering.[10])

Table 7-5. Charactistics of Diagnostic Tests for Cushing Syndrome

Test	Characteristics[a]
Overnight dexamethasone suppression test (low dose)	Sensitivity 98% Specificity 87% Likelihood ratio Positive 7.5 Negative 0.02
24-Hour urine free cortisol	Sensitivity 94% Specificity 95% Likelihood ratio Positive 18.8 Negative 0.06
24-Hour urine 17-OH steroids	Sensitivity 89% Specificity 73% Likelihood ratio Positive 3.3 Negative 0.30
High-dose dexamethasone suppression test for pituitary Cushing syndrome (17-OH steroids)	Sensitivity 93% Specificity 80% Likelihood ratio Positive 4.65 Negative 0.09
Corticotropin-releasing hormone stimulation test for pituitary Cushing syndrome	Sensitivity 91% Specificity 95% Likelihood ratio Positive 18.2 Negative 0.09
Inferior petrosal sinus sampling for adrenocorticotropic hormone concentrations to determine cause of Cushing syndrome	Sensitivity 88% Specificity 83% Likelihood ratio Positive 5.2 Negative 0.14
Combined tests Combination of overnight dexamethasone suppression test and 24-hour urine free cortisol	Both positive Likelihood ratio 141 Both negative Likelihood ratio 0.001

[a]Sensitivity and specificity data from references 11–13.

Table 7-6. Charactistics of Diagnostic Tests for Primary Aldosteronism

Test	Characteristics
Low serum potassium (hypokalemia <3.5 mM/L) after exclusion of diuretic use or gastrointestinal loss	Sensitivity 87% Specificity 95% Likelihood ratio Positive 17.4 Negative 0.14
Low plasma renin activity with usual sodium diet and untreated disease	Sensitivity 95% Specificity 75% Likelihood ratio Positive 3.8 Negative 0.26
Low plasma renin activity with low sodium diet or after diuretic administration	Sensitivity 90% Specificity 70% Likelihood ratio Positive 3.0 Negative 0.14
24-Hour urine aldosterone excretion (metabolite) with usual or high sodium diet	Cannot be interpreted without concurrent plasma renin level to define primary or secondary aldosteronism
Computed tomography scan of adrenal areas (0.5-cm cuts) for adrenal adenoma, Conn's tumor	Sensitivity 75% Specificity 90% Likelihood ratio Positive 7.5 Negative 0.27
Captopril test for plasma renin and aldosterone levels (postcaptopril plasma aldosterone/renin ratio >50 ng/dl/ng/ml/hr[14,15]	Sensitivity 100% Specificity 80% Likelihood ratio Positive 5.0 Negative 0
I[131]-iodo-norcholesterol adrenal scan, for adrenal adenoma, Conn's tumor[a]	Sensitivity Specificity Likelihood ratio Positive Negative
Adrenal venous studies for imaging (venography) and samples for aldosterone and cortisol to test for adrenal adenoma, Conn's tumor	Sensitivity 100% Likelihood ratio Specificity unknown Positive unknown Negative unknown

[a]No data available.

in decision analysis now support the concept, once thought wasteful, that more than one test is a better strategy for initial detection than relying on a single evaluation,[4] as long as the tests are noninvasive and reasonably inexpensive.

The following chapters review the characteristics of the various forms of secondary hypertension and strategies for detecting these disorders. The chapters proceed from the initial screening modalities to definitive diagnostic techniques. To emphasize the pathophysiologic disturbances that account for these disorders, they are grouped by mechanism rather than more conventional classification (Table 7-7).

Table 7-7. Reversible Causes of Hypertension Classified by Hypertensive Mechanism

Adrenergic (catecholamine-related) hypertension
    Pheochromocytoma
    Anxiety states, panic disorder
    Overdose of sympathomimetic drugs
        Amphetamines
        Phenylpropanolamine ("diet pill")
        Cocaine?
    Monoamine oxidase inhibitor/tyramine syndrome
    α_2-Agonist (clonidine-like) withdrawal
    Alcohol withdrawal
    Brain tumor (posterior fossa)
    Spinal cord transection
    Other neurologic syndromes
Adrenocortical hypertension and related syndromes
    Mineralocorticoid excess
        Primary aldosteronism (Conn syndrome)
        Idiopathic (pseudoprimary) aldosteronism
        Dexamethasone suppressible aldosteronism
        Primary desoxycorticosterone (DOC) excess
        11-OH hydroxylase deficiency (DOC excess)
        17-OH hydroxylase deficiency (DOC excess)
        Glucocorticoid receptor deficiency syndrome
    Apparent mineralocorticoid excess
        11-OH dehydrogenase deficiency
        Licorice-induced "pseudoaldosteronism"
    Glucocorticoid excess
        Cushing syndrome
        Exogenous glucocorticoid administration
Reversible renal hypertension—renin dependent
    Renal artery stenosis, renovascular hypertension
        Fibromuscular dysplasias of renal arteries
        Atherosclerosis of renal arteries
        Takayasu-type granulomatous arteritis
        Compression of renal arteries by tumor
        Dissection of renal arteries, trauma, aneurysm
        Neurofibromatosis (Von Recklinghausen's disease)

(Continues)

Table 7-7. *(Continued)*

Renal infarction
Renin-secreting tumors
  Hemangiopericytoma of the kidney
  Other renal and non-renal renin-secreting tumors
  Obstructive renal disease, hydronephrosis, and reflux nephropathy
Secondary renal hypertension, partially or not reversible with mixed mechanisms—
  volume and renin related
  Glomerulonephritis syndromes
  Interstitial renal diseases
  Diabetic nephropathy
  Hemolytic uremia syndrome
  Polycystic renal disease
  Atheroembolic renal disease
  Collagen-vascular diseases
    Scleroderma renal crisis
    Polyarteritis nodosa
    Systemic lupus erythematosus with nephritis
Coarctation of the aorta
  Congenital anomalies
  Inflammatory (granulomatous) aortitis (Takayasu)
Other reversible hypertensive syndromes
  Oral contraceptive pill–induced hypertension
  Toxemia of pregnancy or pregnancy-induced hypertension
Hypertension related to transplantation
  Cyclosporine hypertension
  Steroid hypertension
Sleep apnea syndrome

Diagnosis of Secondary and/or Reversible Hypertension

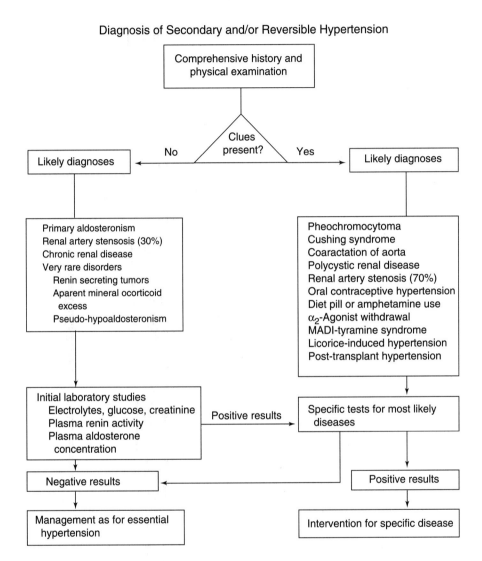

REFERENCES

1. Parfrey PS, Bear JC, Morgan J et al: The diagnosis and prognosis of autosomal dominant polycystic kidney disease. N Engl J Med 323:1085, 1990

2. Harris PC, Thomas S, Ratcliffe PJ et al: Rapid genetic analysis of families with polycystic kidney disease 1 by means of a microsatellite marker. Lancet 338:1484, 1991

3. Mathew CGP, Easton DF, Nakamura Y, Ponder BAJ, and the MEN 2A International Collaborative Group: Presymptomatic screening for multiple endocrine neoplasia type 2A with linked DNA markers. Lancet 337:7, 1991

4. Pauker SG, Kopelman RI: Interpreting hoofbeats: can Bayes help clear the haze? N Engl J Med 327:1009, 1992

5. Swenson SJ, Brown ML, Sheps SG et al: Use of 131 I-MIBG scintigraphy in the evaluation of suspected pheochromocytoma. Mayo Clin Proc 60:29, 1985

6. Shapiro B, Sisson JC, Lloyd R et al: Malignant phaeochromocytoma: clinical, biochemical and scintigraphic characterization. Clin Endocrinol 20:189, 1984

7. Ackery DM, Tippett PA, Condon BR et al: New approach to the localisation of phaeochromocytoma: imaging with iodine-131-meta-iodobenzylguanidine. BMJ 288:1587, 1984

8. Krakoff LR, Garbowit D: Adeno-medullary hypertension: a review of syndromes, pathophysiology, diagnosis and treatment. Clin Chem 37:1849, 1991

9. Bravo EL, Tarazi RC, Gifford RW, Stewart BH: Circulating and urinary catecholamines in pheochromocytoma: diagnostic and pathophysiologic implications. N Engl J Med 301:682, 1979

10. Mann SJ, Pickering TG: Detection of renovascular hypertension: state of the art 1992. Ann Intern Med 117:845, 1992

11. Crapo L: Cushing's syndrome: a review of diagnostic tests. Metabolism 28:955, 1979

12. Gold EM: The Cushing syndromes: changing views of diagnosis and treatment. Ann Intern Med 90:829, 1979

13. Kaye TB, Crapo L: The Cushing syndrome: an update on diagnostic tests. Ann Intern Med 112:435, 1990

14. Lyons DF, Kem DC, Brown RD et al: Single dose captopril as a diagnostic test for primary aldosteronism. J Clin Endocrinol Metab 57:892, 1983

15. Hambling C, Jung RT, Gunn A et al: Re-evaluation of the captopril test for the diagnosis of primary hyperaldosteronism. Clin Endocrinol (Oxf) 36:499, 1992

8

ADRENERGIC OR ADRENOMEDULLARY HYPERTENSION

Adrenergic or adrenomedullary hypertension includes all the forms of secondary or reversible hypertension that are primarily due to increased activity of the sympathetic nervous system.[1] These disorders may be caused by several mechanisms: (1) overproduction of catecholamines, the neurotransmitters and neurohormones of this system; (2) excessive release of these amines by disease states, exogenous drugs, or drug withdrawal syndromes; or (3) use or abuse of agents that mimic sympathoadrenal action. Adrenergic hypertension is associated with highly variable arterial pressure and with symptoms due either to sudden changes in pressure or to other manifestations of sympathoadrenal excess. Symptoms, however, may not be specific and, in fact, may lead the physician away from the correct diagnosis. Despite the sophistication of modern technology, the detection of adrenergic or adrenomedullary hypertension still depends on a keen sense of suspicion leading to a perceptive medical history. The laboratory or imaging tests then confirm the hypothesis that has been generated by astute observation.

PHEOCHROMOCYTOMA

Pheochromocytoma is the best known form of hypertension due to excess production and secretion of catecholamines by neoplastic chromaffin cells.[2] While often considered a disease of children and young adults, pheochromocytoma may be found in middle-aged patients and should not be dismissed as a possibility in the elderly.[3] Less than 0.5 percent of all hypertensive patients have pheochromocytoma. These tumors may be solitary or multiple. Pheochromocytoma may occur as a sporadic tumor or as part of the so-called birthmark syndromes (phacomatoses) of neurofibromatosis (von Recklinghausen),[4] or the von Hippel-Lindau syndrome. The type II form of multiple endocrine neoplasia (MEN-II) is well known to include pheochromocytoma.

More than 80 percent of pheochromocytomas originate in the adrenal medullae. Chromaffin cell rests along the aorta in periaortic ganglia, including the organ of Zuckerkandl at the bifurcation, account for most of the nonadrenal pheochromocytomas. Occasionally, these tumors occur within the wall of the urinary bladder. Intrathoracic pheochromocytomas (less than 10 percent) are usually found in the posterior mediastinum; intra- and pericardial chromaffin tumors have recently been reported. Paragangliomas (chemodectomas) of the carotid body, on rare occasions, may produce and secrete catecholamines.

87

The clinical lore of pheochromocytoma is extensive and has given rise to such clinical "pearls" as "The Rule of 10" (i.e., "10 percent of pheochromocytomas are nonadrenal, 10 percent are outside the abdomen, 10 percent are malignant, and so forth). Individual series suggest that these approximations are acceptable if one adds ±10 percent to each of the categories.

Hypertension in pheochromocytoma is due to the effects of elevated circulating catecholamines. Increased norepinephrine, an agonist for α_1- and α_2-receptors, raises peripheral resistance. This will cause elevations of diastolic pressure that may reach 200 mmHg in some patients during paroxysmal episodes. High plasma levels of epinephrine may stimulate both β_1- and β_2-receptors, increasing heart rate, but reducing peripheral resistance. β-Receptor–stimulated release of renin from renal juxtaglomerular cells may lead to high concentrations of plasma renin activity, increasing arterial pressure by the action of angiotensin II.[5] In benign pheochromocytoma, plasma dopamine levels are not increased. However, in malignant tumors, elevations of dopamine and its precursor L-dopa may be observed. The former may contribute to the cardiovascular manifestations of the disease.

Initial detection of pheochromocytoma depends on recognizing the symptoms and signs that are usually present. Hypertension may be of a widely fluctuating type or have a more sustained pattern. Lack of a highly variable blood pressure is not a basis for excluding this disease. Paroxysmal hypertension without symptoms occasionally occurs as the sole manifestation of pheochromocytoma. This may be recorded during general anesthesia for surgery (perhaps due to ganglionic stimulation by anesthetic agents), during pregnancy, after administration of sympathomimetic amines, or by chance occurrence. However, if questioned carefully, nearly all patients with pheochromocytoma have symptoms such as headache, sweating, palpitations, apprehension, constipation, and weight loss. The symptoms, however, are nonspecific and may be misleading. Hyperthyroidism, coronary heart disease, cardiac arrhythmias, mitral valve prolapse, anxiety states, and carcinoid and other diseases may be suggested by the initial clinical picture. For those patients with pheochromocytoma as part of a familial syndrome (i.e., neurofibromatosis or MEN-II), the presenting manifestations may be due to the other features of their disorder. Regardless of the initial symptoms or signs, once suspected, pheochromocytoma must be confirmed by appropriate biochemical tests and imaging. By contrast, the absence in an *accurate history* of either *compatible symptoms* or one of the predisposing *familial syndromes* is highly specific for exclusion of pheochromocytoma. Extensive diagnostic testing is not needed in this circumstance.

Pheochromocytomas may produce a variety of noncatecholamine substances. Whether these substances cause any symptoms is uncertain. The substances include peptides (e.g., enkephalins, neuropeptide Y,[6] and atrial natriuretic peptides[7]) and proteins (e.g., chromogranin A).[8]

Once suspected, the initial test for pheochromocytoma is measurement of urinary excretion of catecholamine metabolites, in particular, total metanephrine or vanillylmandelic acid (VMA). This test is widely available and performed in a reliable manner. Total metanephrine and VMA may be measured in first voided morning urine samples (expressed as micrograms per milligrams creatinine) or timed urine samples (4 to 6 hours or 24-hour collections). In most series, total metanephrine excretion is the most sensitive initial screening test; it is available from many clinical laboratories. VMA excretion may be less sensitive, but is highly specific if performed correctly. When these do not give a clear-cut diagnosis, measurement of plasma catecholamine concentrations or excretion of catecholamines in the urine[9,10] may be helpful (Table 8-1).

When catecholamine metabolite excretion or the plasma catecholamine level, or both, are markedly elevated (e.g., plasma norepinephrine concentration above 2,000 ng/L [pg/ml]), the likelihood of pheochromocytoma is definite enough to proceed to imaging. For intermediate elevations, 600 to 2,000 ng/L, the clonidine suppression test may be useful to distinguish between pheochromocytoma and a nonspecific elevation of plasma catecholamine level, such as occurs in some patients with essential hypertension or undue anxiety.[11] Clonidine administration suppresses plasma catecholamine concentration in cases of nonspecific adrenergic excess, but fails to do so in chromaffin cell neoplasms, which presumably secrete catecholamines independently of sympathetic tone transmitted from the central nervous system. The method used for performance of the clonidine suppression test is given in Appendix 2.

Occasionally, plasma catecholamine concentrations are normal when the tumor is strongly suspected (e.g., in MEN-II). In such cases, suppression of plasma norepinephrine may be indeterminate. Instead, these patients may have a large increase in plasma catecholamine concentration in response to intravenous glucagon.[12]

Table 8-1. Laboratory Tests for Pheochromocytoma

Test	Comments
Urine metanephrine excretion, timed or per milligram creatinine	Widely available and well standardized; very useful for first screening test
Urine vanillylmandelic acid excretion, timed or per milligram creatinine	Widely available; perhaps less specific in some series due to false-positive results if chemical method is nonspecific
Urine catecholamines: norepinephrine and epinephrine excretion, timed or 24-hour collection	Excessive sensitivity; many false-positive results, slightly above normal range, hence less specific
Supine plasma catecholamines: norepinephrine and epinephrine	Lack of sensitivity and specificity (70–80%); useful during clonidine suppression test or glucagon stimulation for additional tests
Serum chromogranin A	Similar test characteristics to plasma catecholamine concentrations; may have increased false-positive results in renal insufficiency
Plasma neuropeptide Y	Primarily a research probe at present

Following confirmation by biochemical determinations, localization of pheochromocytoma is necessary. Adrenal and periaortic masses may be detected by sonography or conventional computed tomography scanning[13] (Fig. 8-1 and Table 8-2).

Recent studies suggest that greater specificity for the diagnosis may be conferred by T_2-weighted magnetic resonance imaging[14,15] (Fig. 8-2). Radioisotope scanning with meta-iodo-benzylguanidine (MIBG) may be helpful, especially for detection of recurrent or metastatic tumors[16,17] (Fig. 8-3).

Rarely, sampling the superior and inferior vena cava at several levels for plasma catecholamine concentrations will be needed to localize a pheochromocytoma when the tumor is too small to be visualized or is located where the radiologic techniques are insensitive (bladder wall and pelvis). The very rare cardiac pheochromocytoma should be identified by transthoracic or transesophageal echocardiography, if suspected.

Definitive treatment of pheochromocytoma is surgery. However, medical management should be started as soon as the diagnosis is likely, to protect the patient from hypertensive crises. Hypertensive crises of pheochromocytoma should be prevented or treated with receptor blockade. Intravenous phentolamine is effective for emergencies. Therapy with oral α-blockers, phenoxybenzamine, or $α_1$-blockers (prazosin, terazosin, or doxazosin[18]) is useful for

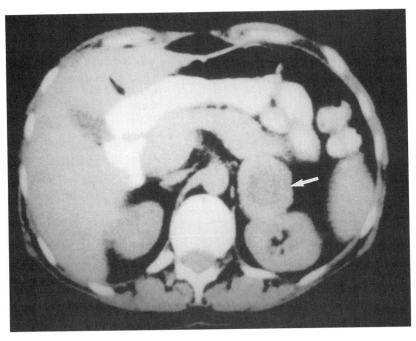

Fig. 8-1. Computed tomography scan of a pheochromocytoma (arrow).

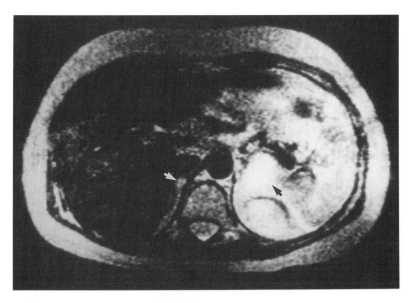

Fig. 8-2. T_2-weighted magnetic resonance imaging of a pheochromocytoma. The T_2-weighted spin resonance has enhanced the image of the pheochromocytoma, anterior to the upper pole of the left kidney *(black arrow)*. A small right adrenal pheochromocytoma was also found by enhancement *(white arrow)*.

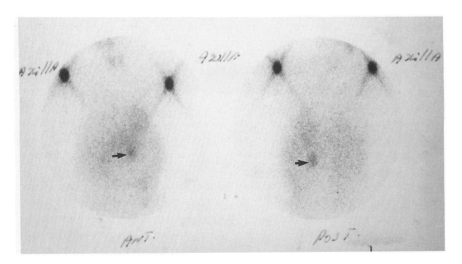

Fig. 8-3. ^{131}I-mono-iodo-benzylguanidine scan of a left adrenal pheochromocytoma *(arrows)* seen on both anterior and posterior views. The patient was from a family with multiple endocrine neoplasia, type II. Markers for reference are placed in the axillae.

Table 8-2. Imaging for Pheochromocytoma

Method	Comments
Chest radiograph	Will occasionally detect posterior mediastinal tumor
Abdominal radiograph	Will occasionally detect large suprarenal mass; very low sensitivity and specificity
Intravenous urography	May detect large suprarenal or para-aortic mass; low sensitivity and specificity
Abdominal sonography	May detect large suprarenal mass (>4 cm); less accurate for para-aortic masses; cannot detect small tumors; no tissue characterization
Abdominal and/or thoracic computed tomography scanning	Highly (90–95%) sensitive for >1–2-cm adrenal tumors; little tissue characterization
Magnetic resonance imaging	Highly sensitive and specific for pheochromocytoma; T_2-weighted mode highlights chromaffin tumors
^{131}I meta-iodo-benzylguanidine (MIBG) imaging	Useful to characterize known tumors, such as chromaffin cell tumors; may detect adrenomedullary hyperplasia in MEN-II

sustained control of pressure before surgery. If tachycardia or arrhythmias are present, addition of β_1-selective β-blockers may be helpful. In some patients, use of the combined α/β-blocker labetalol may be effective. For inoperable pheochromocytoma, reduced catecholamine synthesis can be achieved by administration of α-methyl-*p*-tyrosine, an inhibitor of tyrosine hydroxylase, the rate-limiting enzyme for catecholamine production (Table 8-3).

Malignant pheochromocytomas may produce massive amounts of catecholamines from large, multicentric tumor masses. Very high levels of other tumor markers, such as neuropeptide Y, may also be found.[19] Control of catecholamine production by α-methyl-*p*-tyrosine has no effect on the tumor itself. However, chemotherapeutic regimens combining vincristine and dacarbazine may be effective.[20] Tumor ablation with high doses of radioactive ^{131}I-MIBG has also been reported.[17,21]

After a single or solitary pheochromocytoma has been discovered and removed by surgery, long-term surveillance of the patient is necessary. Recurrence of multicentric pheochromocytoma occurs in 10 to 15 percent of cases in many series. Recurrence as malignant pheochromocytoma may occur and requires surgery and consideration of chemotherapy (see above). I recommend that all patients with a history of apparently cured pheochromocytoma be seen once a year and that a urine metanephrine excretion measurement be obtained annually or whenever symptoms occur that raise the question of recurrent tumor.

In summary, pheochromocytoma should be considered in all hypertensive patients whether the elevation in pressure is evanescent or stable. Those with no clinical features of the tumor can be managed without extensive diagnostic assessment. Symptoms and signs compatible with pheochromocytoma require diagnostic evaluation for catecholamine excess; when found, search for a tumor is necessary.

DRUG-INDUCED ADRENERGIC HYPERTENSION

Paroxysmal or episodic hypertension may occur as a result of several drugs that either directly or indirectly stimulate adrenergic mechanisms. The usual clinical presentation is the sudden appearance of hypertension, often associated with severe headache. Tachycardia may be present. Overdosage with amphetamine or one of its analogues may cause this syndrome. An over-the-counter appetite suppressant, phenylethanolamine, may also produce this disorder.[22,23] It has been suggested that the latter is more likely to raise pressure in the presence of a cyclo-oxygenase inhibitor, such as indomethacin, which reduces production of vasodilatory prostaglandins.[22] Patients taking monoamine oxidase inhibitors (e.g., tranylcypromine, phenelzine) are at risk of hypertensive episodes if they consume food or drink (wine) containing tyramine. In all these examples, the increase in pressure or heart rate, or both, is due to activation of adrenergic receptors by direct action of the drug or by its release of catecholamines from nerve terminals. Blockade of α- and β-adrenergic receptors is appropriate therapy with such drugs as (1) prazosin, a postsynaptic α_1-antagonist; (2) phentolamine, an α_1- and α_2-antagonist; and (3) labetalol, a combined α- and β-receptor antagonist.

Clonidine withdrawal hypertension occurs as a rapid increase in blood pressure after stopping the centrally acting α_2-receptor agonist. This "overshoot" hypertension may be observed after cessation of other central α_2-receptor agonists: methyldopa, guanabenz, or guanfacine. The mechanism

Table 8-3. Specific Pharmacologic Therapy for Adrenomedullary Hypertension

Agent	Comments
Intravenous α-receptor blockade	Phentolamine, blocks α_1- and α_2-receptors; fall in pressure not specific to pheochromocytoma
Oral α-receptors (phenoxybenzamine, prazosin, terazosin, doxazosin)	Useful for reduction of systemic vascular resistance, vasoconstriction, in hyperadrenergic states
Intravenous or oral β_1-selective receptor blockade (metoprolol, atenolol, esmolol)	Caution in using alone, as paradoxical rise in pressure may occur, if α-receptors not blocked
Combined α/β-receptor blockade (labetalol)	May be used intravenously or orally; β-blockade greater than α-blockade
Catecholamine synthesis inhibition (α-methyl-p-tyrosine)	Slow onset, suitable only for nonoperable pheochromocytoma; side effects include pseudo-Parkinson syndrome, crystalluria

for the sudden increase in blood pressure in this syndrome is activation of peripheral sympathetic tone, adrenergic excess. This is in response to the increased central drive caused by cessation of treatment with the α_2-agonist. Re-starting clonidine or another α_2-agonist will reduce arterial pressure. In patients who cannot take oral medication, intravenous administration of peripheral adrenergic receptor antagonists such as phentolamine with or without a β-blocker (intravenous propranolol, metoprolol, or esmolol) or a combined α/β-blocker (labetalol) may be necessary.

Occasionally, severe hypertension may be seen in patients during withdrawal from alcohol. Associated cardiac arrhythmias (particularly atrial fibrillation) and cardiomyopathy may be present. These patients are often treated initially with benzodiazepines and may respond well. However, the elevation in pressure is presumably due to sympathoadrenal activation. β-Receptor blockers or clonidine may then be effective. If parenteral medication is needed, intravenous labetalol may be helpful.

Cocaine

Recent case reports and series document the cardiac toxicity of cocaine, emphasizing the occurrence of myocardial infarction and cardiac arrhythmias.[24] Cocaine has a well-established adrenergic action by preventing neuronal uptake and inactivation of catecholamines. It has been suggested that the adrenergic effects of cocaine may also cause sudden increases in arterial pressure, accounting for intracranial hemorrhage[25] and abruptio placentae in pregnancy.[26] Administration of the β-receptor propranolol may paradoxically increase arterial pressure in cocaine toxicity due to enhanced or unopposed stimulation of vascular α-adrenergic receptors.[27] Cocaine use has been associated with renal infarction, which might raise pressure through release of renin.[28] These observations suggest that hypertension associated with cocaine use should be treated with combined α- and β-receptor blockade. Converting enzyme inhibitors may have a theoretical benefit if the renin system is stimulated by adrenergic mechanisms or renal ischemia.

Transient Endogenous Adrenergic Hypertension

Brief episodes of elevated arterial pressure (greater than 140 mmHg systolic or greater than 90 mmHg diastolic pressure) may occur as often as 10 percent of the day in normal subjects. Aerobic exercise raises systolic pressure physiologically. Isometric exertion, as in lifting weights, mental stress, or challenge may briefly increase both systolic and diastolic pressure. Two specific syndromes, however, have recently been characterized and are briefly described: panic disorder syndrome and "white coat" hypertension.

In the panic disorder syndrome, regularly recurring panic or anxiety attacks occur that may be triggered by a wide variety of circumstances. During these attacks, ambulatory blood pressure monitoring has revealed a significant increase in heart rate and systolic and diastolic pressures. Between attacks arterial pressure is normal.[29] The cardiovascular risk of these episodic elevations in pressure is uncertain. While the anxiety element may respond to treatment with benzodiazepines, the effect of this treatment on arterial pressure is unknown. The transient increases in arterial pressure and heart rate imply that both α- and β-adrenergic receptors are stimulated by neurally released and circulating catecholamines. Therapy with combined α- and β-receptor blockade might be effective.

White coat hypertension is the transient elevation of arterial pressure due to the presence of a physician,[30] as may occur on teaching rounds.[31] Twenty-four hour ambulatory blood pressure monitoring defines this syndrome by establishing that average daytime pressures outside the medical setting or when physicians are not present are entirely normal.[32] Various behavioral challenges have little power to predict the presence of white coat hypertension.[33,34] It is uncertain whether such patients are at risk; hence, the effect of treatment is unknown.

NEUROLOGIC SYNDROMES

Hypertension may be observed in patients with brain tumors, particularly those neoplasms occurring in the posterior fossa and near vasomotor pathways of the medulla.[35] It is not known whether reduction of arterial pressure in such patients is beneficial (reducing the likelihood of brain hemorrhage) or harmful (because of ischemia in jeopardized areas with reduced blood flow due to local edema). Cautious decrease in arterial pressure using reversible agents (intravenous nitroprusside) should be considered when necessary, as during neurosurgery.

High spinal cord transection or diseases that interrupt cord tracts in the cervical or high thoracic levels may cause rapidly changing and erratic blood pressure patterns from low to high in minutes. Bladder distention is a well-known stimulus for intraspinal reflexes, which may trigger sudden and large increases in arterial pressure in these patients. In part these fluctuations are due to lack of central buffering by baroreflex efferent pathways, which cannot communicate with lower neurons because of interruption of spinal tracts above the thoracolumbar outflow of the sympathetic nervous system. Despite the large variations in minute to minute pressure, average pressure may be normal.[36] It is not apparent that, in the absence of sustained hypertension, antihypertensive therapy is necessary.

SUMMARY

The various syndromes of adrenergic and adrenomedullary hypertension form a group of reversible disorders that should be considered readily detectable. They require specific pharmacologic treatment with adrenergic receptor antagonists (or, rarely, catecholamine synthesis inhibition) and are correctable. It is somewhat ironic that the progress made in safe and accurate diagnosis of pheochromocytoma and the sophisticated pharmacology that has led to specific receptor antagonists has been paralleled by the increasing appearance of new forms of adrenergic hypertension due to an expanding and uncontrolled access to sympathomimetic substances such as amphetamines, phenylpropanolamine, and cocaine. All physicians, particularly those in emergency departments, should be wary of these disorders.

REFERENCES

1. Krakoff LR, Garbowit D: Adeno-medullary hypertension: a review of syndromes, pathophysiology, diagnosis and treatment. Clin Chem 37:1849, 1991

2. Manger WM, Gifford RW Jr: Pheochromocytoma. Springer-Verlag, New York, 1977

3. Cooper ME, Goodman D, Frauman A et al: Pheochromocytoma in the elderly: a poorly recognized entity? BMJ 293:1474, 1986

4. Kalff V, Shapiro B, Lloyd R et al: The spectrum of pheochromocytoma in hypertensive patients with neurofibromatosis. Arch Intern Med 142:2092, 1982

5. Lenz T, Thiede HM, Nussberger J et al: Hyperreninemia and secondary hyperaldosteronism in a patient with pheochromocytoma and von Hippel-Lindau disease. Nephron 62:345, 1992

6. Helman LJ, Cohen PS, Averbuch SD et al: Neuropeptide Y expression distinguishes malignant from benign pheochromcytoma. J Clin Oncol 7:1720, 1989

7. Vesely DL, Arnold WC, Winters CJ et al: Increased circulating concentration of the N-terminus of the atrial natriuretic factor prohormone in persons with pheochromocytomas. J Clin Endocrinol Metab 71:1138, 1990

8. O'Conner DT, Bernstein KN: Radioimmunoassay of chromogranin A in plasma as a measure of exocytotic sympathoadrenal activity in normal subjects and patients with pheochromocytoma. N Engl J Med 311:764, 1984

9. Bravo EL, Tarazi RC, Gifford RW, Stewart BH: Circulating and urinary catecholamines in pheochromocytoma: diagnostic and pathophysiologic implications. N Engl J Med 301:682, 1979

10. Duncan MW, Compton P, Lazarus L, Smythe GA: Measurement of norepinephrine and 3,4-dihydroxyphenylglycol in urine and plasma for the diagnosis of pheochromocytoma. N Engl J Med 319:136, 1988

11. Bravo EL, Tarazi RC, Fouad FM et al: Clonidine-suppression test: a useful aid in the diagnosis of pheochromocytoma. N Engl J Med 305:623, 1981

12. Grossman E, Goldstein DS, Hoffman A, Keiser HR: Glucagon and clonidine testing in the diagnosis of pheochromocytoma. Hypertension 17:733, 1991

13. Bravo EL, Gifford RW Jr: Pheochromocytoma: diagnosis, localization and management. N Engl J Med 311:1298, 1984

14. Quint LE, Glazer GM, Francis IR et al: Pheochromocytoma and paraganglioma: comparison of MR imaging with CT and I-131 MIBG scintigraphy. Radiology 165:89, 1987

15. Schmedtje JF Jr, Sax S, Pool JL et al: Localization of ectopic pheochromocytomas by magnetic resonance imaging. Am J Med 83:770, 1987

16. Shapiro B, Sisson JC, Lloyd R et al: Malignant phaeochromocytoma: clinical, biochemical and scintigraphic characterization. Clin Endocrinol 20:189, 1984

17. Ackery DM, Tippett PA, Condon BR et al: New approach to the localisation of phaeochromocytoma: imaging with iodine-131-meta-iodobenzylguanidine. BMJ 288:1587, 1984

18. Miura Y, Yoshinaga K: Doxazosin: a newly developed, selective alpha-1-inhibitor in the management of patients with pheochromocytoma. Am Heart J 116:1785, 1988

19. Grouzman E, Comoy E, Bohoun C: Plasma neuropeptide Y concentrations in patients with neuroendocrine tumors. J Clin Endocrinol Metab 68:808, 1989

20. Averbuch SD, Steakley CS, Young RC et al: Malignant pheochromocytoma: effective treatment with a combination of cyclophosphamide, vincristine, and dacarbazine. Ann Intern Med 109:267, 1988

21. Sisson JC, Shapiro B, Beierwaltes WH et al: Radiopharmaceutical treatment of malignant pheochromocytoma. J Nucl Med 24:197, 1993

22. Louis WJ, Horwitz JD: Hypertensive responses to phenylpropanolamine. p. 199. In Morgan JP, Kagan D, Brody JS (eds): Phenylpropanolamine: Risks, Benefits, and Controversies. Praeger, New York, 1985

23. Lake CR, Zaloga G, Clymer R et al: A double dose of phenylpropanolamine causes transient hypertension. Am J Med 85:339, 1988

24. Isner JM, Estes NAM, Thompson PD et al: Acute cardiac events temporally related to cocaine abuse. N Engl J Med 315:1438, 1986

25. Wojak JC, Flamm ES: Intracranial hemorrhage and cocaine use. Stroke 18:712, 1987

26. Acker D, Sachs BP, Tracey KJ, Wise WE: Abruptio placentae associated with cocaine use. Am J Obstet Gynecol 146:220, 1983

27. Ramoska E, Sachetti AD: Propranolol-induced hypertension in treatment of cocaine intoxication. Ann Emerg Med 14:1112, 1985

28. Scharff JA: Renal infarction associated with intravenous cocaine use. Ann Emerg Med 13:1145, 1984

29. White WB, Baker LH: Ambulatory blood pressure monitoring in patients with panic disorder. Arch Intern Med 147:1973, 1987

30. Mancia G, Bertinieri G, Grassi G et al: Effects of blood pressure measurement by the doctor on patient's blood pressure and heart rate. Lancet 2:695, 1983

31. Simons RJ, Baily RG, Zelis R, Zwillich CW: The physiologic and psychologic effects of the bedside presentation. N Engl J Med 321:1273, 1989

32. Pickering TG, James GD, Boddie C et al: How common is white coat hypertension? JAMA 259:225, 1988

33. Floras JS, Hassan MO, Jones JV, Sleight P: Pressor responses to laboratory stresses and daytime blood pressure variability. J Hypertens 5:715, 1987

34. Siegel WC, Blumenthal JA, Divine GW: Physiological, psychological, and behavioral factors and white coat hypertension. Hypertension 16:140, 1990

35. Yagil Y, Futterweit W, Krakoff LR et al: Cerebellar tumor causing hypertensive crisis and simulating pheochromocytoma and Cushing's syndrome. Mount Sinai J Med 56:5, 1989

36. Krum H, Howes LG, Brown DJ, Louis WJ: Blood pressure variability in tetraplegic patients with autonomic hyperreflexia. Paraplegia 27:284, 1989

9

ADRENOCORTICAL HYPERTENSION

Hypertension may be caused by an excess of either mineralocorticoid or glucocorticoid action. Several well-defined forms of clinical secondary hypertension have been identified and characterized. These may be the consequence of endogenous overproduction of cortisol (Cushing syndrome), aldosterone (Conn syndrome), congenital abnormalities of adrenal steroid synthesis, impairment of steroid metabolism, or exposure to exogenous steroids.

Adrenocortical hypertension due to excess production or administration of the glucocorticoid cortisol (Cushing syndrome) or synthetic glucococorticoids is associated with characteristic and, to some extent, specific symptoms and signs that are detectable by an accurate history and physical examination. Several of the congenital disorders of steroidogenesis, the congenital adrenal hyperplasias, also produce a unique set of physical findings (e.g., abnormal development of gender characteristics). By contrast, mineralocorticoid excess in the form of primary aldosteronism, or the recently defined syndrome of apparent mineralocorticoid excess, may only be suspected on the basis of hypokalemia and suppressed plasma renin activity. Thus, secondary hypertension due to abnormal adrenocortical function represents a diverse spectrum and requires familiarity with the endocrinology of the adrenal steroid pathways.

PATHOGENESIS

Adminstration of exogenous steroids having either a mineralocorticoid or glucocorticoid action will cause elevation of arterial pressure in experimental animals, causing experimental hypertension. However, important differences exist between the mechanisms accounting for mineralocorticoid- and glucocorticoid-induced hypertension, as summarized in Table 9-1.

Experimental mineralocorticoid hypertension is easily induced by giving rats exogenous desoxycorticosterone plus a high salt diet. This form of experimental hypertension is clearly salt dependent and will not develop if salt intake is restricted to low or normal levels.[1] Elevation of arterial pressure in this model is associated with an expanded extracellular volume due to mineralocorticoid action.[2] Since systemic vascular resistance is increased in mineralocorticoid hypertension, the relationship of salt retention, hypervolemia, and the hemodynamic state of increased vascular resistance has not been entirely explained. Various studies have suggested the following: (1) expan-

99

Table 9-1. Comparison Between Experimental Glucocorticoid and Mineralocorticoid Hypertension

Mineralocorticoid Hypertension	Glucocorticoid Hypertension
Requires high salt intake for hypertension to occur	Can be induced on low salt intake
Renin system: plasma and renal renin are suppressed	Renin level is normal or increased, as determined by plasma renin activity
Hypokalemia and salt/water retention	Serum potassium is normal, plasma volume may be increased due to shift from intracellular to extracellular space
No change in plasma renin substrate-angiotensinogen	Increased hepatic production and serum concentration of angiotensinogen
No effect of angiotensin antagonism or converting enzyme inhibition	Reduction of arterial pressure by angiotensin antagonists and converting enzyme inhibition
Increased sensitivity to injected catecholamines or angiotensin II in some studies	Increased sensitivity to injected catecholamines or angiotensin II in some studies
No known reduction in activity of the vasodilator prostaglandins or kinins	Some studies suggest reduced production of prostaglandin E or kinins

sion of extracellular volume leads to autoregulatory changes, increasing resistance in many tissues due to an initial phase of increased cardiac output followed by the slow phase of autoregulation of local blood flow, the Guyton mechanism[3,4]; (2) altered turnover of neuronal catecholamine stores; and (3) induced release of natriuretic hormones with vasoconstrictor activity, which inhibit Na/K-ATPase and exhibit ouabain-like activity.[5,6] Not all these mechanisms have been studied in human mineralocorticoid excess syndromes. However, the clinical disorders of mineralocorticoid excess are characterized by excess blood and extracellular fluid volume, low serum potassium, and profound suppression of plasma renin activity. There is a tendency for increased plasma concentrations of atrial natriuretic peptide in clinical mineralocorticoid excess as an expression of hypervolemia.[7]

Increased arterial pressure due to glucocorticoid excess (as in Cushing syndrome) can also be produced in animal models by administration of corticosterone (the natural glucocorticoid of rodents) or the synthetic steroids dexamethasone or prednisolone.[8,9] Low salt intake does not prevent glucocorticoid hypertension.[1] However, increased plasma volume may occur in glucocorticoid hypertension due to a shift of fluid from intracellular to extracellular and intravascular compartments.[10,11] Despite the increase in these volumes, the renin system is not suppressed in experimental or clinical glucocorticoid hypertension, and plasma renin activity may be normal or increased.[9,12,13] Part of the reason for increased plasma renin activity is the elevation of plasma angiotensinogen caused by a direct of effect of glucocorticoid action on hepatic synthesis and release of this protein.[14] Other suggested mechanisms to account for glucocorticoid-induced hypertension are increased vascular responsiveness to vasoconstrictor agonists such as norepinephrine[15–17] and/or a reduction in vasodilator kinins and prostaglandins.[18,19]

CLINICAL FORMS

Mineralocorticoid Excess Syndromes

Primary Aldosteronism

Hypertension due to primary aldosteronism is a rare disorder, occurring in less than 1 percent of all hypertensive persons, but is one of the more common forms of curable secondary hypertension. It is usually detected by the presence of hypokalemia, often less than 3.5 mEq/L, in the absence of any provoking cause.[20] Diuretic use or gastrointestinal losses from vomiting, diarrhea, or use of cathartics should be excluded. The history is usually unremarkable, but symptoms of hypokalemia such as muscle cramps, weakness, polyuria, or cardiac arrhythmias may be detected (usually in retrospect). Muscle irritability and symptoms with Chvostek and Trousseau signs may occasionally be found owing to the alkalosis accompanying extreme degrees of hypokalemia. Physical examination is usually unimpressive; signs of glucocorticoid excess are not present.

Diagnosis of primary aldosteronism depends on demonstration that the renin system is suppressed and aldosterone production is increased.[21] Measurements of plasma renin activity, 24-hour urine aldosterone excretion, and plasma aldosterone concentrations on both low and high salt intake are desirable to establish suppression of the renin system. The elevated plasma aldosterone level is not normally reduced by either a high salt diet or saline infusion. Similarly, suppressed plasma renin activity in primary aldosteronism is not significantly increased by either a low salt diet or diuresis with agents such as furosemide.

Aldosteronoma Versus Bilateral Secretion of Aldosterone: Idiopathic or Pseudoprimary Aldosteronism

Once primary aldosteronism is established, the cause must be determined. The most common entities responsible for the combination of hypertension, hypokalemia, suppressed renin, and increased production of aldosterone are (1) true primary aldosteronism due to an aldosterone-secreting adenoma (Conn syndrome), and (2) bilateral hypersecretion of aldosterone (idiopathic or pseudoprimary aldosteronism or primary adrenal hyperplasia). These two disorders together account for more than 90 percent of cases of primary aldosteronism. In various series, Conn syndrome (aldosteronoma) varies from 50 to 70 percent of all those with primary aldosteronism. Most cases of primary aldosteronism occur as isolated events, without any familial syndrome evident. Familial primary aldosteronism has recently been characterized in several genetically related family members who had either aldosteronomas or bilateral adrenal hyperplasia.[22,23] This was designated *familial aldosteronism II* by Gordon et al.,[22] since the first form of familial hyperaldosteronism to be described was glucocorticoid-remediable aldosteronism, now called *familial aldosteronism I* (see the section, *Glucocorticoid-Remediable Aldosteronism*).

There are important clinical and pathophysiologic distinctions between the two major forms of primary aldosteronism; most notable is the difference in likelihood of surgical cure. If an aldosterone-producing adenoma is found, it may be removed by unilateral adrenalectomy (preserving a normal adrenal gland) with the potential for cure (60 to 70 percent) of both the endocrine disorder and the hypertension. If bilateral oversecretion of aldosterone causes the clinical picture of primary aldosteronism, the case for surgery is much less strong, as a bilateral adrenalectomy would be required to correct the metabolic defect; cure of hypertension is unusual (Table 9-2).

Patients with aldosteronomas usually have a more severe endocrinologic disturbance than those with idiopathic aldosteronism, as reflected by lower serum potassium concentrations, lower or undetectable levels of plasma renin activity (often less than 0.5 ng/ml/hr), and greater secretion of aldosterone (plasma or serum greater than 20 ng/dl) and 18-OH corticosterone (greater than 50 ng/dl), a precurser of aldosterone.[24–26] Plasma atrial natriuretic peptide is increased in primary aldosteronism. However, levels tend to be higher after saline infusion or when patients are supine in patients with aldosteronomas than in patients with idiopathic aldosteronism.[7] The level of arterial pressure is, however, not a good basis for distinguishing between the two syndromes.

Several studies suggest that most aldosterone-secreting adenomas behave as if the tumor secretion of aldosterone is primarily controlled by adrenocorticotropic hormone (ACTH). This is supported by the parallel variation between plasma cortisol and aldosterone in such patients that decreases from early morning (typically 8:00 AM) to noon, despite the assumption of upright posture. By contrast, most patients with idiopathic aldosteronism have the usual increase (associated with standing) in plasma aldosterone concentration during this interval. In some cases, there is a small but detectable increase in plasma renin activity in parallel with the rise in plasma aldosterone. Exceptions, however, occur ("renin-dependent adenomas") so that the posture test is not entirely reliable in classifying the cause of primary aldosteronism.[27] The response to angiotensin converting enzyme (ACE) inhibition may be helpful. Patients with primary aldosteronism due to aldosterone-producing adenomas have no change in plasma aldosterone concentration after captopril. By contrast, normal subjects, those with essential hypertension, and some, but not all, patients with idiopathic aldosteronism suppress plasma aldosterone concentration after ACE inhibition.[28,29]

It was once suggested that idiopathic aldosteronism might be due to trophic stimulation of the adrenal glomerulosa zone by γ-melanocyte stimulating hormone (γ-MSH), an aldosterone-stimulating factor of pituitary origin[25,30,31] or a serotonin pathway.[32] It now seems more likely that idiopathic aldostero-

Table 9-2. Comparison Between True Primary Aldosteronism (Conn Syndrome) and Bilateral Hyperaldosteronism

Conn Syndrome (Aldosteronoma)	Bilateral Hyperaldosteronism (Idiopathic or Pseudoprimary Aldosteronism)
Serum potassium often <3.5 mEq/L and frequently <3.0 mEq/L	Serum potassium tends to be low normal or slightly low (3.0–3.9 mEq/L)
Plasma renin activity (PRA) levels very low or undetectable by sensitive assays	PRA levels low normal to moderately suppressed, usually detectable by sensitive assays
Posture study: plasma aldosterone and cortisol fall from 8:00 AM (supine) to noon (standing); no change in very low PRA	Posture study: plasma aldosterone increases from 8:00 AM (supine) to noon (standing) with a small increase in PRA
Captopril test: no change in plasma aldosterone; very high plasma aldosterone/PRA ratio (>50 ng/dl/ng/ml/hr postcaptopril)	Captopril test: variable change in plasma aldosterone, may fall as in essential hypertension; plasma aldosterone/PRA ratio variable but lower than with Conn's tumor
Plasma 18-OH DOC usually >50 ng/dl	Plasma 18-OH DOC 20–40 ng/dl
Plasma atrial natriuretic peptide supine or after saline infusion usually >40 pg/ml (75%)[7]	Plasma atrial natriuretic peptide supine or after saline infrequently >40 pg/ml (20%)

nism represents one end of the spectrum of low renin essential hypertension in which the adrenal response to angiotensin II is increased. This results in a persistently high ratio of plasma aldosterone to plasma renin activity, despite lower than average renin levels. The latter view is supported by the observation that occasional patients with idiopathic aldosteronism have amelioration of their hypokalemia and reduction of plasma aldosterone and arterial pressure during long-term treatment with ACE inhibitors.

Once endocrinologic studies have led to a presumptive diagnosis of the Conn syndrome, curative surgery should be considered. Removal of a Conn's tumor will certainly eliminate the biochemical abnormalities, but may not always reduce arterial pressure to normal. One strategy used to predict the blood pressure response to surgery is the pharmacologic blockade of aldosterone action by giving high doses of the mineralocorticoid antagonist spironolactone (200 to 400 mg/day), for 4 to 6 weeks. If blood pressure falls to normal during this interval, the likelihood that surgery will cure the hypertension is increased.

Localization of Aldosteronomas

Once an aldosterone-producing adenoma is suspected on the basis of hormone measurements, localization by appropriate imaging is necessary to guide surgical management. The usual Conn's tumor or aldosteronoma is a small, benign adrenal cortical tumor with a diameter of 0.5 to 2.0 cm. From 60 to 80 percent may be seen on computed tomography scans, but thin sections of 5 mm are necessary for optimal visualization (Fig. 9-1).

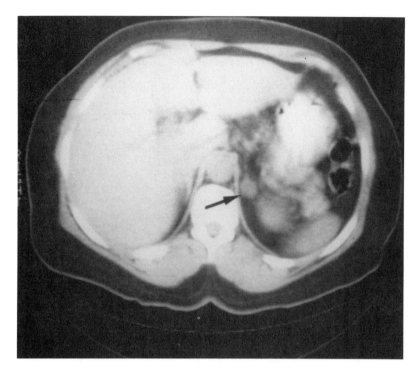

Fig. 9-1. Abdominal computed tomography scan of a left adrenal aldosterone-producing adenoma (Conn's tumor) approximately 2 cm (*arrow*).

Magnetic resonance imaging of the adrenal areas may also detect aldosteronomas; T_2-weighted imaging does not enhance the image as it does with pheochromocytoma. ^{131}I-iodocholesterol scans have also been helpful in detection.[33,34] Since 20 to 30 percent of all aldosteronomas are small, less than 1.0 cm, imaging by current techniques may not reveal the diagnosis. False-negative results must be considered but false-positive results are also possible. Nodular adrenal hyperplasia may be misinterpreted on computed tomography scan as unilateral adrenal adenoma.[35]

Definitive localization of a Conn's tumor requires not only that a tumor be present (if found) but that it be the single source of excessive secretion of aldosterone. Therefore adrenal vein catheterization for venography, with blood samples for steroid determination, is necessary (Fig. 9-2). Use of ACTH or angiotensin II to enhance lateralization of aldosterone secretion have been reported to be valuable. Since most aldosteronomas behave as if the secretion was controlled by ACTH, it is not surprising that adrenal venous aldosterone concentration from the side with the tumor is enhanced by infusion of ACTH. However, the few "renin-dependent" aldosteronomas may respond better to angiotensin II as a secretogogue for diagnosis.

Aldosterone-Secreting Adrenal Carcinomas

Aldosterone-producing adrenal carcinomas are rare (less than 5 percent of cases of primary aldosteronism). Hypokalemia is profound and plasma aldosterone concentrations are markedly elevated even when compared with benign aldosteronomas. These neoplasms are much larger than Conn's tumors and may have intratumoral calcification.[36]

Peri- and Postsurgical Management. Patients undergoing surgery for removal of a Conn's tumor may be treated with spironolactone to reduce arterial pressure and correct hypokalemia. This approach may also stimulate the suppressed renin system, causing aldosterone secretion from the opposite adrenal gland, which will be needed in the postoperative phase. Following removal of an aldosteronoma, there may be a brief (3- to 7-day) period of hypoaldosteronism, with its risk of hyperkalemia and hypotension due to volume losses and an inadequate response by the renin system. This postoperative complication can be avoided by intramuscular injection of deoxycorticosterone (DOC) during the 1 to 3 days after surgery with close evaluation of serum potassium and volume status.

Medical Treatment. Sustained pharmacologic treatment of primary aldosteronism may be needed for patients with idiopathic or pseudoprimary aldosteronism and patients with aldosteronomas who have contraindications to surgery or who refuse it, preferring a noninvasive strategy. Spironolactone is the obvious choice and is the only mineralocorticoid antagonist available for this approach. However, the high doses (100 to 400 mg/day) needed for effec-

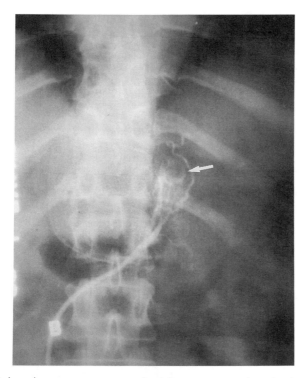

Fig. 9-2. Adrenal venous contrast study delineating an adrenal adenoma (*arrow*) that was confirmed by analysis of plasma adrenal vein aldosterone concentrations.

tive blockade of aldosterone action may cause adverse reactions, particularly painful gynecomastia in men, menstrual disorders in premenopausal women, and abdominal cramps. The other potassium-sparing agents amiloride or triamterene can be used and may be effective for correcting hypokalemia. Addition of other diuretic drugs may be helpful, as the presumed basis for hypertension due to excess aldosterone is volume retention. Since all these patients have low renin levels, control of arterial pressure may be achieved with calcium channel blocking agents. As indicated above, some patients with idiopathic aldosteronism have a pathophysiology suggestive of excessive adrenocortical sensitivity to angiotensin II. Therapy with ACE inhibitors may be beneficial in such individuals.

Other Forms of Mineralocorticoid Excess

Several rare syndromes may mimic primary aldosteronism and should be considered in the differential diagnosis of hypertension associated with hypokalemia and suppressed renin. These entities are briefly described.

Inherited Disorders of Steroid Synthesis

Glucocorticoid-Remediable Aldosteronism. The original description of this disorder reported hypertension with features of primary aldosteronism in a father and son. Both hypertension and hypokalemia were ameliorated by administration of low (replacement level) doses of dexamethasone, suggesting that the hyperaldosteronism was dependent on ACTH secretion by the pituitary. However, there were no signs of Cushing syndrome or other evidence of overproduction of the pituitary hormone. Excess aldosterone production was subsequently found to be accompanied by high levels of 18-OH cortisol, implying formation of 18-oxo steroids in the fascicular zone of the adrenal cortex.[37] Explanation for this unusual pattern has recently been provided by contemporary human genetic studies. Analysis of the genes that control adrenal steroidogenesis from families with glucocorticoid-remediable aldosteronism reveals an unusual chimeric crossover of the aldosterone synthase gene (CYPB11B2) with the ACTH regulatory portion (CYPB11B1). Both of these genes code for a steroid 11-OH hydroxylase. Extra copies of this chimeric gene are present and are presumably controlled by ACTH in the adrenal fasciculata zone, resulting in formation of aldosterone by an ACTH-dependent enzyme. Cortisol and adrenal androgens are produced in normal amounts. There is, then, no abnormal phenotype; gender development and growth are normal. When suspected, as in young hypertensive persons with features of primary aldosteronism, individual patients and their families can be screened by analysis of leukocyte DNA for classification and diagnosis.[38–40]

11-OH Hydroxylase Deficiency. Several forms of congenital adrenal hyperplasia occur that have abnormalities in the genetic control of synthetic enzymes for the adrenocortical steroids.[41,42] In some of these disorders, the defective enzyme impairs cortisol synthesis, leading to excessive ACTH secretion by the pituitary, increased adrenal androgen production, and either virilization of female genotypes or precocious puberty of the male; these are the adrenogenital syndromes. Ninety percent of those with the adrenogenital syndrome have a defect in steroid 21-hydroxylase (P450c21) and are salt wasters due to reduced production of aldosterone. Hypertension is obviously not part of their pathophysiology. By contrast, 5 to 6 percent of those with congenital adrenal hyperplasia have a deficiency of 11-OH hydroxylase (P450c11). This defect leads to increased desoxycorticosterone secretion, hypokalemia, and suppressed plasma renin activity, causing signs and symptoms of mineralocorticoid hypertension.[42] It is now known that the deficiency of 11-OH hydroxylase may be due to either one of two true mutations in the gene (CYP11B1) located on the long arm of chromosome 8.[43,44] Management of congenital adrenal hyperplasia is dependent on replacement with dexamethasone at levels sufficient to keep ACTH secretion close to normal, reducing stimulation of the adrenal cortex and diminishing secretion of DOC.

17-OH Hydroxylase Deficiency. The 17-steroid hydroxylase deficiency syndrome also leads to excess DOC secretion in association with an inability to form cortisol, estrogens, and androgens. In this disorder, failure of 17-hydroxylation and resultant low cortisol production leads to increased ACTH secretion; in markedly driving the adrenal to overproduce DOC and corticosterone, the latter serves as a substitute glucocorticoid. Hypertension is due to mineralocorticoid (DOC) excess with hypokalemia and suppression of plasma renin. These patients typically fail to develop secondary gender characteristics at puberty due to an inability to form the sex steroids dependent on 17-hydroxylation. Dexamethasone, given at replacement doses, reduces DOC secretion by suppressing ACTH, thus normalizing serum potassium and arterial pressure.

Desoxycorticosterone Excess Syndromes. DOC is nearly as potent a mineralocorticoid as aldosterone. Normally DOC is hydroxylated at the 11 position to form corticosterone. If this step is unimpaired, DOC is secreted at very low levels under control of ACTH by the pituitary rather than the renin-angiotensin system. Excess DOC secretion may occur in adrenal carcinomas accompanying massive cortisol secretion. In some adrenal carcinomas, there is a relative block in 11-steroid hydroxylase, leading to disproportionate hypersecretion of DOC.[45,46] DOC-secreting adrenal adenomas have also been described.[47,48]

Glucocorticoid Receptor Deficiency. Glucocorticoid receptor deficiency is a rare syndrome defined by the presence of markedly increased cortisol secretion without the features of Cushing syndrome.[49] Reduced numbers of glucocorticoid receptors have been demonstrated in some patients. Despite evidence for reduced glucocorticoid action in these patients, their arterial pressure is usually normal or elevated. They may be hypokalemic. It has been suggested that, in response to functional central glucocorticoid deficiency, ACTH secretion is increased, which drives the adrenal cortex to secrete increased cortisol and DOC.[50] Excess of both steroids may act on renal mineralocorticoid receptors (presumably normal) to cause salt and water retention, as in other forms of mineralocorticoid excess. Theoretically, spironolactone should be an effective antihypertensive therapy.

Synthetic Mineralocorticoid Hypertension

Several synthetic steroids have mineralocorticoid action. The best known is 9-α-fluoro-cortisone, which is often used as a replacement hormone for those with documented mineralocorticoid deficiency. 9-Fluoro-cortisone is also given as therapy to patients with orthostatic hypotension as a volume-retaining intervention to raise pressure. Overdosage of this steroid may cause hypertension. Other synthetic steroids developed as antiallergy remedies for intranasal or topical use have been found to cause mineralocorticoid hypertension when absorbtion sufficient to cause renal retention of salt and water occurs, mimicking primary aldosteronism. Both plasma renin activity and aldosterone production will be suppressed in the patients with synthetic mineralocorticoid excess.

Apparent Mineralocorticoid Excess

Patients (children and young adults) have been described with hypertension, hypokalemia, and suppressed plasma renin activity *without* overproduction of known mineralocorticoids, use of steroid medications, or signs of Cushing syndrome. Hypertension and hypokalemia can be corrected by replacement doses of dexamethasone (suggesting dependency on normal pituitary adrenal relationships) and by treatment with spironolactone, implying that stimulation of mineralocorticoid receptors is required for expression of the syndrome. Thus, these patients have "apparent mineralocorticoid excess" without increased steroid secretion.[51]

The pathogenesis of apparent mineralocorticoid excess is understandable through recognition that (1) cortisol is a potent mineralocorticoid that binds to type I steroid receptors with an affinity similar to aldosterone and DOC, whereas cortisone has a much lower affinity,[52] and that (2) in the kidney, cortisol is normally inactivated by conversion to cortisone by 11-OH steroid dehydrogenase (11-OH DHA) and possibly other pathways, reducing availability to the mineralocorticoid receptor.[53] It is likely that a deficiency in 11-OH DHA, presumably on a genetic basis, leads to increased urinary free cortisol excretion without excess adrenocortical secretion. The half-life of plasma cortisol is extended due to reduced inactivation; cortisol secretion rates may be less than normal. The excess free urinary cortisol causes retention of salt and water, wasting of potassium, and the pathogenetic sequence of mineralocorticoid hypertension. Since cortisol secretion remains dependent on normal pituitary stimulation by ACTH, the ameliorating effect of dexamethasone is explained.

Licorice-Induced Pseudoaldosteronism

The hypertension and hypokalemia associated with prolonged ingestion of the natural licorice used to flavor candies or chewing tobacco are now understood to be part of an acquired form of apparent mineralocorticoid excess syndrome.[54] Glycerrhyzic acid, the culprit in this disorder, is a very weak mineralocorticoid agonist, but an effective inhibitor of 11-OH DHA. Licorice administration increases urinary free cortisol and its metabolites, while reducing the excretion of cortisone and 11-OH DHA–dependent metabolites of cortisone. This mimics the patterns of urinary steroid metabolism in the naturally occurring form of apparent mineralocorticoid excess.[55]

Cushing Syndrome

Nearly 80 percent of patients with Cushing syndrome have hypertension, but only 20 percent have hypokalemia. Plasma renin activity may be increased, normal, or suppressed in this disorder and is not correlated with cortisol secretion. Plasma renin substrate (angiotensinogen) may be increased.[56] Thus, the pathogenesis of hypertension due to glucocorticoid excess differs from that caused by mineralocorticoid excess. Naturally occurring Cushing syndrome may be due to hypercortisolism as a result of an adrenal adenoma, carcinoma, pituitary adenoma, or ACTH-producing nonpituitary (ectopic) neoplasm. Long-term exposure to excess exogenous glucocorticoids may raise arterial pressure, but the incidence of hypertension appears to be less frequent than that observed in the Cushing syndrome of natural origin.

Diagnosis of hypertension due to glucocorticoid excess depends on the history and physical examination for recognition of either exogenous steroid use or the typical signs and symptoms of hypercortisolism. Once suspected, increased cortisol secretion may be confirmed by 24-hour urine excretion of free cortisol and the overnight low-dose dexamethasone suppression test.[57] Thereafter, the precise cause of Cushing syndrome may be defined by the various stimulation and suppression tests of cortisol and ACTH regulation, combined with appropriate imaging techniques.[58]

Hypertension in Cushing syndrome may vary from a minimal elevation to excessively high pressures (above 110 mmHg diastolic). Usually pressure levels are substantially decreased by removal of the cause of the syndrome by curative surgery. For inoperable conditions, adrenolytic therapy with such agents as o,p-DDD may be helpful. Transient inhibition of glucocorticoid receptors can be achieved through administration of RU 486, a glucocorticoid receptor antagonist.[59] Given the diversity of pathogenetic mechanisms present in Cushing syndrome, antihypertensive drug therapy may require a combination of agents. For patients with normal or elevated plasma renin levels, ACE inhibition may be effective.[60] When plasma renin activity is suppressed due to the mineralocorticoid effect of massive secretion of cortisol or excess DOC production (as in adrenocortical carcinomas or the ectopic ACTH syndrome), spironolactone administration may be helpful to inhibit steroid action at mineralocorticoid receptor sites. The excessive α-receptor responsiveness suggested in cortisol excess[15,16] should theoretically respond well to α_1-receptor antagonists.

REFERENCES

1. Knowlton AI, Loeb EN: Depletion of carcass potassium in rats made hypertensive with dexoxycorticosterone acetate (DCA) and with cortisone. J Clin Invest 36:1295, 1957

2. Haak D, Mohring J, Mohring B et al: Comparative study on development of corticosterone and DOCA hypertension in rats. Am J Physiol 233:F403, 1977

3. Guyton AC, Coleman TG, Cowley AW et al: Arterial pressure regulation: overriding dominance of the kidneys in long-term regulation and in hypertension. Am J Med 52:584, 1972

4. Guyton AC: Blood pressure control—special role of the kidneys and body fluids. Science 252:1813, 1991

5. Haddy FJ: Sodium-potassium pump in low-renin hypertension. Annu Rev Physiol 93(Pt. 2):781, 1983

6. Hamlyn JM, Blaustein MP, Bova S et al: Identification and characterization of a ouabain-like compound from human plasma. Proc Natl Acad Sci USA 88:6259, 1991

7. Opocher G, Rocco S, Carpene G et al: Usefulness of atrial natriuretic peptide assay in primary aldosteronism. Am J Hypertens 5:811, 1992

8. Elijovich F, Krakoff LR: Effect of converting enzyme inhibition on glucocorticoid hypertension in the rat. Am J Physiol 238:H844, 1980

9. Krakoff LR, Selvadurai R, Sutter E: Effect of methylprednisolone upon arterial pressure and the renin angiotensin system in the rat. Am J Physiol 228:613, 1975

10. Connell JMC, Whitworth JA, Davies DL et al: Haemodynamic, hormonal and renal effects of adrenocorticotrophic hormone in sodium-restricted man. J Hypertens 6:17, 1988

11. Connell JMC, Whitworth JA, Davies DL et al: Effects of ACTH and cortisol administration on blood pressure, electrolyte metabolism, atrial natriuretic peptide and renal function in normal man. J Hypertens 5:425, 1987

12. Krakoff LR: Measurement of plasma renin substrate by radioimmunoassay of angiotensin I: concentration in syndromes associated with steroid excess. J Clin Endocrinol Metab 37:608, 1973

13. Krakoff L, Nicolis G, Amsel B: Pathogenesis of hypertension in Cushing's syndrome. Am J Med 58:216, 1975

14. Krakoff LR, Eisenfeld AJ: Hormonal control of plasma renin substrate (angiotensinogen). Circ Res, suppl. II. 41:4, 1977

15. Whitworth JA, Connell JMC, Lever AF, Fraser R: Pressor responsiveness in steroid induced hypertension in man. Clin Exp Pharmacol Physiol 13:353, 1986

16. Sudhir K, Jennings GL, Esler MD et al: Hydrocortisone-induced hypertension in humans: pressor responsiveness and sympathetic function. Hypertension 13:416, 1989

17. Pirpiris M, Krishnankutty S, Yeung S et al: Pressor responsiveness in corticosteroid-induced hypertension in humans. Hypertension 19:567, 1992

18. Handa M, Kondo K, Suzuki H, Saruta T: Dexamethasone hypertension in rats: role of prostaglandins and pressor sensitivity to norepinephrine. Hypertension 6:236, 1984

19. Saruta T, Suzuki H, Handa M et al: Multiple factors contribute to the pathogenesis of hypertension in Cushing's syndrome. J Clin Endocrinol Metab 62:275, 1986

20. Bravo EL, Tarazi RC, Dustan HP et al: The changing clinical spectrum of primary aldosteronism. Am J Med 74:641, 1983

21. Lim RC Jr, Nakayama DK, Biglieri EG et al: Primary aldosteronism: changing concepts in diagnosis and management. Am J Surg 152:116, 1986

22. Gordon RD, Klemm SA, Tunny TJ, Stowasser M: Primary aldosteronism: hypertension with a genetic basis. Lancet 340:159, 1992

23. Stowasser M, Gordon RD, Tunny TJ et al: Familial hyperaldosteronism type II: five families with a new variety of primary aldosteronism. Clin Exp Pharmacol Physiol 19:319, 1992

24. Kem DC, Tang K, Hanson CS et al: The prediction of anatomical morphology of primary aldosteronism using serum 18-hydroxycorticosterone levels. J Clin Endocrinol Metab 60:67, 1985

25. Melby JC: Endocrine hypertension. J Clin Endocrinol Metab 69:697, 1989

26. Biglieri EG, Schambelan M, Hirai J et al: The significance of elevated levels of plasma 18-hydroxycorticosterone in patients with primary aldosteronism. J Clin Endocrinol Metab 49:87, 1979

27. Fontes RG, Kater CE, Biglieri EG, Irony I: Reassessment of the predictive value of the postural stimulation test in primary aldosteronism. Am J Hypertens 4:786, 1991

28. Lyons DF, Kem DC, Brown RD et al: Single dose captopril as a diagnostic test for primary aldosteronism. J Clin Endocrinol Metab 57:892, 1983

29. Hambling C, Jung RT, Gunn A et al: Re-evaluation of the captopril test for the diagnosis of primary hyperaldosteronism. Clin Endocrinol (Oxf) 36:499, 1992

30. Griffing GT, McIntosh T, Berelowitz B et al: Plasma beta-endorphin levels in primary aldosteronism. J Clin Endocrinol Metab 60:315, 1985

31. Griffing GT, Berelowitz B, Hudson M et al: Plasma immunoreactive gamma melanotropin in patients with idiopathic hyperaldosteronism, aldosterone-producing adenomas, and essential hypertension. J Clin Invest 76:163, 1985

32. Gross MD, Grekin RJ, Gniadek TC, Villareal JZ: Suppression of aldosterone by cyproheptadine in idiopathic aldosteronism. N Engl J Med 305:181, 1981

33. White EA, Schambelan M, Rost CR et al: Use of computed tomography in diagnosing the cause of primary aldosteronism. N Engl J Med 303:1503, 1980

34. Hogan MJ, McRae J, Schambelan M, Biglieri EG: Location of aldosterone-producing adenomas with 131-I-19-iodocholesterol. N Engl J Med 294:410, 1976

35. Doppman JL, Gill JR Jr, Miller DL et al: Distinction between hyperaldosteronism due to bilateral hyperplasia and unilateral aldosteronoma: reliability of CT [see comments]. Radiology 184:677, 1992

36. Farge D, Chatellier G, Pagny JY et al: Isolated clinical syndrome of primary aldosteronism in four patients with adrenocortical carcinoma. Am J Med 83:635, 1987

37. Ulick S, Chan CK, Gill JR et al: Defective fasciculata zone function as the mechanism of glucocorticoid-remediable aldosteronism. J Clin Endocrinol Metab 71:1151, 1990

38. Lifton RP, Dluhy RG, Powers M et al: A chimaeric 11 beta-hydroxylase/aldosterone synthase gene causes glucocorticoid-remediable aldosteronism and human hypertension. Nature 355:262, 1992

39. Lifton RP, Dluhy RG, Powers M et al: Heredity hypertension caused by chimaeric gene duplications and ectopic expression of aldosterone synthase. Nature Genet 2:66, 1992

40. Rich GM, Ulick S, Cook S et al: Glucocorticoid-remediable aldosteronism in a large kindred: clinical spectrum and diagnosis using a characteristic biochemical phenotype. Ann Intern Med 116:813, 1992

41. White PC, New MI, Dupont B: Congenital adrenal hyperplasia (first of two parts). N Engl J Med 316:1519, 1987

42. White PC. New MI, Dupont B: Congenital adrenal hyperplasia (second of two parts). N Engl J Med 316:1580, 1987

43. Helmberg A, Ausserer B, Kolfer R: Frame shift by insertion of 2 basepairs in codon 394 of CYP11B1 causes congenital adrenal hyperplasia due to steroid 11-beta-hydroxylase deficiency. J Clin Endocrinol Metab 75:1278, 1992

44. White PC, Dupont J, New MI et al: A mutation in CYP11B1 (arg-448-his) associated with steroid 11-beta-hydroxylase deficiency in Jews of Moroccan origin. J Clin Invest 87:1664, 1991

45. Schambelan M, Slaton PE, Biglieri EG: Mineralocorticoid production in hyperadrenocorticism. Am J Med 51:299, 1971

46. Hogan MJ, Schambelan M, Biglieri EG: Concurrent hypercortisolism and hypermineralocorticoidism. Am J Med 62:777, 1977

47. Irony I, Biglieri EG, Perloff D, Rubinoff H: Pathophysiology of deoxycorticosterone-secreting adrenal tumors. J Clin Endocrinol Metab 65:836, 1987

48. Biglieri EG, Kater CE, Arteaga EA: Mineralocorticoid hypertension due to hyperaldosteronism and hyperdeoxycorticosteronism. J Hypertens, suppl. 4:61, 1986

49. Chrousos GP, Vingerhoeds A, Brandon D et al: Primary cortisol resistance in man. A glucocorticoid receptor-mediated disease. J Clin Invest 69:1261, 1982

50. Iida S, Gomi M, Moriwaki K et al: Primary cortisol resistance accompanied by a reduction in glucocorticoid receptors in two members of the same family. J Clin Endocrinol Metab 60:967, 1985

51. Stewart PM, Corrie JET, Shackleton CHL, Edwards CRW: Syndrome of apparent mineralocorticoid excess: a defect in the cortisol-cortisone shuttle. J Clin Invest 82:340, 1988

52. Arriza JL, Weinberger C, Cerelli G et al: Cloning of human mineralocorticoid receptor complementary DNA: structural and functional kinship with the glucocorticoid receptor. Science 237:268, 1987

53. Edwards CRW, Stewart PM, Burt D et al: Localization of 11-beta-hydroxysteroid dehydrogenase-tissue specific protector of the mineralocorticoid receptor. Lancet 2:986, 1988

54. Stewart PM, Wallace AM, Valentino R et al: Mineralocorticoid activity of liquorice: 11-beta-hydroxysteroid dehydrogenase deficiency comes of age. Lancet 2:821, 1987

55. Farese RV, Biglieri EG, Shackleton CHL et al: Licorice-induced hypermineralocorticoidism. N Engl J Med 325:1223, 1991

56. Krakoff LR, Garbowit D: Hypertension of Cushing's syndrome. p. 113. In Biglieri EG, Melby JC (eds): Endocrine Hypertension. Raven Press, New York, 1990

57. Crapo L: Cushing's syndrome: a review of diagnostic tests. Metabolism 28:955, 1979

58. Kaye TB, Crapo L: The Cushing syndrome: an update on diagnostic tests. Ann Intern Med 112:435, 1990

59. Nieman LK, Chrousos GP, Kellner C et al: Successful treatment of Cushings's syndrome with the glucocorticoid antagonist RU 486. J Clin Endocrinol Metab 61:536, 1985

60. Greminger P, Vetter W, Groth H et al: Captopril in Cushing's syndrome. Klin Wochenschr 62:855, 1984

10

REVERSIBLE RENAL HYPERTENSION

Many disorders of the kidneys may cause hypertension. This section focuses primarily on those that are reversible by intervention such as balloon angioplasty or surgery. The form of reversible renal hypertension identified most often is renal artery stenosis. However, other entities considered in this section include obstructive renal disease and certain renal tumors that, although exceedingly rare, are curable and fascinating lessons in pathophysiology.

RENAL ARTERY STENOSIS: RENOVASCULAR HYPERTENSION

Hypertension due to narrowing of one or more renal arteries may be the most common form of reversible secondary hypertension. Moreover, the pathogenetic mechanisms by which narrowing of the renal arteries leads to increased arterial pressure have been well delineated in a large series of experimental and clinical studies. The lessons learned from the study of experimental renal artery stenosis not only apply to the human forms of renovascular hypertension, but may well account for more common forms of hypertension whenever intrarenal nephrosclerosis (i.e., microvascular renal arteriolar disease) is present.

Pathogenesis of Renovascular Hypertension

The increase in arterial pressure following impairment of the arterial supply to one or both kidneys has been one of the best studied forms of both experimental and clinical hypertension, since it was originally defined by Goldblatt and colleagues in the 1930s. A profusion of reports from the experimental literature led to recognition that elevated arterial pressure caused by impaired perfusion of one or both kidneys, or portions of them, can be understood in terms of two separate, but linked mechanisms. The first mechanism is the salt- and water-retaining functions of glomerular filtration and tubular reabsorption (i.e., the kidney as filter and tubular pump) that control extracellular fluid volume. The second mechanism is the primary endocrine apparatus of the kidney, the juxtaglomerular apparatus of the afferent arterioles, which secretes active renin into the circulation and also controls efferent arteriolar vasoconstriction to maintain intraglomerular pressure. These two separate mechanisms explain both Goldblatt kidney models (the two-kidney and one-kidney model) of experimental renovascular hypertension[1,2] (Fig. 10-1).

113

Goldblatt Two-Kidney Hypertension

Experimental narrowing of one renal artery without any alteration of the opposite kidney in a laboratory animal is referred to as the *Goldblatt two-kidney model*, unilateral renal artery stenosis with an initially normal opposite kidney (Fig. 10-2). Renin secretion from the ischemic kidney leads to angiotensin II formation and vasoconstriction, with elevated arterial pressure as a direct effect. Angiotensin II–stimulated secondary aldosteronism elicits hypokalemia from renal potassium loss. The elevated pressure and activated renin system affect the opposite kidney by reducing its renin secretion and causing a pressure natriuresis and volume loss, despite secondary aldosteronism. The natriuresis of the normal opposite kidney is probably limited because of the actions both of aldosterone at tubular sites and of circulating angiotensin II on afferent arterioles, the glomerulus, and tubular function. In brief, hypertension in the early phases of the two-kidney Goldblatt model is due entirely to an activated renin system from the ischemic kidney. Plasma renin activity (PRA) is elevated; its origin is also the ischemic kidney. Normalization of arterial pressure follows either angiotensin II antagonism or angiotensin converting enzyme (ACE) inhibition. Removing the stenosis from the affected kidney or performing unilateral nephrectomy will, of course, also cure this form of experimental hypertension at this stage.

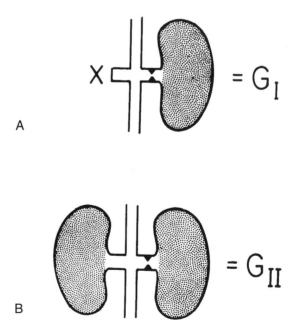

Fig. 10-1. Schematic depiction of the two Goldblatt models of renovascular hypertension. **(A)** Two-kidney model of unilateral renal artery stenosis with a normal opposite kidney. **(B)** One-kidney model with unilateral renal artery stenosis and removal of the opposite kidney.

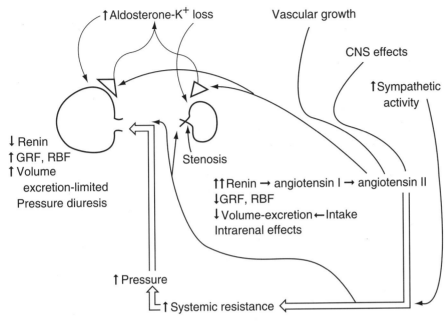

$\uparrow$ Aldosterone-K^+ loss

Vascular growth

CNS effects

$\uparrow$ Sympathetic activity

$\downarrow$ Renin
$\uparrow$ GRF, RBF
$\uparrow$ Volume
  excretion-limited
Pressure diuresis

Stenosis

$\uparrow\uparrow$ Renin $\rightarrow$ angiotensin I $\rightarrow$ angiotensin II
$\downarrow$ GRF, RBF
$\downarrow$ Volume-excretion $\leftarrow$ Intake
Intrarenal effects

$\uparrow$ Pressure

$\uparrow$ Systemic resistance

Fig. 10-2. Pathogenetic scheme for Goldblatt two-kidney hypertension: unilateral renal artery stenosis with unaffected opposite kidney. Volume loss of unaffected kidney limited by angiotensin II (secondary aldosteronism). The limited pressure diuresis of the nonstenotic side is evident. GFR, glomerular filtration rate; RBF, renal blood flow; CNS, central nervous system.

If the early phase of experimental Goldblatt two-kidney hypertension is not reversed and arterial pressure remains elevated, the pathologic changes of nephrosclerosis, due to sustained hypertension, evolve in the previously normal kidney. With progressive afferent arteriolar and glomerular sclerosis, the previously normal kidney begins to acquire a prohypertensive action. The preglomerular afferent arteriolar narrowing reduces the kidney's filtering ability and stimulates its renin-secreting activity. After a varying period (usually several months in rats), the hypertension is no longer due to an activated renin system alone, but to the combination of both the renin system and the secondary pathologic changes described. Relief of the stenosis, unilateral nephrectomy, angiotensin II antagonism, or ACE inhibition will no longer normalize arterial pressure. However, the kidney distal to the renal artery stenosis is protected from hypertension. If the stenosis is removed along with nephrectomy of the *opposite* kidney (once normal, now nephrosclerotic), blood pressure may return to normal. The clinical counterpart to this strategy has occasionally been reported, but is now rarely needed, as less radical alternatives are available for treatment.

The exact time periods for the early and late phases of experimental Goldblatt two-kidney hypertension that correspond to those for human hypertension due to unilateral renal artery stenosis are not precisely defined.

The consensus is that unilateral renovascular hypertension is most curable (by either balloon angioplasty or surgery) within 5 years of its onset. The response to these interventions in patients with more long-standing hypertension tends to be less favorable.

Patchy or focal intrarenal arteriolar pathology, as may be seen in periarteritis nodosa, scleroderma (renal crisis), malignant hypertension, or even more routine nephrosclerosis, may be viewed as a form of the Goldblatt two-kidney phenomenon when such patients have elevated renin levels and respond well to ACE inhibition. The implication is that areas of normal or relatively spared renal tissue are mixed in between the focal ischemic regions—counterparts to the two kidneys, one normal and one ischemic, of the model. Perhaps the activated circulating renin-angiotensin system in such conditions causes enough angiotensin II–mediated constriction of the remaining normal renal tissue for it to become ischemic. This hormone-induced ischemia may be relieved by ACE inhibition, which interrupts the activated renin-angiotensin system. Improvement in renal function during treatment with ACE inhibitors has certainly been observed in several of these diseases.

Goldblatt One-Kidney Hypertension

If an animal undergoes unilateral nephrectomy and narrowing of the artery to the remaining kidney, the model of Goldblatt one kidney is produced—the entire renal mass will become ischemic or underperfused (Fig. 10-3). Two mechanisms begin immediately: activation of the renin system and increased retention of salt and volume. These are caused by the combined effects of decreased glomerular filtration and increased tubular reabsorption. Unless salt intake is restricted, volume retention will proceed, raising arterial pressure via the mechanisms described by Guyton and colleagues.[3–5] The arterial pressure will eventually increase enough to reperfuse the single kidney at a pressure high enough to suppress renin secretion. In the salt-replete state, the role of the renin system will be hidden; PRA will be normal or low, and blockade of the renin system will have no effect on pressure. However, if salt intake is prevented or a salt and water diuresis is caused by diuretic administration, the renin system remains activated and accounts for the persistently elevated pressure. Thus, the Goldblatt one-kidney model of experimental hypertension is characterized by the reciprocal interplay of these two mechanisms.

It is evident that in the Goldblatt one-kidney model, reduction of arterial pressure by the *combination* of salt depletion and blockade of the renin system reduces renal perfusion as arterial pressure falls. In addition, the renin system acts as an intrarenal mechanism for maintaining glomerular pressure (by efferent arteriolar constriction) in the presence of impaired arterial perfusion caused by stenosis of the main renal artery. It is no wonder, then, that interruption of the renin system in this model leads to disproportionate glomerular hypotension (the result of efferent arteriolar dilation) and diminished glomerular filtration. This affects the entire functional renal mass

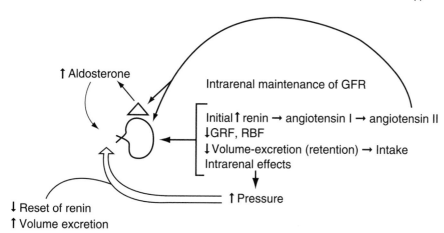

Fig. 10-3. Pathogenetic scheme for Goldblatt one-kidney hypertension: unilateral stenosis with removal of opposite kidney. Compare the lack of the "escape valve" function of normal renal tissue with the two-kidney model. GFR, glomerular filtration rate; RBF, renal blood flow.

because normally perfused renal tissue is not available as it is in the Goldblatt two-kidney model.

The clinical counterpart for the Goldblatt one-kidney model includes patients with bilateral renal artery stenosis, found in 10 to 20 percent of those with either fibromuscular dysplasia or atherosclerotic renal artery stenosis. The human renal transplant is susceptible to the Goldblatt one-kidney mechanism should the transplant artery become narrowed. Occasionally, a patient with a solitary kidney due to a congenital abnormality or to prior nephrectomy will develop renal artery stenosis. In all these situations, reversal of the renal arterial obstruction is necessary not only to control the hypertension but also to prevent progression of renal insufficiency. It is likely that some patients with advanced nephrosclerosis due to the combination of prior hypertension and other forms of intrarenal disease have a Goldblatt one-kidney–like pathophysiology (i.e., virtually all of their afferent arterioles are narrowed). This may explain why occasionally renal function deteriorates when ACE inhibitors are administered to patients with moderate renal insufficiency who are undergoing volume depletion therapy.[6] For these patients, primary emphasis on relief of vasoconstriction, which includes afferent arteriolar dilation (calcium channel entry blockers), may be beneficial.

Clinical Renovascular Hypertension

Diagnostic Assessment

The optimal technique for initial screening of patients for renovascular hypertension is controversial because of differences in sensitivity, specificity, risk, and cost of the various modalities available (Table 10-1 and Table 7-4).

Table 10-1. Tests for Renovascular Hypertension

Test	Characteristics and Features
Plasma renin activity (PRA) measured at mid-day, with patient off medication $\geq$1 wk; related to 24-hr sodium excretion (renin-sodium profile); widely available, relatively inexpensive	Tends to be elevated or normal in renovascular hypertension, almost never low; fair sensitivity and specificity
Oral captopril test with measurement of PRA before and 60 min after dose	Requires standardized conditions; fair sensitivity and specificity, but improves on PRA test
Postcaptopril or ACE inhibitor radioisotope renal scan	Highly sensitive for unilateral renal artery stenosis; may be limited in some with bilateral stenosis
Intravenous contrast urography with early (rapid-sequence) films and tomography	Still has some adherents,[55] but largely replaced by isotope renal scans; some risk of dye, less sensitive than isotope renal scan
Renal sonography	Limited sensitivity; excellent for determination of renal size, cysts, outflow tract obstruction
Doppler flow measurement of renal arterial flow	Useful when arteriography is too risky; highly operator dependent for accuracy and reliability; high false-positive rates for <50% stenoses[60]
Digital subtraction venous angiography	Once promising, now infrequent; requires large dye volume; poor visualization of renal arterial anatomy
Renal vein renin determination: baseline and stimulated	Theoretically, the required basis for established unilateral renal ischemia; practically, many misleading studies

Assessing the Renin System. Activation of the renin-angiotensin system because of impaired renal perfusion is the basis for several clinical tests to detect renovascular hypertension. Elevation of PRA, alone, when measured in a resting state or after stimulation by upright posture, low salt intake, or diuresis has been found to have poor accuracy for detection of renovascular hypertension. Interruption of the renin system by inhibition of converting enzyme offers a potentially valuable approach. Muller et al.[7] evaluated the immediate effect of the ACE inhibitor captopril for diagnosis of secondary hypertension, particularly renovascular hypertension, in a large retrospective analysis. Of the 246 patients studied, 56 had renovascular hypertension, 122 had essential hypertension, and 68 had other forms of secondary hypertension. The single-dose captopril test they employed was performed under the following conditions: (1) normal salt intake and (2) if possible, withdrawal of all antihypertensive medications for 3 weeks. Patients were tested while sitting. During a baseline period of 30 minutes, blood pressure was measured repeatedly and a venous sample for PRA measurement was obtained. Next,

50-mg oral captopril (dissolved in water for a few minutes to improve absorption) was administered. Blood pressure was measured every 10 to 15 minutes afterward for 60 minutes. A second venous blood sample for PRA was obtained to determine the stimulated PRA. Blood pressure responses, alone, were not well correlated with the diagnosis of renovascular hypertension. However, evaluation of baseline and stimulated PRA (including both absolute and percentage increases) led to a set of criteria highly predictive for this diagnosis, nearly 100 percent sensitivity and specificity for untreated subjects without renal insufficiency. The criteria included high stimulated PRA and high absolute increases in PRA. Also, an increase of the PRA of 150 percent or more if the baseline PRA was above normal (1.4 to 3.0 ng/ml/hr) or an increase of 400 percent or more if the baseline PRA was within the normal range was highly predictive. The normal range for PRA differs somewhat between laboratories due to variations in the methods used.

Single-dose captopril tests have been evaluated in two prospective trials.[8,9] Fredrickson et al.[9] studied 100 patients, 29 with renovascular hypertension and 71 with essential hypertension. Patients were tested when sitting and given 50 mg of captopril. Baseline and stimulated PRA levels were obtained (60 minutes after captopril). A detailed sensitivity/specificity analysis was performed, with the conclusion that the most accurate measurement for diagnosis of renovascular hypertension was the postcaptopril (stimulated) PRA. When post-captopril PRA was more than 5.7 ng/ml/hr, the test was 100 percent sensitive and 86 percent specific for patients not receiving diuretics and 100 percent sensitive, 70 percent specific for those taking diuretics.

Far less accuracy was found by Postma et al.[8] using a variation of the single-dose captopril test. A prospective study was conducted with 149 patients, of whom 44 had renovascular hypertension (angiographic criteria). The protocol differed from that used in the two other studies in that patients were studied in the supine position and the dose of captopril was 25 mg. Several analyses were used, but in all cases the sensitivity and specificity for both captopril-stimulated PRA and the absolute percentage of increase in PRA were far less than described in the other two studies.[7,9] This was largely due to the high proportion of patients with renal artery stenosis who had false-negative tests (i.e., stimulated PRA levels that overlapped those found in the comparison group with essential hypertension). While no explanation for these differences is certain, it is likely that sitting, which partially stimulates renin secretion, and more complete inhibition of converting enzyme action by the higher (50 mg) dose of captopril account for the greater accuracy described in the studies by Muller et al.[7] and Frederickson et al.[9]

For the single-dose captopril test to be maximally useful in predicting the diagnosis of renovascular hypertension, patients should be tested after withdrawal from antihypertensive medication, when seated, and using a 50-mg dose of captopril. False-positive and false-negative results occur, implying that additional diagnostic tests must be performed if it is necessary to be certain of the diagnosis. There is some risk of excessive hypotension after captopril in elderly patients[10] and in those who are kept on antihypertensive drugs, especially the diuretics or α-receptor blockers.

Measurement of PRA in samples from the renal veins will help to reveal the functional significance of unilateral renal artery stenosis.[11] Increased renin secretion from the side of the stenosis may be stimulated by upright tilting, diuretic administration, or ACE inhibition.[12,13] Ideally, the patient with unilateral renal artery stenosis will have a high ratio (greater than 1.4) of affected renal vein renin activity to that of the unaffected side *and* no significant gradient between the unaffected renal vein and peripheral vein renin activity (i.e., no renin production from the kidney with a normal renal artery). However, false-negative and false-positive renal vein renin studies do occur. These misleading studies may be due to antihypertensive agents, particularly continued use of ACE inhibitors or β-blockers, and technical problems with sampling or the assay. Once a favorite for early investigation of possible renal artery stenosis, renal vein renin determination has become a less attractive choice due to its invasive requirement and limited sensitivity and specificity for predicting either renal artery anatomy or likelihood of the value of balloon angioplasty or surgery. In my view, a lateralizing renal vein renin study is not a necessary prerequisite for considering correction of renal artery stenosis when an activated renin-angiotensin system causing the hypertension and unequivocal renal artery stenosis is evident by arteriography.

Assessing Renal Perfusion. Radioisotope renography (the renal scan) is perhaps the most widely used and best characterized method for noninvasive detection of renal artery stenosis (Fig. 10-4). Diagnostic specificity may be

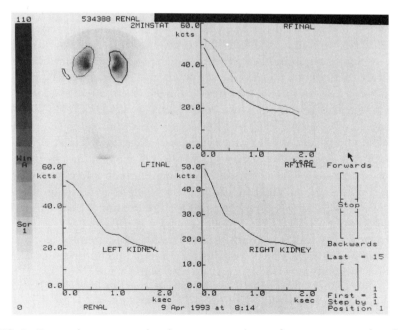

Fig. 10-4. Pre- and postcaptopril radioisotope renal scan from a patient with right renal artery stenosis. **(A)** Precaptopril renal scan. Excretion patterns are similar in the right and left kidney. *(Figure continues.)*

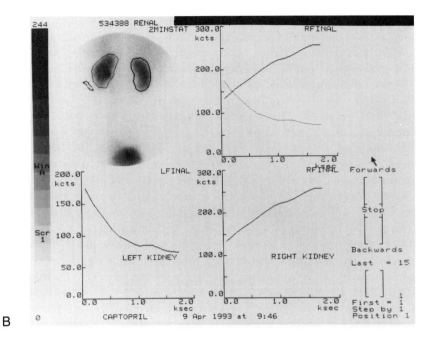

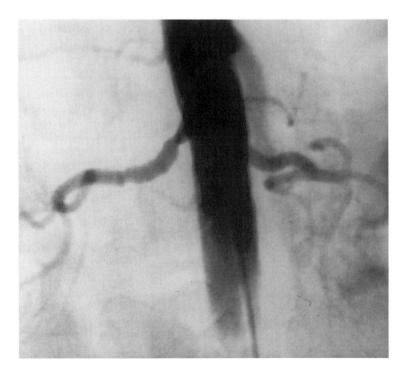

Fig. 10-4 *(Continued)*. **(B)** Postcaptopril renal scan. Excretion is markedly delayed in the right kidney. **(C)** Arteriogram of the same patient that clearly reveals right artery stenosis with poststenotic dilation.

enhanced by administration of an ACE inhibitor.[14–16] Isotope renal scans have largely replaced intravenous urography for detection of renal artery stenosis because of concerns about the adverse effects (particularly renal injury) of contrast media necessary for the latter procedure.

Renal dimensions can be estimated least invasively by abdominal sonography. Doppler assessment of flow in the renal arteries has been used to detect renal artery stenosis. The sensitivity and specificity of this technique are promising: sensitivity was 93 percent and specificity 98 percent for those with single renal arteries in one study.[17] The renal arteries can be visualized by magnetic resonance imaging; atherosclerotic renal artery stenosis has been demonstrated by this modality with high sensitivity and specificity.[18]

Renal arteriography remains the gold standard for detection of renal artery stenosis. Digital imaging of arterial injections requires much less contrast material, important for patients with renal insufficiency for whom contrast-induced impairment of renal function may be more likely. At one time, digital vascular imaging of the renal arteries after intravenous dye injection was thought to be a promising, less invasive modality. This approach has become little used in recent years because of poor sensitivity and specificity for diagnosis and the large volume of dye needed for arterial imaging because of dilution of the dye with intravenous administration.

Table 10-2. Clinical Characteristics of Fibromuscular Dysplasias and Atherosclerotic Renal Artery Stenosis

Fibromuscular Dysplasias	Atherosclerosis
Children to young adults	Middle aged to elderly
No unusual features in the history	Often a history of mild hypertension; smoking and other risk factors; coronary, cerebrovascular, or peripheral arterial disease
Subcostal systolic/diastolic high-pitched bruit is characteristic and highly predictive, when present	Harsh systolic abdominal bruit often found but not sensitive or specific
Typically normal glucose tolerance, serum lipids	Typically have elevated low-density lipoprotein cholesterol, low high-density lipoprotein fraction, noninsulin-dependent diabetes
Renal function (urea nitrogen, creatinine) usually normal	Mild to severe reduction in renal function at diagnosis
Findings usually limited to renal arteries; carotid or mesenteric stenoses occasionally found, but rarely symptomatic	Evidence of multifocal atherosclerotic disease: carotid bruits, evidence of coronary heart disease, claudication, peripheral arterial occlusions, aortic aneurisms
Excellent cure rate for hypertension (70–80%) after balloon angioplasty	Cure rate for hypertension 30–50% after balloon angioplasty; arterial surgery better in some series, but high risk of complications

Individual Forms

The different forms of renovascular hypertension are often related to different age groups. Atherosclerotic renal artery stenosis is a disease of the elderly, whereas the other forms of renovascular hypertension tend to occur in young adults or children. The major features distinguishing the two most common causes of clinical renovascular hypertension, the fibromuscular dysplasias and atherosclerosis, are given in Table 10-2. Descriptions of these and the other clinical forms of renovascular hyperplasia follow.

Fibromuscular Dysplasias

Fibromuscular dysplasia is a group of disorders that includes several anatomic variations whereby disordered growth of the intimal, medial, or adventitial layers of the main or branch renal arteries (individually or separately) obstruct blood flow. These nonatherosclerotic and noninflammatory stenoses tend to be the cause of moderate to severe hypertension, with diastolic pressures often higher than 100 mmHg, in young adults or children. In reported series, women are more often affected than men, and persons of white or Latin origin are affected more often than blacks. These are statistical trends; exceptions have been reported.

The typical patient with fibromuscular dysplasia as a cause of renovascular hypertension is a young woman with moderate to severe hypertension, perhaps in the malignant phase, and a high-pitched, nearly continuous, upper abdominal, subcostal bruit. Renal function, blood urea nitrogen, or creatinine are nearly always normal, even when bilateral renal artery stenosis is present. Hypokalemia may be present due to secondary aldosteronism of the high renin state. The response to antihypertensive therapy is not specific, but a substantial fall in pressure after ACE inhibition is often observed. If measured before treatment, PRA will be elevated. The oral captopril test will often be diagnostic (significant rapid fall in pressure, excessive rise in PRA). The radioisotope renal scan after ACE inhibition should be conclusive. Renal vein renin studies add some useful information, but can be misleading as to the likelihood of the diagnosis.

When the clinical picture favoring fibromuscular dysplasia is well defined, as described above, one may proceed directly to renal arteriography with the expectation that balloon angioplasty can be done at the same session. High cure rates are expected for initial balloon angioplasty for fibromuscular dysplasia (Fig. 10-5). However, 20 to 30 percent of patients may need repeat angioplasty within 6 to 12 months for optimal relief of residual stenoses. As interventional radiologic skills have advanced, the need to consider vascular surgery for renovascular hypertension due to fibromuscular dysplasia has receded.

Atherosclerotic Renal Artery Stenosis

The development of atherosclerotic renal artery stenosis should be viewed not merely as a form of secondary hypertension, but as a phase in the evolution of a multiarterial pathologic expression of the atherosclerotic process. The diagnosis and treatment of renal artery obstruction are only a part of the overall management. In fact, atherosclerotic renal artery disease should be viewed, in part, as a complication of aggressive atherogenesis due to the same confluence of risk factors that account for coronary, carotid, aortic, and

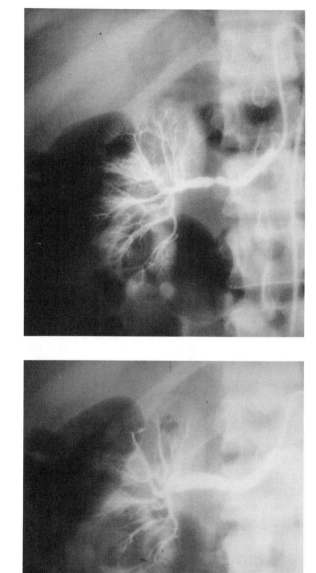

A

B

Fig. 10-5. Selective renal arteriogram from a patient with fibromuscular hyperplasia of a main renal artery. Arteriograms were taken **(A)** before and **(B)** after balloon angioplasty.

peripheral atherosclerotic pathology. As atherosclerotic manifestations are being delayed or prevented in middle-aged patients through progressive control of the cardiovascular risk factors, it is not surprising that there appears to be an increase of complications of a persisting silent arterial pathology in those surviving to an older age. Atherosclerotic renal artery stenosis, accounting for the more difficult to manage hypertension and progressive renal insufficiency, is, more often than not, a disease of the elderly.[19–21]

The typical patient with atherosclerotic renal artery stenosis is a 60- to 80-year-old individual with a past history of risk factors, usually smoking, hyperlipidemia, noninsulin-dependent diabetes, and drug-treated hypertension (Fig. 10-6). In addition, at the time renal artery stenosis is considered, the patient often already has evidence of coronary heart disease, cerebrovascular disease, including carotid stenosis, and/or peripheral arterial occlusive phenomena—bruit, reduced pulses, or claudication. With this background, clinical clues to advancing atherosclerotic renal arterial occlusion include (1) more difficult to treat hypertension; (2) appearance of retinal hemorrhage or exudate in association with the elevation of pressure[22]; (3) an increase in serum creatinine, especially if related to ACE inhibition; and (4) sudden unexplained pulmonary congestion.[23]

Thus, most patients with atherosclerotic renal artery stenosis will have evidence of advanced multifocal arterial pathology; target organ damage of

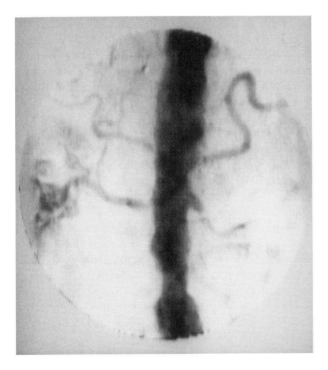

Fig. 10-6. Digital vascular venous angiogram from a patient with bilateral atherosclerotic renal artery stenosis and extensive aortic atheromatosis. This 65-year-old woman had a known history of prior smoking, hypercholesterolemia, and noninsulin-dependent diabetes.

varying significance; already be taking several medications for control of blood pressure, other risk factors, ischemic heart disease, and possibly cerebrovascular disease (including anticoagulants); and be at high risk of aggressive interventions. Arteriography can induce further renal insufficiency (although newer contrast agents offer promise in this regard). There is the risk that arteriography or attempted balloon angioplasty can disrupt aortic plaques, leading to the syndrome of cholesterol embolization.[24]

Aggressive intervention, balloon angioplasty, or vascular surgery can, without doubt, improve patients with atherosclerotic renal artery stenosis in several ways: reduction of arterial pressure, greater ease in gaining drug control of arterial pressure, and stabilization or improvement in renal function.[19,20,23,25–30] Balloon angioplasty may be effective for those with noncalcified renal arterial occlusions. However, if calcification or occlusion by osteal lesions that begin in the aorta adjacent to the renal artery orifice are present, vascular surgery may be more effective.[25] In any one case, however, the risk versus predicted benefit of either intervention needs careful consideration; increased age and more advanced and widespread pathology increase the likelihood of an adverse outcome.[30]

The medical management of atherosclerotic renal artery stenosis includes at least two components. First, appropriate antihypertensive medication is needed. For unilateral renal artery stenosis with well-preserved renal function, ACE inhibitors may be effective and beneficial for both reduction in arterial pressure and prevention of cardiac failure. In cases of bilateral renal artery occlusion, calcium channel entry blockers may reduce pressure with less risk of impairing renal perfusion (compared with ACE inhibitors). Perhaps this is due to direct dilation of narrowed renal arteries (analogous to the effect of these agents on atherosclerotic coronary arteries). The second component needed for treatment is attempted regression of the atherosclerotic renal artery plaque. In an oft-quoted case report, regression of such a narrowing has been documented by arteriography following cholesterol-lowering therapy with cholestyramine and clofibrate.[31] Whether calcium channel entry blockers have the ability to prevent progress of the atherosclerotic process in the renal arteries, as has been suggested for the coronary arteries,[32–34] remains unknown. At this time, the role of antithrombotic agents or anticoagulants (aspirin, ticlopidine, or coumadin) for preventing progression of atherosclerotic renal artery stenosis is unexplored.

Medical management of patients with atherosclerotic renal artery stenosis requires ongoing surveillance of their complex overall pathology. They need reassessment of the control of arterial pressure, therapy of ischemic disease wherever present, monitoring of renal function, and adjustment of medication and other therapy on a frequent and judicious basis. Such patients are best managed by a skilled and experienced physician who is knowledgeable in the relevant areas of internal medicine, cardiology, nephrology, endocrinology, and neurology.

Other Forms of Renovascular Hypertension

Unilateral or bilateral renal artery stenosis may rarely be found as a cause of secondary hypertension either in patients with neurofibromatosis in its full-blown form or in those with only multiple café-au-lait spots. We have seen one such case, a 16-year-old girl having many café-au-lait pigmentations, no cutaneous tumors, and left renal artery stenosis due to a fibromatous narrowing.

The granulomatous arteritis syndromes, known as the *Takayasu type*, involving the aorta and large arteries may cause inflammatory narrowing of the renal arteries.[35–37] Most often the patients are children, young adults, or in middle age. Evidence of an inflammatory process may be suggested by a mild normochromic anemia and elevated erythrocyte sedimentation rate. The tuberculin skin test (purified protein derivative of tuberculin) is often positive.[37] In adults, however, the initial inflammatory phase may be no longer evident. The appearance of the renal artery narrowing is smooth and tapered with poststenotic dilation, distinct from the features of fibromuscular dysplasia or atherosclerotic disease. When active inflammation is evident, patients with granulomatous arteritis are treated with a course of steroids. Although the stenoses are highly fibrotic and resistant to dilation, successful balloon angioplasty has been reported.[36] Vascular surgery is also an alternative, but restenosis and thromboses tend to develop with time.[37] Management of arterial pressure by appropriate drug therapy can certainly be attempted and may be all that is needed if pressure is controlled and renal function is well maintained.

Dissections of the renal artery, most often due to trauma, are known causes of stenosis. Occlusion due to aortic dissections wending their way into the wall of the renal artery have also been reported. Solid retroperitoneal tumors may compress the renal artery; pheochromocytoma has been known to achieve this effect.

RENIN-SECRETING TUMORS

Nature's experiment proved that excess renin could be the cause of hypertension with secondary aldosteronism, not requiring stenosis of the renal arteries, when Robertson et al.[38] described the first patient with a known renin-secreting neoplasm, a hemangiopericytoma of the renal cortex. Since then, this very rare cause of renin-dependent hypertension (sometimes called *primary reninism*[39]) has occasionally been found, usually in severely hypertensive patients with the combination of high PRA levels, secondary aldosteronism reflected by hypokalemia, and normal renal arteries.[40,41] Erythrocytosis has also been reported.[42] Usually renal vein renin levels will lateralize to the side of the neoplasm, but selective intrarenal sampling from upper and lower pole veins may be needed for localization. Careful imaging of the kidney by sonography, computed tomography or magnetic resonance imaging may detect these small tumors. Abdominal aortography may not visualize the smaller renal arteries in sufficient detail for diagnosis; selective arteriography may be necessary for adequate definition. Proof that a renal mass is a renin-producing tumor, before surgery, has been provided in one case by positive immunohistochemical localization in tissue obtained by computed tomography–directed needle biopsy.[43] With the availability of ACE inhibitors, the hypertension due to renin-secreting neoplasms should be controlled by drug treatment. However, the definitive cure requires removal of the tumor, ideally by subtotal nephrectomy.

Other renin- or prorenin-producing tumors have been reported. Wilms tumor or nephroblastoma of infancy and childhood has been associated with elevated active renin levels and hypertension.[44–46] Prorenin levels may be ele-

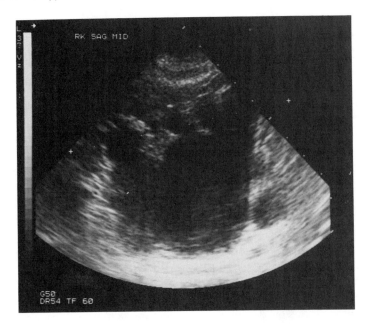

Fig. 10-7. Abdominal sonogram of a patient with unilateral hydronephrosis and atrophic kidney. The arrow indicates a rim of remaining renal cortex.

vated without hypertension and can be used as a marker for tumor recurrence with these cancers.[47]

Adult renal cancers have also been reported to be associated with renin production, probably of tumor origin, as suggested by renal vein renin studies or immunostaining of the neoplastic tissue.[48] Adult renal cancers do not produce enough renin to cause increased peripheral PRA or reversible secondary hypertension.

Nonrenal neoplasms have also been shown to form and secrete renin. Prorenin production and secretion has been found in several ovarian cancers,[49–51] a pancreatic neoplasm,[49] and even an ileal carcinoma.[52] Renin secretion has been demonstrated from the pulmonary metastasis from a rare glomangiosarcoma.[53] Usually, the ratio of prorenin to renin produced by these nonrenal tumors far exceeds the normal ratio. This suggests a reduced "processing" from prorenin to active renin, the circulating form that normally occurs in physiologic renin secretion by the kidney.[49] Morphologic studies of a prorenin-producing ovarian tumor has implied that renin production was maintained by a constitutive rather than a regulated pathway.[50]

OBSTRUCTIVE RENAL DISEASE

Hypertension has been associated with obstructive processes of the ureters and outflow tracts. The cause of the obstruction may be congenital or acquired strictures of the ureteropelvic junction, ureter, or ureterovesical junction. Flank pain, or a history of back or flank trauma should raise this possibility.[54] Such disorders are now readily detected by abdominal sonography (Fig. 10-7) or, if unavailable, by intravenous contrast urography.[55] Unilateral hydronephrosis has been associated with a high renin state with lateralization of renin secretion to the affected side.[56–58] Erythrocytosis may also be present with markedly elevated hemoglobin concentrations.[54] In these cases, relief of the urinary tract obstruction is not always associated with cure of hypertension. However, excision of the renin-secreting atrophic hydronephrotic kidney may correct the hypertension.[56,57] A nonsurgical approach that has had recent success is the use of intrarenal embolizaton[58] to cause necrosis of residual renal cortical tissue, the source of renin secretion. A medical alternative is ACE inhibition for reduction of arterial pressure by pharmacologic interruption of the activated renin-angiotensin system. Our group has successfully treated several patients of this type with ACE inhibitor monotherapy and achieved excellent long-term control of their arterial pressure.

In children, reflux nephropathy may cause dilation of the ureters and renal pelvis with scarring and distortion of renal parenchyma. In this disorder, hypertension may be caused by several mechanisms, including renal retention of extracellular fluid and loss of renal vasodilator or antihypertensive secretions without increased secretion of renin.

Urinary retention due to benign prostatic hypertrophy in elderly men may occasionally cause secondary hypertension. This possibility should be considered in men with symptoms of prostatic disease or evidence of urinary retention on physical examination (enlarged bladder) or sonography. Usually, such patients have unilateral or bilateral hydronephrosis due to high intravesical pressures resulting from chronic urinary outflow tract obstruction. Patients may not always have symptoms to suggest the degree of urinary retention, yet relief of the prostatic obstruction can reduce arterial pressure.[59]

REFERENCES

1. Brunner HR, Kirshman JD, Sealey JE, Laragh JH: Hypertension of renal origin: evidence of two different mechanisms. Science 174:1344, 1971

2. Gavras H, Brunner HR, Vaughan ED, Laragh JH: Angiotensin-sodium interaction in blood pressure maintainence of renal hypertensive rats and normotensive rats. Science 180:1369, 1973

3. Coleman TG, Granger HJ, Guyton AC: Whole body circulatory autoregulation and hypertension. Circ Res, suppl. II. 28:76, 1971

4. Guyton AC, Coleman TG, Cowley AW et al: Arterial pressure regulation: overriding dominance of the kidneys in long-term regulation and in hypertension. Am J Med 52:584, 1972

5. Guyton AC: Blood pressure control—special role of the kidneys and body fluids. Science 252:1813, 1991

6. Toto RD, Mitchell HC, Lee HC et al: Reversible renal insufficiency due to angiotensin converting enzyme inhibitors in hypertensive nephrosclerosis. Ann Intern Med 115:513, 1991

7. Muller FB, Sealey JE, Case DB et al: The captopril test for identifying renovascular disease in hypertensive patients. Am J Med 80:633, 1986

8. Postma CT, van der Steen PHM, Hoefnagels WHL et al: The captopril test in the detection of renovascular disease in hypertensive patients. Arch Intern Med 150:625, 1990

9. Frederickson ED, Wilcox CS, Bucci CM et al: A prospective evaluation of a simplified captopril test for the detection of renovascular hypertension. Arch Intern Med 150:569, 1990

10. Postma CT, Dennesen PJ, de Boo T, Thien T: First dose hypotension after captopril; can it be predicted? A study of 240 patients. J Hum Hypertens 6:205, 1992

11. Pickering TG, Sos TA, Vaughan ED Jr et al: Predictive value and changes of renin secretion in hypertensive patients with unilateral renovascular disease undergoing successful renal angioplasty. Am J Med 76:398, 1984

12. Thibonnier M, Joseph A, Sassano P et al: Improved diagnosis of unilateral renal artery lesions after captopril administration. JAMA 251:56, 1984

13. Tunny TJ, Klemm SA, Hamlet SM, Gordon RD: Diagnosis of unilateral renovascular hypertension: comparative effect of intravenous enalaprilat and oral captopril. J Urol 140:713, 1988

14. Setaro JF, Saddler MC, Chen CC et al: Simplified captopril renography in diagnosis and treatment of renal artery stenosis. Hypertension 18:289, 1991

15. Mann SJ, Pickering TG, Sos TA et al: Captopril renography in the diagnosis of renal artery stenosis: accuracy and limitations. Am J Med 90:30, 1991

16. Mann SJ, Pickering TG: Detection of renovascular hypertension: state of the art 1992. Ann Intern Med 117:845, 1992

17. Hansen KJ, Tribble RW, Reavis SW et al: Renal duplex sonography: evaluation of clinical utility. J Vasc Surg 12:227, 1990

18. Kent KC, Edelman RR, Steinman TI et al: Magnetic resonance imaging: a reliable test for the evaluation of proximal aortic atherosclerotic renal arterial stenosis. J Vasc Surg 13:311, 1991

19. Olin JW, Vidt DG, Gifford RW Jr, Novick AC: Renovascular disease in the elderly: an analysis of 50 patients. J Am Coll Cardiol 5:1232, 1985

20. Vidt DG: Geriatric hypertension of renal origin: diagnosis and management. Geriatrics 42:59, 1987

21. Rimmer JM, Gennari FJ: Atherosclerotic renovascular disease and progressive renal failure. Ann Intern Med 118:712, 1993

22. Davis BA, Crook JE, Vestal RE, Oates JA: Prevalence of renovascular hypertension in patients with grade III or IV hypertensive retinopathy. N Engl J Med 301:1273, 1979

23. Pickering TG, Herman L, Devereux RB et al: Recurrent pulmonary oedema in hypertension due to bilateral renal artery stenosis: treatment by angioplasty or surgical revascularization. Lancet 2:551, 1988

24. Dahlberg PJ, Frecentese DF, Cogbill TH: Cholesterol embolism: experience with 22 histologically proven cases. Surgery 105:737, 1989

25. Ying CY, Tifft CP, Gavras H, Chobanian AV: Renal revascularization in the azotemic hypertensive patient resistant to therapy. N Engl J Med 311:1070, 1984

26. Martin LG, Price RB, Casarella WJ et al: Percutaneous angioplasty in clinical management of renovascular hypertension: initial and long term results. Radiology 155:629, 1985

27. Sos TA, Pickering TG, Sniderman K et al: Percutaneous transluminal renal angioplasty in renovascular hypertension due to atheroma or fibromuscular dysplasia. N Engl J Med 309:274, 1983

28. Beraud J-J, Calvet B, Durand A, Mimran A: Reversal of acute renal failure following percutaneous translumenal recanalization of an atherosclerotic renal artery occlusion. J Hypertens 7:909, 1989

29. Messina LM, Zelenock GB, Yao KA, Stanley JC: Renal revascularization for recurrent pulmonary edema in patients with poorly controlled hypertension and renal insufficiency: a distinct subgroup of patients with arteriosclerotic renal artery occlusive disease. J Vasc Surg 15:73, 1992

30. Hansen KJ, Starr SM, Sands RE et al: Contemporary surgical management of renovascular disease. J Vasc Surg 16:319, 1992

31. Basta LL, Williams C, Kioschos JM, Spector AA: Regression of atherosclerotic stenosing lesions of the renal arteries and spontaneous cure of systemic hypertension through control of hyperlipidemia. Am J Med 61:420, 1976

32. Lichtlen PR, Hugenholtz PG, Rafflenbeul W et al: Retardation of angiographic progression of coronary artery disease by nifedipine. Lancet 335:1109, 1990

33. Waters D, Lesperance J, Francetich M et al: A controlled clinical trial to assess the effect of a calcium channel blocker on the progression of coronary atherosclerosis. Circulation 82:1940, 1990

34. Henry PD: Calcium antagonists for the treatment of atherosclerosis. Contemp Intern Med Nov/Dec:33, 1992

35. Lall SB, Dave V, Dash SC, Bhargava S: Peripheral and renal vein renin activity in patients with renovascular hypertension due to nonspecific aortoarteritis. Angiology 42:979, 1991

36. Sharma S, Saxena A, Talwar KK et al: Renal artery stenosis caused by nonspecific arteritis (Takayasu disease): results of treatment with percutaneous transluminal angioplasty. Am J Roentgenol 158:417, 1992

37. Milner LS, Jacobs DW, Thomson PD et al: Management of severe hypertension in childhood Takayasu's arteritis. Pediatr Nephrol 5:38, 1991

38. Robertson PW, Klidjian A, Harding LK et al: Hypertension due to a renin-secreting renal tumor. Am J Med 43:963, 1967

39. Conn JW, Cohen EL, Lucas CP et al: Primary reninism. Hypertension, hyperreninemia, and secondary aldosteronism, due to renin-producing juxtaglomerular cell tumours. Arch Intern Med 130:682, 1972

40. Baruch D, Corvol P, Alhenc-Gelas F et al: Diagnosis and treatment of renin-secreting tumors. Report of 3 cases. Hypertension 6:760, 1984

41. Corvol P, Pinet F, Galen FX et al: Seven lessons from seven renin secreting tumors. Kidney Int S38, 1988

42. Remynse LC, Begun FP, Jacobs SC, Lawson RK: Juxtaglomerular cell tumor with elevation of serum erythropoietin. J Urol 142:1560, 1989

43. Schonfeld AD, Jackson JA, Somerville SP et al: Renin-secreting juxtaglomerular tumor causing severe hypertension: diagnosis by computerized tomography-directed needle biopsy. J Urol 146:1607, 1991

44. Malone PS, Duffy PG, Ransley PG et al: Congenital mesoblastic nephroma, renin production, and hypertension. J Pediatr Surg 24:599, 1989

45. Silberman TL, Blau EB: Wilms' tumor, the hyponatremic/hypertension syndrome, and an elevated atrial natriuretic factor. Am J Pediatr Hematol Oncol 14:273, 1992

46. Khan AB, Carachi R, Leckie BJ, Lindop GB: Hypertension associated with increased renin concentrations in nephroblastoma. Arch Dis Child 66:525, 1991

47. Johnston MA, Carachi R, Lindop GB, Leckie B: Inactive renin levels in recurrent nephroblastoma. J Pediatr Surg 26:613, 1991

48. Steffens J, Bock R, Braedel HU et al: Renin-producing renal cell carcinomas—clinical and experimental investigations on a special form of renal hypertension. Urol Res 20:111, 1992

49. Atlas SA, Hesson TE, Sealey JE et al: Characterization of inactive renin ("prorenin") from renin-secreting tumors of nonrenal origin. Similarity to inactive renin from kidney and normal plasma. J Clin Invest 73:437, 1984

50. Anderson PW, Macaulay L, Do YS et al: Extrarenal renin-secreting tumors: insights into hypertension and ovarian renin production. Medicine (Baltimore) 68:257, 1989

51. Anderson PW, d'Ablaing G, Penny R et al: Secretion of prorenin by a virilizing ovarian tumor. Gynecol Oncol 45:58, 1992

52. Saito T, Fukamizu A, Okada K et al: Ectopic production of renin by ileal carcinoma. Endocrinol Jpn 36:117, 1989

53. Morris BJ, Pinet F, Michel JB et al: Renin secretion from malignant pulmonary metastatic tumour cells of vascular origin. Clin Exp Pharmacol Physiol 14:227, 1987

54. Meulman NB, Farebrother TD, Collett PV: Unilateral hydronephrosis secondary to blunt ureteral trauma, presenting with hypertension and erythrocytosis. Aust NZ J Surg 62:592, 1992

55. Cameron HA, Close CF, Yeo WW et al: Investigation of selected patients with hypertension by the rapid-sequence intravenous urogram. Lancet 339:658, 1992

56. Mizuiri S, Amagasaki Y, Hosaka H et al: Hypertension in unilateral atrophic kidney secondary to ureteropelvic junction obstruction. Nephron 61:217, 1992

57. Hirsch DJ, Jindal KK: Hypokalemic hypertension associated with unilateral hydronephrosis. Can Med Assoc J 142:1261, 1990

58. Pezzulli FA, Purnell FM, Dillon EH: Post-traumatic unilateral hydronephrosis with hypertension treated by embolization. Urology 33:70, 1989

59. Ghose RR, Harindra V: Unrecognised high pressure chronic retention of urine presenting with systemic arterial hypertension. BMJ 298:1626, 1989

60. Dondi M, Fanti S, Barozzi L et al: Evaluation by captopril renal scintigraphy and echo-Doppler flowmetry of hypertensive patients at high risk for renal artery stenosis. J Nucl Biol Med 36:309, 1992

11

OTHER FORMS OF RENAL HYPERTENSION

Many forms of chronic renal disease are associated with elevated blood pressure. The pathogenesis of hypertension in these disorders is complex and is most often due to a mixture of components, including, but not limited to, volume retention, activation of the renin-angiotensin system, abnormal sympathetic dysfunction,[1] and/or loss of endothelial cell–mediated vasodilation.[2]

Whatever the specific mechanisms operating in a given patient, it seems most likely that effective treatment of hypertension in those with chronic renal disease will be beneficial. The benefit will be derived in two ways. First, reduction of arterial pressure should diminish risk of stroke, heart failure, and (to some extent) coronary heart disease, as it does in those without renal disease. Second, some evidence shows that the progression of renal disease itself (reflected by estimates of albuminuria, proteinuria, or glomerular filtration rate) can be slowed or even reversed through antihypertensive therapy for the more common forms of chronic renal disease, particularly diabetic nephropathy and nephrosclerosis.[3–6] However, the reduction of arterial pressure by antihypertensive drug treatment does not invariably improve renal function. It has been found that the progression of renal insufficiency in black hypertensive patients is particularly resistant to antihypertensive drug therapy.[5,7]

It is a vastly oversimplified approach to consider hypertension in chronic renal disease as a single entity when there are so many specific renal diseases in which hypertension may occur. These include the various forms of genetic disorders, glomerulonephritis syndromes, interstitial renal diseases, diabetic nephropathy, and renal involvement by the collagen-vascular diseases (particularly polyarteritis nodosa, scleroderma, and systemic lupus erythematosus). Although a wealth of literature is available on the various characteristics of each of these diseases, most of them occur infrequently enough for there to be little experience with regard to the causative mechanisms for elevated arterial pressure or response to specific drug therapies. The remainder of this chapter focuses on the forms of chronic renal disease that are relatively well characterized or, in the case of diabetic nephropathy, assume much importance within the hypertensive population.

DIABETIC NEPHROPATHY

The relationship between hypertension and diabetes is not a simple one. Typically, those with insulin-dependent diabetes mellitus (IDDM; formerly, juvenile onset or type I diabetes mellitus) are normotensive for many years before the appearance of an elevated arterial pressure. When they do become hypertensive, those with IDDM ordinarily already have diabetic nephropathy as manifested by either microalbuminuria or proteinuria. Red cell membrane transport characteristics may help to predict which patients with diabetes are more likely to develop both hypertension and nephropathy on the basis of a predisposition to essential hypertension.[8,9] Past studies have demonstrated that nonselective antihypertensive drug treatment can retard the progression of diabetic nephropathy.[10–12]

Activation of the intrarenal renin-angiotensin system, as a basis for preserving intraglomerular hyperfiltration due to efferent arteriolar constriction, has been linked to diabetic nephropathy in experimental studies in insulin-deficient rats.[13] Subsequent clinical studies of angiotensin converting enzyme (ACE) inhibitors for treatment of hypertension with diabetic nephropathy show definite promise.[4,14,15] Several calcium channel entry blockers may also be effective in reducing the proteinuria of diabetic nephropathy, notably diltiazem and verapamil.[15,16] Short-term studies with the dihydropyridine calcium entry blockers suggest that these agents may be less effective in decreasing diabetic proteinuria.[16,17] However, the goals of antihypertensive therapy in diabetic patients are to reduce the risk of stroke and cardiovascular disease and to retard the progression of nephropathy. If ACE inhibition does not adequately reduce arterial pressure, the addition of a calcium entry blocker (initially diltiazem or verapamil) may be helpful. Should these calcium entry blockers be inadequate for reduction of pressure, my own preference is to try the combination of ACE inhibition with the more potent dihydropyridine agents, such as nifedipine-GITS, isradipine, or felodipine. Finally, it should not be forgotten that metabolic control of glucose metabolism by appropriate administration of insulin may also be necessary for optimal prevention of renal insufficiency.[18] Strict metabolic control by keeping plasma glucose and amino acids closer to the normal range may minimize the glomerular hyperperfusion and renal enlargement that mark the early phase of diabetic nephropathy.

The relationship between diabetic renal disease and hypertension in adult populations with non-IDDM (NIDDM) is more complex. Approximately 6 to 7 percent of those with essential hypertension have NIDDM.[19,20] Many of these patients have microalbuminuria or mild proteinuria (less than 600 mg/24 hr) and modest reductions in creatinine clearance. There is no doubt that these patients are at risk of progression of renal disease, particularly if they are black.[5,7] Studies are insufficient to determine the degree to which antihypertensive therapy, per se, or any specific agent may prevent progression of renal insufficiency in such patients. There is, however, concern that thiazide diuretic agents, in particular, may not be beneficial due to their potential for impairing glucose tolerance.[21] β-Blockers are suspect as well, but this is offset by their value in preventing ischemic heart disease.[22–24]

A recent report indicates that ACE inhibition can reduce microalbuminuria and prevent an increase in serum creatinine in normotensive adult patients with NIDDM.[6] These results suggest that hypertensive persons with NIDDM and any degree of albuminuria or proteinuria may benefit from ACE inhibition, as well. However, the dominant risk in such patients is of stroke and coronary heart disease. Effective and safe reduction of arterial pressure using other appropriate agents (calcium channel entry blockers and β-receptor blockers) is often necessary.

FAMILIAL POLYCYSTIC RENAL DISEASE

The best-characterized form of congenital inherited chronic renal disease associated with hypertension is familial polycystic renal disease. In patients with polycystic kidneys, bilateral flank masses are often palpated. The condition is easily detected or confirmed by sonography (Fig. 11-1). Some families with this syndrome display specific DNA genetic markers that are associated with an earlier onset of hypertension and renal insufficiency compared with those families without this trait.[25] In familial polycystic renal disease, the renin-angiotensin system is inappropriately activated; treatment with ACE inhibitors may be quite effective without impairment of renal function.[26] It is advisable to screen family members of patients with polycystic renal disease to detect early hypertension, renal functional impairment, and silent urinary tract infection.[27]

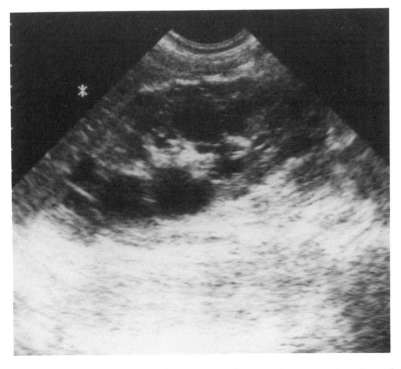

Fig. 11-1. Abdominal sonogram of a 35-year-old man with hypertension due to familial polycystic kidneys. His mother and several siblings are affected. Renal function at this time is normal. Blood pressure was normalized on an ACE inhibitor as monotherapy.

TYPE II PSEUDOHYPOALDOSTERONISM

Renal tubular disorders may be linked to elevated arterial pressure. One of the more recently characterized syndromes is type II pseudohypoaldosteronism. Ordinarily, low aldosterone secretion is associated with hypotension and salt wasting, as occurs in adrenal insufficiency. Type I pseudoaldosteronism—salt wasting, low blood pressure, and elevated plasma renin and aldosterone levels—have been attributed to an inherited resistance to the action of mineralocorticoids. However, in type II pseudoaldosteronism (a rare disorder), elevated blood pressure is associated with hyperkalemia, low plasma renin levels, and normal aldosterone production. Studies of renal tubular function in affected patients have revealed excessive reabsorption of sodium and chloride ion in the distal renal tubule (suggesting an overactive reabsorptive chloride pump). The resultant volume retention leads to compensatory suppression of renin secretion and angiotensin II formation with decreased aldosterone secretion.[28] Hyperkalemia ensues and may independently maintain aldosterone production at near-normal levels. Diuretics that prevent sodium and chloride reabsorption at distal renal tubular sites correct the hyperkalemia and reduce arterial pressure.

COLLAGEN-VASCULAR DISEASES

Systemic arterial hypertension is clearly associated with several of the collagen diseases, most notably systemic lupus erythematosus, polyarteritis nodosa and other vasculitis syndromes, and scleroderma. The pathogenesis of elevated arterial pressure, however, differs among these disorders.

Systemic Lupus Erythematosus

In systemic lupus erythematosus, hypertension tends to occur late in the course of the disease after the development of lupus nephritis and often following the institution of steroid therapy. In such patients, the appearance of hypertension worsens the prognosis, increasing the risk of cardiovascular morbidity and progression to renal failure.[29–32] Smoking also adds to the risk of renal progression.[29] It is likely that the elevated pressure in patients with lupus nephritis is due to a combination of several factors. Volume retention due to impaired glomerular filtration, activation of the renin system by intrarenal vasculitis,[32] or increased systemic vascular resistance due to widespread vascular lesions may all participate.

ACE inhibition may have some value for reduction of proteinuria in patients with lupus nephritis[33] and (based on experimental studies) for preventing steroid-induced hypertension.[34–36] The comparative values of different antihypertensive agents have not been established in treating hypertension in systemic lupus erythematosus with or without nephritis. Nonetheless, aggressive reduction of arterial pressure should be attempted to reduce overall risk. Our experience suggests that ACE inhibitors and calcium entry blockers can be effective. Centrally acting agents (methyldopa, reserpine, and the α_2-agonists) should be avoided because their adverse effects of sedation may be confused with cerebral vasculitis in unstable patients.

Polyarteritis and Vasculitis Syndromes

Hypertension may occur as a progressive or fulminant disorder in the vasculitis syndromes—polyarteritis nodosa, the Churg-Strauss variant of small vessel arteritis, or Wegener's granulomatosis.[37–39] The elevation in arterial pressure is due to renal ischemia as a result of inflammatory stenosis, which may involve the main renal arteries[40] or small branches. As a consequence, impaired perfusion activates the renin-angiotensin system as it does in other forms of renal artery stenosis.[41] Renal arteriography may be helpful as a diagnostic measure in polyarteritis nodosa, since the appearance of intrarenal visceral artery aneurisms is characteristic.[42] On occasion, renal infarctions may be observed distal to totally occluded arteries. Given that the pathogenesis of the hypertension is due to an activated renin system, antihypertensive therapy with ACE inhibitors is indicated, along with the appropriate anti-inflammatory or immunosuppressive measures.

Scleroderma

There are, to me, two relationships between systemic arterial hypertension and scleroderma. Systemic scleroderma, as a chronic disorder of the skin and intestinal tract, often affects older patients in whom the age-related increase in arterial pressure of essential hypertension often occurs with the frequency expected in aging populations. In this situation, the significance of an elevated arterial pressure is no different from that in anyone else of the same age. Antihypertensive drug therapy is justified, and, if Raynaud syndrome is present, the vasodilator calcium channel entry blockers may be useful.

Much more ominous is the occasional appearance of severe hypertension with renal insufficiency, often in younger patients with systemic scleroderma or progressive systemic sclerosis, now called *scleroderma renal crisis*.[43,44] In this unique complication of scleroderma, the degree of skin or gastrointestinal manifestations may be mild or even barely symptomatic. An abrupt increase in arterial pressure occurs that may be sufficient to cause hypertensive encephalopathy and/or pulmonary congestion. There is early evidence of a nephropathy manifested by proteinuria, hematuria, and increasing serum urea nitrogen and creatinine levels. Microangiopathic anemia may be present, and thrombocytopenia is not unusual. Plasma renin activity is elevated, a clue to renal ischemia as a consequence of vascular pathology of intrarenal arteries with evidence of fibrinoid degeneration and necrosis of afferent arterioles. Secondary aldosteronism with hypokalemia may be present, an expected consequence of the activated renin-angiotensin system. In other words, this syndrome is a variation of malignant hypertension and shares its pathogenesis.

The advent of the ACE inhibitors, for specific interruption of the renin-angiotensin system in the treatment of hypertension, has had major beneficial effects on the treatment and outcome of scleroderma renal crisis. Prior to the availability of ACE inhibitors, most patients progressed rapidly to renal failure with uncontrollable hypertension. Bilateral nephrectomy reduced arterial pressure to normal, but then required renal replacement therapy. In the past decade, use of the ACE inhibitors to treat scleroderma renal crisis has often led to control of arterial pressure and improvement, even normalization, of renal function in long-term follow-up.[45] These observations indicate the need for starting ACE inhibitor therapy as soon as hypertensive scleroderma renal crisis is recognized. If renal function worsens on ACE inhibitor therapy, alternate diagnoses should be considered; bilateral renal artery stenosis has been recorded as occurring in a patient with scleroderma.[46] Some patients with scleroderma renal crisis will progress to renal failure and require dialysis; there is the chance, however, that they may recover renal function and be able to discontinue dialysis. Complete remission is possible for occasional patients who may become normotensive and not require continuous drug treatment. I have observed such a patient who was able to undergo a successful pregnancy years after ACE inhibitor therapy for scleroderma renal crisis was discontinued.[47]

About 10 percent of those with scleroderma renal crisis develop renal failure without being significantly hypertensive, even though they have other features of severe microvascular disease, microangiopathic anemia, and thrombocytopenia.[48] At this time, the lack of hypertension in these individuals has not been adequately explained.

RENAL INFARCTION AND RENAL ARTERY EMBOLISM

An increase in pressure to hypertensive levels or further elevation of pressure in an established hypertensive patient may occur with sudden segmental or total renal ischemia due to thrombotic or embolic occlusion of the main renal artery or its branches. When sufficient ischemia is present for renal infarction to occur, flank pain and hematuria are often present, sometimes with fever and leukocytosis, suggesting either renal calculi or infection. The serum lactate dehydrogenase may be substantially elevated; high concentrations of the enzyme detected in the urine will confirm a suspected diagnosis. Renal infarcts are visualized readily by computed tomography. Magnetic resonance imaging may also demonstrate renal infarction.[49] Renal arteriography visualizes the occluded vessels.

Renal artery thrombosis is often due to atherosclerotic renal artery stenosis. However, any cause of reduced blood flow (sickle cell anemia, polycythemia, hypotension) or renal artery narrowing (fibromuscular dysplasia, arteritis, or distortion [aneurysm]) may participate in thrombus formation. Renal artery thrombosis and renal infarction have been associated with oral contraceptive use.

Occlusive emboli to renal arteries may cause renal ischemia or infarction and hypertension (Table 11-1). Such events may occur in the course of infective endocarditis, as a result of intracardiac thrombi (as in patients with chronic atrial fibrillation or the dilated chambers of a cardiomyopathy) or the sterile endocarditis syndromes (systemic lupus erythematosus, disseminated cancer). Cholesterol emboli may be the result of ulcerating suprarenal artery aortic atherosclerosis or the consequence of arteriography. The syndrome of cholesterol embolization should be considered when renal failure, purpura of the lower extremities, and a vasculitis-like picture (fever, eosinophilic leukocytosis) occur following any form of arteriography.[50] Cholesterol embolism has been reported during anticoagulant use and after thrombolytic therapy for acute coronary thrombosis.[51,52]

Where there is total renal artery occlusion causing oliguric or anuric renal insufficiency, aggressive intervention by vascular surgery may reverse renal failure, even after days or weeks of support by dialysis. For segmental renal infarctions, hypertension may be transient and renal function is usually well preserved. Hence medical management, through use of antihypertensive agents (especially ACE inhibitors when elevated renin levels are found), is justified.[53] Anticoagulation may be considered when there are no contraindications. Thrombolytic therapy, via selective intrarenal arterial injections of either urokinase or streptokinase, has been reported to improve renal perfusion and (in one of four cases) reverse acute renal failure.[54]

HYPERTENSION DUE TO SUBCAPSULAR PERIRENAL HEMATOMA

Hypertension appearing after blunt trauma to the flank or back may be due to a subcapsular hematoma of the kidney compressing the renal cortex, leading to renin secretion and angiotensin II–dependent hypertension. This has been referred to in the older literature as the *Page kidney* due to its similarity to an experimental model of hypertension, described by Page and colleagues, caused by wrapping one kidney with silk or cellophane to produce unilateral perinephritis. It is not unusual for elevated blood pressure to be discovered

Table 11-1. Sources of Renal Emboli

Cardiac valvular vegetations	Infective endocarditis, systemic lupus erythematosus (Libman-Sachs endocarditis), marantic endocarditis (disseminated cancer)
Intracardiac thrombi	Left atrial dilation due to chronic atrial fibrillation, mitral valve disease; left ventricle: ventricular aneurism, dilated cardiomyopathy
Aortic aneurism or atherosclerosis	Emboli from ulcerating lesion; cholesterol emboli after arteriography, vascular surgery, or anticoagulant or thrombolytic therapy

long after the traumatic effect, allowing time for calcification of the hematoma and considerable scarring and distortion of the underlying renal cortex. An example of a perirenal hematoma found on computed tomographic scan is shown in Figure 11-2.

The opposite kidney is usually normal unless long-standing hypertension has led to nephrosclerosis. In my experience, blood pressure is often well controlled in these patients with an ACE inhibitor, as expected for a renin-dependent form of hypertension. If the hematoma is discovered soon after trauma, aspiration might be attempted. There is too little information to know whether hypertension can be prevented by a more aggressive surgical approach. Nephrectomy is not advised in these patients, as renal function does continue in the kidneys.

POST-LITHOTRIPSY HYPERTENSION

The appearance of new hypertension following extracorporeal lithotripsy for treatment of renal calculi has been reported. A case report has documented renin-dependent hypertension due to an intrarenal hematoma.[55] However, such complications are rare. The possibility of either intrarenal hematoma or fibrosis as a consequence of ultrasonic renal injury has prompted scrutiny of blood pressure patterns in those treated with renal lithotripsy.[56] Several large series suggest that the appearance of new hypertension after lithotripsy is no different from that expected for an age-matched comparison group.[57,58]

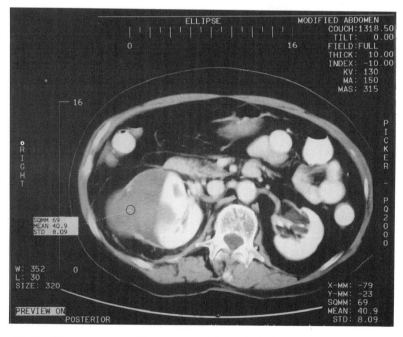

Fig. 11-2. Obvious perirenal hematoma of the right kidney, detected several months after an auto accident with blunt trauma to the right flank.

However, if hypertension does appear after lithotripsy, renal injury should be suspected. Even if a renal hematoma is later found, the primary management will be antihypertensive therapy. Measurement of plasma renin activity and a trial of ACE inhibitor therapy might unmask the renin-angiotensin–dependent mechanism expected in these patients.

HYPERTENSION IN ADVANCED OR END-STAGE RENAL DISEASE

All too many hypertensive patients are still detected at an advanced stage of renal insufficiency (i.e., when the creatinine clearance is less than 30 percent of normal). In the absence of characteristics of a reversible or specific form of renal pathology, these patients comprise a heterogeneous population of those who may have had chronic glomerulonephritis or interstitial nephropathies intermixed with nephrosclerosis, related to prior hypertension. As the serum creatinine increases, these patients will acquire the other characteristics of chronic renal insufficiency, including anemia, hypocalcemia, acidosis, and a tendency to hyperkalemia. Reduction of arterial pressure remains necessary for these patients, as the risk of stroke and ischemic heart disease persist. However, it is less certain that progression of renal failure can be diminished by antihypertensive therapy at this stage.

Treatment of hypertensive patients with advanced renal disease should take into account that arterial disease and the increased likelihood of cardiac ischemia may be present due to chronic anemia, left ventricular hypertrophy, and dilation. Judicious use of β-receptor blockers and coronary vasodilating calcium channel entry blockers should be considered. For those with a tendency to retain fluid, a loop active diuretic such as furosemide may be useful also. The role of ACE inhibitors in patients with advanced renal insufficiency is unclear. Many have low plasma renin activity. Mild hyperkalemia may be present, implying that a risk of a further increase in serum potassium is present, should ACE inhibition decrease aldosterone secretion. Since recent studies indicate that sympathetic neuron activity may be increased in these patients,[1] α-receptor blockers may be useful. My own preference, however, is to avoid centrally acting antiadrenergic agents (methyldopa, clonidine, reserpine) because of their lesser performance in quality of life studies.[59,60]

Once patients require dialysis for supplemental support of renal function, control of their hypertension may improve markedly, principally due to the volume-unloading effects of either hemodialysis or peritoneal dialysis.[61] The need for antihypertensive medications may diminish or cease altogether. In recent years, the use of erythropoietin for treatment of the anemia of chronic renal failure has become widespread. A tendency for increased arterial pressure during erythropoietin therapy has been noted.[62] However, the hypertensive risk of gradual increases in hematocrit to about 30 percent seems to be minimal.[63,64] Except for diuretic agents, for which there is no longer a rationale for use, there is no contraindication for the use of any antihypertensive agent (even ACE inhibitors) for optimal management of arterial pressure of patients on dialysis.

REFERENCES

1. Converse RL Jr, Jacobsen TN, Toto RD et al: Sympathetic overactivity in patients with chronic renal failure. N Engl J Med 327:1912, 1992

2. Vallance P, Leone A, Calver A et al: Accumulation of an endogenous inhibitor of nitric oxide synthesis in chronic renal failure. Lancet 339:572, 1992

3. Keane WF, Anderson S, Aurell M et al: Angiotensin converting enzyme inhibitors and progressive renal insufficiency. Ann Intern Med 111:503, 1990

4. Kasiske BL, Kalil RSN, Ma JZ et al: Effect of antihypertensive therapy on the kidney in patients with diabetes: a meta-regression analysis. Ann Intern Med 118:129, 1993

5. Walker GW, Neaton JD, Cutler JA et al: Renal function change in hypertensive members of the Multiple Risk Factor Intervention Trial: racial and treatment effects. JAMA 268:3085, 1992

6. Ravid M, Savin H, Jutrin I et al: Long-term stabilizing effect of angiotensin-converting enzyme inhibition on plasma creatinine and on proteinuria in normtensive type II diabetic patients. Ann Intern Med 118:577, 1993

7. Rostand SG, Brown G, Kirk KA et al: Renal insufficiency in treated essential hypertension. N Engl J Med 320:684, 1989

8. Krowlewski AS, Canessa M, Warram JH et al: Predisposition to hypertension and susceptibility to renal disease in insulin-dependent diabetes mellitus. N Engl J Med 318:140, 1988

9. Mangili R, Bending JJ, Scott G et al: Increased sodium-lithium countertransport activity in red cells of patients with insulin-dependent diabetes and nephropathy. N Engl J Med 318:146, 1988

10. Parving H-H, Andersen AR, Smidt et al: Aggressive antihypertensive treatment reduces rate of decline in kidney function in diabetic nephropathy. Lancet 1:1175, 1983

11. Mogensen CE: Long-term antihypertensive treatment inhibits progression of diabetic nephropathy. BMJ 285:285, 1982

12. Parving HH, Andersen AR, Smidt UM: Effect of antihypertensive treatment on kidney function in diabetic nephropathy. BMJ 294:1443, 1987

13. Zatz R, Dunn R, Meyer T et al: Prevention of diabetic glomerulonephropathy by pharmacological amelioration of glomerular capillary hypertension. J Clin Invest 77:1925, 1986

14. Bjorcks S, Nyberg G, Mulec H et al: Beneficial effects of ACE inhibition on renal function in patients with diabetic nephropathy. BMJ 293:471, 1986

15. Bakris GL: Effects of diltiazem or lisinopril on massive proteinuria associated with diabetes mellitus. Ann Intern Med 112:701, 1990

16. Demarie BK, Bakris GL: Effects of different calcium antagonists on proteinuria associated with diabetes mellitus. Ann Intern Med 113:987, 1991

17. Bakris GL: Angiotensin-converting enzyme inhibitors and progression of diabetic nephropathy. Ann Intern Med 118:643, 1993

18. Tuttle KR, Bruton JL, Perusek MC et al: Effect of strict glycemic control on renal hemodynamic response to amino acids and renal enlargement in insulin-dependent diabetes mellitus. N Engl J Med 324:1626, 1991

19. Hypertension Detection and Follow-up Program Cooperative Group: Five-year findings of the Hypertension Detection and Follow-up Program. I. Reduction in mortality of persons with high blood pressure, including mild hypertension. JAMA 242:2562, 1979

20. Tuck ML, Bravo EL, Krakoff LR, et al: Modern Approach to the Treatment of Hypertension (MATH) Study Group: endocrine and renal effects of nifedipine gastrointestinal therapeutic system in patients with essential hypertension: results of a multicenter trial. Am J Hypertens 3:333S, 1991

21. Pandit MK, Burke J, Gustafson AB et al: Drug-induced disorders of glucose tolerance. Ann Intern Med 118:529, 1993

22. Wikstrand J, Warnold I, Olsson G et al: Primary prevention with metoprolol in patients with hypertension: mortality results from the MAPHY study. JAMA 259:1976, 1988

23. Goldman L, Sia STB, Cook EF et al: Costs and effectiveness of routine therapy with long-term beta-adrenergic antagonists after acute myocardial infarction. N Engl J Med 319:152, 1988

24. Psaty BM, Koepsell TD, LoGerfo JP et al: Beta-blockers and primary prevention of coronary heart disease in patients with hypertension. JAMA 261:2087, 1989

25. Parfrey PS, Bear JC, Morgan J et al: The diagnosis and prognosis of autosomal dominant polycystic kidney disease. N Engl J Med 323:1085, 1990

26. Chapman AB, Johnson A, Gabow PA, Schrier RW: The renin-angiotensin-aldosterone system and autosomal dominant polycystic kidney disease. N Engl J Med 323:1091, 1990

27. Ravine D, Walker RG, Gibson RN et al: Treatable complications in undiagnosed cases of autosomal dominant polycystic kidney disease. Lancet 337:127, 1991

28. Take C, Ikeda K, Kurasawa T, Kurokawa K: Increased chloride reabsorption as an inherited renal tubular defect in familial type II pseudohypoaldosteronism. N Engl J Med 324:472, 1991

29. Ward MM, Studenski S: Clinical prognostic factors in lupus nephritis. The importance of hypertension and smoking. Arch Intern Med 152:2082, 1992

30. Lupus nephritis: prognostic factors and probability of maintaining life-supporting renal function 10 years after the diagnosis. Gruppo Italiano per lo Studio della Nefrite Lupica (GISNEL). Am J Kidney Dis 19:473, 1992

31. Esdaile JM, Federgreen W, Quintal H et al: Predictors of one year outcome in lupus nephritis: the importance of renal biopsy [see comments]. Q J Med 81:907, 1991

32. Banfi G, Bertani T, Boeri V et al: Renal vascular lesions as a marker of poor prognosis in patients with lupus nephritis. Gruppo Italiano per lo Studio della Nefrite Lupica (GISNEL). Am J Kidney Dis 18:240, 1991

33. Shapira Y, Mor F, Friedler A et al: Antiproteinuric effect of captopril in a patient with lupus nephritis and intractable nephrotic syndrome. Ann Rheum Dis 49:725, 1990

34. Kohlman O Jr, Ribeiro AB, Marson O et al: Methylprednisolone-induced hypertension: role for the autonomic and renin-angiotensin system. Hypertension, suppl. II. 3:107, 1981

35. Elijovich F, Krakoff LR: Effect of converting enzyme inhibition on glucocorticoid hypertension in the rat. Am J Physiol 238:H844, 1980

36. Garcia DL, Rennke HG, Brenner BM, Anderson S: Chronic glucocorticoid therapy amplifies glomerular injury in rats with renal ablation. J Clin Invest 80:867, 1987

37. Hoffman GS, Kerr GS, Leavitt RY et al: Wegener granulomatosis: an analysis of 158 patients. Ann Intern Med 116:488, 1992

38. O'Meara Y, Green A, Carmody M et al: Systemic vasculitis with renal involvement—a review. Ir J Med Sci 158:300, 1989

39. Guillevin L, Le Thi Huong Du, Godeau P et al: Clinical findings and prognosis of polyarteritis nodosa and Churg-Strauss angiitis: a study in 165 patients. Br J Rheumatol 27:258, 1988

40. Hoover LA, Hall Craggs M, Dagher FJ: Polyarteritis nodosa involving only the main renal arteries. Am J Kidney Dis 11:66, 1988

41. Graham PC, Lindop GB: The renin-secreting cell in polyarteritis—an immunocytochemical study. Histopathology 16:339, 1990

42. Hekali P, Kajander H, Pajari R et al: Diagnostic significance of angiographically observed visceral aneurysms with regard to polyarteritis nodosa. Acta Radiol 32:143, 1991

43. Traub YM, Shapiro AP, Rodnan GP et al: Hypertension and renal failure (scleroderma renal crisis) in progressive systemic sclerosis. Review of a 25-year experience with 68 cases. Medicine 62:335, 1983

44. Steen VD, Medsger TA Jr, Osial TA Jr et al: Factors predicting development of renal involvement in progressive systemic sclerosis. Am J Med 76:779, 1984

45. Steen VD, Costantino JP, Shapiro AP et al: Outcome of renal crisis in systemic sclerosis: relation to availability of angiotensin converting enzyme (ACE) inhibitors [see comments]. Ann Intern Med 113:352, 1990

46. Haluszka O, Rabetoy GM, Mosley CA, Duke MS: Bilateral renal artery stenosis: presenting as a case of scleroderma renal crisis. Clin Nephrol 32:262, 1989

47. Spiera H, Krakoff L, Fishbane-Mayer J: Successful pregnancy after scleroderma hypertensive renal crisis. J Rheumatol 16:1597, 1989

48. Helfrich DJ, Banner B, Steen VD, Medsger TA Jr: Normotensive renal failure in systemic sclerosis. Arthritis Rheum 32:1128, 1989

49. Kim SH, Park JH, Han JK et al: Infarction of the kidney: role of contrast enhanced MRI. J Comput Assist Tomogr 16:924, 1992

50. Dahlberg PJ, Frecentese DF, Cogbill TH: Cholesterol embolism: experience with 22 histologically proven cases. Surgery 105:737, 1989

51. Gupta BK, Spinowitz BS, Charytan C, Wahl SJ: Cholesterol crystal embolization-associated renal failure after therapy with recombinant tissue-type plasminogen activator. Am J Kidney Dis 21:659, 1993

52. Queen M, Biem HJ, Moe GW, Sugar L: Development of cholesterol embolization syndrome after intravenous streptokinase for acute myocardial infarction. Am J Cardiol 65:1042, 1990

53. Lessman RK, Johnson SF, Coburn JW, Kaufman JM: Renal artery embolism: clinical features and long-term follow-up of 17 cases. Ann Intern Med 89:477, 1978

54. Salam TA, Lumsden AB, Martin LG: Local infusion of fibrinolytic agents for acute renal artery thromboembolism: report of ten cases. Ann Vasc Surg 7:21, 1993

55. Lemann J Jr, Taylor AJ, Collier BD, Lipchik EO: Kidney hematoma due to extracorporeal shock wave lithotripsy causing transient renin mediated hypertension. J Urol 145:1238, 1991

56. Smith LH, Drach G, Hall P et al: High Blood Pressure Education Program (NHBPEP) review paper on complications of shock wave lithotripsy for urinary calculi. Am J Med 91:635, 1991

57. Yokoyama M, Shoji F, Yanagizawa R et al: Blood pressure changes following extracorporeal shock wave lithotripsy for urolithiasis. J Urol 147:553, 1992

58. Marberger M, Stackl W, Hruby W et al: Late sequelae of ultrasonic lithotripsy of renal calculi blood pressure changes following extracorporeal shock wave lithotripsy and other forms of treatment for nephrolithiasis. JAMA 263:1789, 1990

59. Croog SH, Levine S, Testa MA et al: The effects of antihypertensive therapy on the quality of life. N Engl J Med 314:1657, 1986

60. Materson BJ, Reda DJ, Cushman WC et al: Single-drug therapy for hypertension in men: a comparision of six antihypertensive agents with placebo. N Engl J Med 328:914, 1993

61. Saldanha LF, Weiler EW, Gonick HC: Effect of continuous ambulatory peritoneal dialysis on blood pressure control. Am J Kidney Dis 21:184, 1993

62. Eschbach JW, Egrie JC, Downing MR et al: Correction of the anemia of end-stage renal disease with recombinant human erythropoietin: results of a combined phase I and phase II clinical trial. N Engl J Med 316:73, 1987

63. Ono K, Hisasue Y: The rate of increase in hematocrit, humoral vasoactive substances and blood pressure changes in hemodialysis patients treated with recombinant human erythropoietin or blood transfusion. Clin Nephrol 37:23, 1992

64. Macia M, Laraudiogoitia E, Hortal L et al: Effect of recombinant human erythropoietin treatment on hemodynamic parameters in continuous ambulatory peritoneal dialysis and hemodialysis patients. Am J Nephrol 12:207, 1992

12

OTHER FORMS OF SECONDARY HYPERTENSION

COARCTATION OF THE AORTA

Hypertension due to aortic coarctation is usually detected in infancy or childhood, but occasionally escapes diagnosis until later in life. Late detection worsens the prognosis and increases risk of left ventricular enlargement, congestive heart failure, aortic rupture, cerebral hemorrhage, and endocarditis. Coarctation may be associated with anomalies of the aortic valve (most often bicuspid valve), the Turner syndrome, and aneurysms of the circle of Willis.[1] Congenital coarctation is usually suspected on the basis of a cardiac murmur, heard best in the back (interscapular area), associated with reduced or absent femoral pulses. Confirming evidence is provided by the chest radiograph (rib notching, the 3 sign of dilated left subclavian artery with poststenotic dilation of the descending aorta beyond the narrowed coarcted segment) (Fig. 12-1). Magnetic resonance imaging is useful for defining the precise location of aortic narrowing (Fig. 12-2). In many instances contrast aortography may be necessary for definitive anatomic characterization of the coarctation and the size and location of the collateral circulation (Fig. 12-3). In congenital coarctation, increased flow throughout the internal mammary system and intercostal arteries may be substantial (and accounts for rib notching on the chest radiograph).

Coarctation causes arterial hypertension of the upper body, due to a direct mechanical effect of a reduced aortic volume during cardiac systole. Impairment of baroreflexes and activation of the renin-angiotensin system may also participate in maintaining the elevated pressure.[2]

Coarctation of the descending aorta may occur within the chest or abdomen and may mimic bilateral renal artery stenosis. Occasionally granulomatous/inflammatory disease of the aorta (Takayasu's disease) may cause acquired coarctation in children, adolescents, or young adults.[3] Rib notching may be absent on chest radiograph in acquired coarctation, perhaps because the intercostal system has already developed.

Definitive therapy of coarctation of the aorta is vascular surgery with relief of the pressure gradient. Postoperative persistence or recurrence of the hypertension may occur and appears to be partly related to the duration of

147

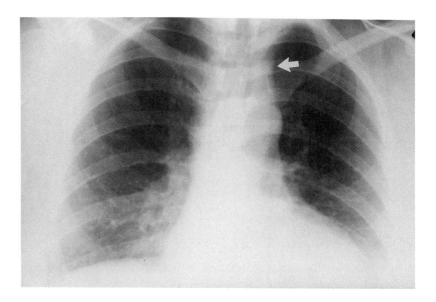

Fig. 12-1. Chest radiograph of a 30-year-old woman with recently discovered hypertension and reduced femoral artery pulses. Dilated left subclavian artery *(arrow)* is indicated. See Figures 12-2 and 12-3 for additional imaging.

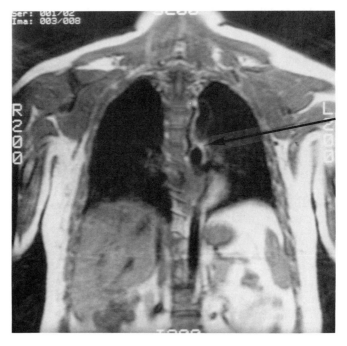

Fig. 12-2. Magnetic resonance imaging of coarctation of the descending thoracic aorta *(arrow)* found in the patient described in Figure 12-1.

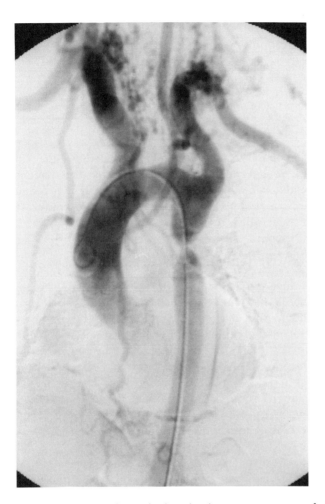

Fig. 12-3. Contrast aortography with digital subtraction imaging of the patient whose magnetic resonance image appears in Figure 12-2. Note the correspondence between the dilated left subclavian artery on the aortogram, magnetic resonance image, and chest radiograph.

hypertension before surgery. In some series, postcoarctation hypertension may be associated with excessive spasm of mesenteric arteries, perhaps because of hyperresponsiveness to the increased arterial pressure. Increased renin has been documented, as has increased arterial pressure response to exercise. For patients in whom persistent hypertension is present after successful surgical repair, long-term antihypertensive drug treatment may be necessary. Balloon angioplasty has been performed for treatment of coarctation of the aorta. It has been suggested that this procedure is less likely than surgery to cause paradoxical hypertension after repair.[4] Balloon aortoplasty does incur the risk of aortic rupture.[5] Series are too small and limited for overall therapeutic appraisal of this technique.

Table 12-1. Causes of Renal Transplant Hypertension

Glucocorticoid excess
Cyclosporine treatment
Renal graft artery stenosis
Chronic graft rejection
Recurrence of primary renal disease

Once coarctation of the aorta is found and treated by either surgery or balloon aortoplasty, long-term follow up is necessary for these patients. The often present bicuspid aortic valve and residual aortic pathology require antibiotic prophylaxis for dental or potentially contaminated procedures. Hypertension may persist or recur, which then requires pharmacologic therapy.

ORAL CONTRACEPTIVE HYPERTENSION

Oral contraceptive pills contain mixtures of synthetic estrogens and progestational agents that may cause small increases in blood pressure within the normal range and, occasionally, mild, moderate, or severe hypertension. The estrogenic component uniformly raises plasma angiotensinogen, the precursor of angiotensin I.[6] This action, however, does not invariably cause hypertension. Plasma renin activity may be increased or normal. It has been suggested that high blood pressure may be due to a failure of normal suppression of renin secretion that should follow the increase in angiotensinogen. Some degree of salt and water retention may also be caused by the oral contraceptives and elicit hypertension in those predisposed to "salt-sensitive" hypertension.

Oral contraceptive pill–induced hypertension is usually reversed within several months of the patient not taking the pill. Hypertension persisting for more than 6 months after cessation of the pill should be re-evaluated for the possibility of another diagnosis. Thrombotic occlusion of a renal artery causing renal infarction with persistent hypertension has been reported. Chronic renal disease and other disorders causing hypertension may be present.

Initial treatment of oral contraceptive hypertension is discontinuation of the pill. Should hypertension persist without a detectable cause, conventional antihypertensive therapy is necessary. At present, no studies can be cited to provide a rationale for choosing a specific antihypertensive agent apart from the speculation that the renin system may be activated in some patients. This observation justifies a trial of angiotensin converting enzyme (ACE) inhibition as monotherapy. If the blood pressure is quickly normalized on drug treatment, later withdrawal of medication may be followed by a period of normal blood pressure.

It is my impression that the incidence of oral contraceptive pill hypertension has decreased substantially since the 1970s. If so, the reduction in incidence may be due to (1) reduced estrogen content of currently available preparations, (2) better screening of those with early hypertension or borderline high pressures to exclude them from use of oral contraceptives, and

(3) earlier detection of minimal elevations in pressure by physicians with a change to alternate forms of contraception.

PREGNANCY-INDUCED HYPERTENSION

A rise in arterial pressure to at least 140 mmHg systolic pressure or at least 90 mmHg diastolic pressure (or both) during pregnancy defines *pregnancy-induced hypertension*. When high blood pressure is present before pregnancy, the term used in obstetric literature is *chronic hypertension*. The increase in pressure during pregnancy may or may not be associated with the syndromes of pre-eclampsia or toxemia. The latter syndromes are considered when edema, increased uric acid, and proteinuria appear. Pregnancy-induced hypertension has recently been associated with hypercalciuria.[7] Further considerations in dealing with hypertension in pregnant women are given in Chapter 21.

HYPERTENSION AFTER TRANSPLANTATION AND CYCLOSPORINE HYPERTENSION

The appearance of new hypertension or worsening of pre-existing hypertension following transplantation of the kidney, heart, or liver is well documented. This has become a major management problem complicating the post-transplant period. The immunosuppressive drugs glucocorticoids and cyclosporine are specifically implicated in the pathogenesis of post-transplant hypertension. Manifestations of glucocorticoid excess have already been presented in Chapter 9. Characteristics of cyclosporine hypertension, however, now extend beyond organ transplantation, as this immunosuppressive agent is being studied in a variety of diseases in which cellular autoimmunity is suspected (see the section, *Cyclosporine Hypertension in Nontransplant Diseases*).

Renal Transplantation

In patients with chronic renal disease, high blood pressure is often present long before transplantation is undertaken. Increased arterial pressure often persists after renal transplantation,[8] despite the hypothesis (and occasional observation) that a kidney from a nonhypertensive subject should normalize blood pressure of a hypertensive subject.[9] Nonetheless, renal graft rejection, immunosuppressive therapy with glucocorticoids or cyclosporine (or both), recurrence of the prior renal disease (on an immunologic basis), or stenosis of the artery supplying the transplanted organ are all implicated in the pathogenesis of renal transplant hypertension (Table 12-1).

It has been reported that average blood pressure in renal transplant patients is related to the dose of glucocorticoid (usually prednisone) needed for immunosuppression.[8] Patients with higher steroid requirements tend to have higher plasma renin activity (partly due to increased renin substrate (angiotensinogen) concentrations. Thus, the level of plasma renin cannot be used to detect graft renal artery stenosis. As with bilateral renal artery stenosis, ACE inhibitor therapy of patients with graft renal artery stenosis may cause reduced glomerular filtration and a rapid increase in serum urea nitrogen and creatinine.[10] The captopril renal scan or Doppler flow measurements of the graft renal artery may be helpful, but, when suspected, there is no substitute for graft renal arteriography for certain diagnosis of stenosis. Balloon angioplasty has been used successfully to dilate graft arteries; vascular surgery may, on occasion, be necessary to restore graft renal blood flow to normal.

A feature of glucocorticoid hypertension is the loss of normal diurnal variation in pressure, such that night or sleep pressures are relatively increased.[11] With the advent of cyclosporine, higher doses of glucocorticoids are used less often for management of renal transplants. However, cyclosporine is associated with higher pressures and a greater left ventricular mass index than noncyclosporine immunosuppressive schedules.[12] Furthermore, in the same study, loss of diurnal variation, as documented by 24-hour ambulatory blood pressure monitoring (whether observed in cyclosporine or noncyclosporine regimens), was associated with a higher left ventricular mass index. There is, then, a rationale for use of ambulatory blood pressure monitoring to determine, with greater accuracy, the effect of antihypertensive drug therapy in these patients.

Heart and Liver Transplantation

Elevated blood pressure has also been noted to occur following cardiac or liver transplantation. Due to the effects of either advanced cardiac failure or hepatic disease, these patients are rarely hypertensive before transplantation. Following successful surgery, hypertension is often present and may be severe. Use of high doses of glucocorticoids and cyclosporine, as immunosuppressive therapy to prevent graft rejection, best accounts for the increase in blood pressure. Hypertension following cardiac[13] or liver[14] transplantation is associated with loss of the normal diurnal variation in pressure; thus, 24-hour monitoring of arterial pressure may be valuable for accurate assessment. As in Cushing syndrome, hypertension after liver transplantation is associated with higher doses of glucocorticoid administration.[14]

Cyclosporine-Related Transplant Hypertension

The exact pathogenesis of cyclosporine-induced hypertension in post-transplant patients is somewhat uncertain. It has been suggested that this agent augments $[Ca^{2+}]$ entry via opened channels in vascular smooth muscle causing vasoconstriction. Renal vasoconstriction has been emphasized for its participation either on a neurogenic basis or as a direct effect of cyclosporine.[15–17] In the renal circulation, afferent arteriolar constriction leads to renin release and angiotensin-dependent hypertension in some settings.[18,19] Abnormal prostaglandin synthesis, systemic vasoconstriction, and abnormal sympathetic nerve function have also been implicated in experimental or clinical studies of post-transplant or cyclosporine-related hypertension.[15,20]

Cyclosporine-induced arteriolar injury may proceed to vascular pathology (i.e., sclerosis), which appears similar to the usual forms of arteriosclerosis in coronary and renal circulations.

The mechanisms described above suggest several approaches either for prevention of cyclosporine and post-transplant hypertension or for specific therapy. Calcium channel entry blockers, especially nifedipine, have been evaluated and in some retrospective and prospective studies appear to be beneficial for reduction of arterial pressure with preservation of renal function.[21-23] In one preliminary report, diltiazem was found to prevent coronary artery disease following cardiac transplantation.[24] Alteration of prostaglandin pathways by high levels of ω-3 fatty acids has been shown to preserve renal function after renal transplantation[25] and decrease arterial pressure (mean arterial pressure fell 18 mmHg) and systemic vascular resistance.[26] Use of ACE inhibitors has also been assessed in post-transplant cyclosporine hypertension with mixed results. A comparison between captopril and nifedipine in cyclosporine-treated renal transplant patients found a similar reduction with both drugs, but a tendency toward reduced renal blood flow and glomerular filtration rate during ACE inhibitor therapy that was not observed with the calcium entry blocker.[27] Another study comparing lisinopril and nifedipine described similar reductions in blood pressure and little difference in renal effects, except for a small reduction of filtration fraction in the ACE inhibitor–treated group.[28] A retrospective study has reported an increase in creatinine clearance when renal transplant patients were changed from an ACE inhibitor to a calcium entry blocker.[23] Perhaps cyclosporine-induced changes in the afferent renal arterioles are so widespread that nearly all functioning glomeruli are underperfused, as in the Goldblatt one kidney model (see Chs. 4 and 10). If so, efferent constriction may be needed to maintain glomerular filtration, unless afferent arteriolar resistance is decreased (i.e., by calcium entry blockers).

Hypertension in post-transplant patients should be treated aggressively. Findings from studies of 24-hour ambulatory blood pressure monitoring imply that the average daily pressure may be higher than the clinic measurements due to the increased night or sleep pressure. For maximal prevention of target organ damage, particularly left ventricular hypertrophy, agents with sustained action that are effective throughout the entire day should be used. In these very special patients, repeated use of noninvasive ambulatory blood pressure monitoring is justified for optimal assessment of antihypertensive management. On the basis of current literature, the calcium entry blockers are preferred. However, more long-term studies are needed. The ACE inhibitors together with calcium entry blockers might be beneficial in selected cases or if cardiac function is reduced and an activated renin system is present. ω-3 Fatty acid supplementation certainly deserves more study, as does the role of adrenergic receptor antagonists, if indeed the sympathetic nervous system participates in pathogenesis.

Cyclosporine Hypertension in Nontransplant Diseases

The immunosuppressive activity of cyclosporine has led to exploration of its effects in several disorders in which T-cell–mediated autoimmune processes are evident. Recent reports describe the effect of cyclosporine on, among others, systemic sclerosis,[29] autoimmune uveitis,[30] membranous nephropathy,[31] and psoriasis.[32] Irrespective of any beneficial effect on the primary disease, hypertension has appeared in 40 to 80 percent of such series, when reported. As one favoring prevention when possible, I hope that consideration is being given to studies evaluating preventive measures in the expanding use of cyclosporine. Short of that, very close observation of blood pressure during cyclosporine therapy is necessary, with introduction of appropriate antihypertensive drug therapy as soon as an elevation in pressure is found. My choice, given all available data, would be the use of a calcium channel blocker as the initial therapy.

SLEEP APNEA HYPERTENSION

Snoring is a fine old tradition as are the unavoidable mid-day naps, often observed when professors dose off at noon and during postlunch rounds and conferences. Lights off, first slide, ZZZZZZZ. Now there is an explanation that includes a recently described form of secondary and reversible hypertension.

The sleep apnea syndrome is comprised of more than the occasional nocturnal buzz. It consists of repeated episodes of true apnea with hypoxia during sleep that is related to obstruction by an enlarged uvula falling by gravity into the pharynx. These patients sleep on their backs. The sleep disturbance and persistent nocturnal hypoxia are believed to trigger chemoreceptive reflexes that increase sympathetic tone and blood pressure, lasting throughout the day.[33] Sleep apnea is most often found in obese, middle-aged men. Their wives eventually complain to the doctor, initiating a workup. However, this syndrome is now found often enough, when one looks for it, that every middle-aged overweight hypertensive man should be questioned carefully about his sleep habits, whether excessive snoring has been noted by his wife or companion, and if unusual sleepiness is present when awake. During the day, prior sleep deprivation leads to somnolence when usual stimulation is at an ebb (e.g., while sitting alone at one's desk or in the car at a traffic light). Complaints of excessive daytime fatigue or somnolence may raise the possibility of depression, underlying neoplasm, anemia, or hypothyroidism. These patients are often hypertensive. When studied by 24-hour ambulatory blood pressure monitoring, the blood pressure in patients with sleep apnea syndrome is consistently higher during the day and night than pressure in control subjects.[34] Once suspected, the diagnosis of sleep apnea syndrome requires special sleep studies (i.e., polysomnography) for a definitive characterization.

Once sleep apnea syndrome is diagnosed in a hypertensive patient, it is possible to decrease the arterial pressure without pharmacologic therapy. In some cases, surgery to reduce the size of the uvula may be needed. However, for the obese patient, weight reduction can be remarkably effective and may even reduce the dimensions of the soft palate and uvula.[35,36] Alternatively, use of nasal inhalation of air under pressure (nasal continuous positive airway pressure) during sleep can also be effective in correcting the nocturnal hypoxia and for reduction of blood pressure.[37,38] Should the previously mentioned interventions not succeed in controlling arterial pressure, antihypertensive medication may be needed. Given the propensity for sleepiness and fatigue in these patients, the centrally acting agents (including the lipophilic β-blockers) should, in my view, be avoided. Since this appears to be a sympathetically mediated form of hypertension, the α_1-receptor blockers, perhaps combined with a nonlipophilic β-blocker, might be effective. No definitive studies provide a basis for the choice of antihypertensive drug therapy in this disorder. Should α/β-antagonism not work, an empirical trial of ACE inhibitors or calcium channel entry blockers seems reasonable.

REFERENCES

1. Friedman WF: Congenital heart disease in infancy and childhood. p. 887. In Braunwald E (ed): Heart Disease. WB Saunders, Philadelphia, 1992

2. Ribeiro AB, Krakoff LR: Angiotensin blockade in coarctation of the aorta. N Engl J Med 295:148, 1976

3. Milner LS, Jacobs DW, Thomson PD et al: Management of severe hypertension in childhood Takayasu's arteritis. Pediatr Nephrol 5:38, 1991

4. Choy M, Rocchini AP, Beekman RH et al: Paradoxical hypertension after repair of coarctation of the aorta in children: balloon angioplasty versus surgical repair. Circulation 75:1186, 1987

5. Balaji S, Oommen R, Rees PG: Fatal aortic rupture during balloon dilatation of recoarctation. Br Heart J 65:100, 1991

6. Krakoff LR: Measurement of plasma renin substrate by radioimmunoassay of angiotensin I: concentration in syndromes associated with steroid excess. J Clin Endocrinol Metab 37:608, 1973

7. Taufield PA, Ales KL, Resnick LM et al: Hypocalciuria in preeclampsia. N Engl J Med 316:715, 1987

8. Popovtzer MM, Pinnggera W, Katz FH et al: Variations in arterial blood pressure after kidney transplantation. Circulation 47:1297, 1973

9. Curtis JJ, Luke RG, Dustan HP et al: Remission of essential hypertension after renal transplantation. N Engl J Med 309:1009, 1983

10. Curtis JJ, Luke RG, Whelchel JD et al: Inhibition of angiotensin-converting enzyme in renal-transplant recipients with hypertension. N Engl J Med 308:377, 1983

11. Imai Y, Abe K, Sasaki S et al: Altered circadian blood pressure rhythm in patients with Cushing's syndrome. Hypertension 12:11, 1988

12. Lipkin GW, Tucker B, Giles M, Raine AEG: Ambulatory blood pressure and left ventricular mass in cyclosporin- and non-cyclosporine-treated renal transplant patients. J Hypertens 11:439, 1993

13. Reeves RA, Shapiro AP, Thompson ME, Johnsen AM: Loss of nocturnal decline in blood pressure after cardiac transplantion. Circulation 73:401, 1986

14. van de Borne P, Gelin M, Van de Stadt J, Degaute J-P: Circadian rhythms of blood pressure after liver transplantation. Hypertension 21:398, 1993

15. Mark AL: Cyclosporine, sympathetic activity and hypertension. N Engl J Med 323:748, 1990

16. Epstein M: Calcium antagonists and the kidney. Implications for renal protection. Am J Hypertens 6:251S, 1993

17. Kaye D, Thompson J, Jennings G, Esler M: Cyclosporine therapy after cardiac transplantation causes hypertension and renal vasoconstriction without sympathetic activation. Circulation 88:1101, 1993

18. Julien J, Farge D, Kreft-Jais C et al: Cyclosporine-induced stimulation of the renin-angiotensin system after liver and heart transplantation. Transplantation 56:885, 1993

19. Clozel JP, Fischli W, Menard J: Effects of the blockade of the renin-angiotensin system in cyclosporin-induced hypertension. J Hypertens 11:75, 1993

20. Scherrer U, Vissing SF, Morgan BJ et al: Cyclosporine-induced sympathetic activation and hypertension after heart transplantation. N Engl J Med 323:693, 1990

21. Hauser AC, Derfler K, Stockenhuber F et al: Effect of calcium-channel blockers on renal function in renal-graft recipients treated with cyclosporine. N Engl J Med 324:1517, 1991

22. Legault L, Ogilvie RI, Cardella CJ, Leenen FH: Calcium antagonists in heart transplant recipients: effects on cardiac and renal function and cyclosporine pharmacokinetics. Can J Cardiol 9:398, 1993

23. Bunke M, Ganzel B: Effect of calcium channel antagonists on renal function in hypertensive heart transplant recipients. J Heart Lung Transplant 11:1194, 1992

24. Schroeder JS, Gao S-Z, Alderman EL et al: A preliminary study of diltiazem in the prevention of coronary artery disease in heart-transplant recipients. N Engl J Med 328:164, 1993

25. Homan van der Heide JJ, Bilo HJG, Donker JM et al: Effect of dietary fish oil on renal function and rejection in cyclosporine-treated recipients of renal transplants. N Engl J Med 329:769, 1993

26. Ventura HO, Milani RV, Lavie CJ et al: Cyclosporine-induced hypertension. Efficacy of omega-3 fatty acids in patients after cardiac transplantation. Circulation 88:II281, 1993

27. Curtis JJ, Laskow DA, Jones PA et al: Captopril-induced fall in glomerular filtration rate in cyclosporine-treated hypertensive patients. J Am Soc Nephrol 3:1570, 1993

28. Mourad G, Ribstein J, Mimran A: Converting-enzyme inhibitor versus calcium antagonist in cyclosporine-treated renal transplants. Kidney Int 43:419, 1993

29. Gisslinger H, Burghuber OC, Stacher G et al: Efficacy of cyclosporin A in systemic sclerosis. Clin Exp Rheumatol 9:383, 1991

30. Deray G, Benhmida M, Le Hoang P et al: Renal function and blood pressure in patients receiving long-term, low-dose cyclosporine therapy for idiopathic autoimmune uveitis. Ann Intern Med 117:578, 1992

31. Guasch A, Suranyi M, Newton L et al: Short-term responsiveness of membranous glomerulopathy to cyclosporine. Am J Kidney Dis 20:472, 1992

32. Fry L: Psoriasis: immunopathology and long-term treatment with cyclosporin. J Autoimmun, suppl. A. 5:277, 1992

33. Carlson JT, Hedner J, Elam M et al: Augmented resting sympathetic activity in awake patients with obstructive sleep apnea. Chest 103:1763, 1993

34. Hla KM, Young TB, Bidwell T et al: Sleep apnea and hypertension. Ann Intern Med 120:382, 1994

35. Kiselak J, Clark M, Pera V et al: The association between hypertension and sleep apnea in obese patients. Chest 104:775, 1993

36. Pi Sunyer FX: Short-term medical benefits and adverse effects of weight loss. Ann Intern Med 119:722, 1993

37. Suzuki M, Otsuka K, Guilleminault C: Long-term nasal continuous positive airway pressure administration can normalize blood pressure in obstructive sleep apnea patients. Sleep 16:545, 1993

38. Wilcox I, Grunstein RR, Hedner JA et al: Effect of nasal continuous positive airway pressure during sleep on 24-hour blood pressure in sleep apnea. Sleep 16:539, 1993

Section III

PREVENTION AND TREATMENT

13

PREVENTION

Until recently, little attention was paid to the possibility that hypertension might be preventable. Instead, effort was primarily aimed at detection of those who were already hypertensive so that treatment could be directed toward the reduction of pressure that had become elevated. The concept that hypertension, as a diagnostic entity, might be delayed or prevented entirely by relatively simple measures is appealing, especially if prevention could be achieved at a low cost. This short chapter summarizes the status of strategies to prevent hypertension.

Recent epidemiologic surveys have found significant relationships between several potentially reversible factors and the tendency for blood pressure to become elevated, particularly in those with a genetic predisposition. The most intensely studied of these predictors for hypertension are given in Table 13-1.

The items listed in Table 13-1 offer opportunities for intervention by reversing or correcting dietary or behavioral patterns before arterial pressure is raised to hypertensive levels. Weight reduction, a lactovegetarian diet, reduction of alcohol intake, increased diet potassium, and increased physical exertion may reduce arterial pressure to within the normal range.[1]

Three studies have been conducted in the United States to determine whether hypertension, defined as sustained pressure of 140/90 mmHg or higher, or the need for antihypertensive medications could be prevented in individuals with high normal pressure or who are likely to become hypertensive.[2–4] Those enrolled in these studies were healthy adults, 30 to 50 years old, often moderately overweight, employed, with high normal diastolic pressures (80 to 89 mmHg) and family histories of hypertension, and were likely to be compliant. Common to all of the trials were attempts at weight reduction and diminution in dietary salt intake. Several other interventions were used in the individual studies, as shown in Table 13-2.

In all these studies, blood pressure tended to fall in both control and intervention groups with time, probably due to the combined effects of acclimatization to clinic measurement and regression to the mean. Weight reduction was the most consistently effective means for either reducing pressure or preventing hypertensive events. Reduced salt intake, alone or in combination with weight reduction or high potassium intake, had either a very small effect or one that was not statistically significant. In other studies, the effect of diminished salt intake on nonhypertensive persons has varied.[5,6] Perhaps the relatively high salt intake in our culture leads to elevated pressure early on in the susceptible subjects[2–4,7–9] (as it does in rats, which are genetically salt sen-

Table 13-1. Characteristics of Healthy Young Adults Who Are Likely To Become Hypertensive

High normal arterial pressure
Family history of hypertension (one or both parents)
Overweight ($\geq$10% above desirable weight) and gaining more
Excessive alcohol intake
High salt intake
Low potassium intake
Low level of regular physical activity

sitive), who then become hypertensive and would not be selected for the prevention trials. In that case, the prevention studies selectively address those less sensitive to salt. In adolescent subjects, salt sensitivity can be detected among the overweight; weight reduction diminishes salt sensitivity.[10] Salt restriction may also be more beneficial in subjects older than those enrolled in the prevention trials.

The various interventions that seem to have had little effect in prevention of hypertension in these three trials include stress management and potassium, calcium, magnesium, and fish oil supplements. However, other reports suggest that fish oil[11,12] or potassium[13] supplementation might be effective, whereas calcium supplementation might not.[14]

Table 13-2. Effects of Various Interventions on Change in Arterial Pressure and Risk of Hypertension, as Defined in Studies

Study	Results
Primary Prevention of Hypertension[2]	Small reductions in pressure due to weight reduction; 55% prevention of incidence of hypertension (hypertension defined as work site pressure of $\geq$90 mmHg diastolic or prescription of antihypertensive drugs)
Hypertension Prevention Trial[3]	Compared with controls, only weight reduction lowered pressure; low sodium with or without high potassium was not significant; hypertensive events (systolic pressure of $\geq$140 mmHg or diastolic pressure of $\geq$90 mmHg or drug treatment) reduced by low calorie or low salt, or both, or low salt, high potassium diet
Trials of Hypertension Prevention Collaborative Research Group[4]	Small but significant reductions in pressure due to weight reduction ($-4/-2$ mmHg systolic/diastolic), low salt ($-2/-1$ mmHg; no effect from stress management or from calcium, magnesium, potassium, or fish oil supplements; only weight reduction associated with significant reduction in hypertension events (-34%)

The three prevention trials described above used a variety of strategies to change the normal behavior of their enrollees regarding diet and exercise patterns. Nutritional and exercise counselors and various educational and follow-up methods by specially trained personnel were required. These measures are not ordinarily available to practicing physicians or to public health agencies. It is not yet known whether the health-related behavior of the large fraction of the public at risk of hypertension can be changed without the intensity of the interventions used in these studies. In other words, what will it cost to achieve these preventive measures on a large scale and for the length of time needed for success? Early education in school-based programs, appropriate use of health advertising, and other health promotional strategies may well be effective.

Despite some limitations of the three prevention trials, the available studies suggest that young adults who are overweight and have a life-style of relatively low physical activity should be counseled to lose weight and increase regular activity, such as with aerobic exercise. If these behaviors are developed into sustained patterns, reduced future cardiovascular disease may be anticipated.[15] If alcohol intake is excessive, reduction to lower levels of drinking may also be beneficial.[16] The case for modest reduction in diet salt or increased potassium intake, or both, as a means to prevent hypertension is less compelling (although presumably harmless). Adolescents and young adults should be aware of all cardiovascular risk factors that can be controlled by their own behavior or life-style. The physician's role in this process is limited primarily to counseling and participation in those public activities that may influence the population at large.

REFERENCES

1. Beilin LJ: The fifth Sir George Pickering memorial lecture: epitaph to essential hypertension—a preventable disorder of known aetiology? J Hypertens 6:85, 1988

2. Stamler R, Stamler J, Gosch FC et al: Primary prevention of hypertension by nutritional-hygienic means. Final report of a randomized controlled trial. JAMA 262:1801, 1989

3. Hypertension Prevention Trial Research Group: The Hypertension Prevention Trial: three-year effects of dietary changes on blood pressure. Arch Intern Med 150:153, 1990

4. The Trials of Hypertension Prevention Collaborative Research Group: The effects of nonpharmacologic interventions on blood pressure of persons with high normal levels. Results of the Trials of Hypertension Prevention. Phase I. JAMA 267:1213, 1992

5. Parker M, Puddey IB, Beilin LJ, Vandongen R: Two-way factorial study of alcohol and salt restriction in treated hypertensive men. Hypertension 16:398, 1990

6. Law MR, Frost CD, Wald NJ: By how much does dietary salt reduction lower blood pressure? III—analysis of data from trials of salt reduction. BMJ 302:819, 1991

7. Intersalt Cooperative Research Group: Intersalt: an international study of electrolyte excretion and blood pressure. Results for 24 hour urinary sodium and potassium excretion. BMJ 297:319, 1988

8. Law MR, Frost CD, Wald NJ: By how much does dietary salt reduction lower blood pressure? I—analysis of observational data among populations. BMJ 302:811, 1991

9. Frost CD, Law MR, Wald NJ: By how much does dietary salt reduction lower blood pressure? II—analysis of observational data within populations. BMJ 302:815, 1991

10. Rocchii AP, Key J, Bondie D et al: The effect of weight loss on the sensitivity of blood pressure to sodium in obese adolescents. N Engl J Med 321:580, 1989

11. Knapp HR, FitzGerald GA: The antihypertensive effects of fish oil: a controlled study of polyunsaturated fatty acid supplements in essential hypertension. N Engl J Med 320:1037, 1989

12. Bonaa KH, Bjerve KS, Straume B et al: Effect of eicosapentaenoic and docosahexaenoic acids on blood pressure in hypertension. N Engl J Med 322:795, 1990

13. Cappucio FP, MacGregor GA: Does potassium supplementation lower blood pressure? A meta-analysis of published trials. J Hypertens 9:465, 1991

14. Cappucio FP, Siani A, Strazullo P: Oral calcium supplementation and blood pressure: an overview of randomized clinical trials. J Hypertens 7:941, 1989

15. Paffenbarger RS Jr, Hyde RT, Wing AL, Hsieh C-C: Physical activity, all-cause mortality, and longevity of college alumni. N Engl J Med 314:605, 1986

16. Hartung GH, Kohl HW, Blair SN et al: Exercise tolerance and alcohol intake: blood pressure relation. Hypertension 16:501, 1990

14

NONPHARMACOLOGIC TREATMENT

As therapeutic interventions, nonpharmacologic therapies have potential benefit for treatment of hypertension.[1] Apart from reduction of arterial pressure, favorable changes in nonhypertensive risk factors—serum lipids and glucose tolerance—may occur. Some interventions (smoking cessation, increased aerobic exercise, and possibly weight reduction) may have benefits independent of arterial pressure by causing favorable changes in known risk factors and other effects. In mild hypertension, nonpharmacologic interventions may be sufficient to reduce arterial pressure without imposition of antihypertensive medication. Even patients who require drug treatment may benefit from some nonpharmacologic or behavioral changes. For example, weight reduction seems to increase the effectiveness of some antihypertensive medications.[2] Salt restriction may augment the effect of those drugs that block the renin-angiotensin system (β-blockers or angiotensin converting enzyme inhibitors).

Many individuals with borderline or high normal blood pressure or defined as hypertensive are overweight. In the United States, a large fraction of the hypertensive population is 15 to 20 percent overweight for their height, based on the body mass index. A sizable fraction are too sedentary, and, despite progress in antismoking campaigns, some still smoke. Salt intake and/or alcohol ingestion may be too high for some. There is then a very sound basis for nonpharmacologic treatment or life-style change in the management of many hypertensive patients either as the only intervention or as a continuing adjunctive measure along with administration of antihypertensive drugs. The following discussion summarizes the current value of these interventions.

WEIGHT REDUCTION

For the overweight hypertensive person, loss of weight decreases arterial pressure. This effect is independent of salt restriction[3,4] and can be as effective as antihypertensive medication.[5] The benefits of sustained weight loss include favorable changes in carbohydrate tolerance, serum lipids, and left ventricular mass.[6] A decrease in salt sensitivity has been shown to accompany weight reduction in obese adolescents in association with lessened insulin resistance.[7,8]

Weight reduction may also enhance responsiveness to antihypertensive agents.[3] In a recent randomized trial in overweight hypertensive persons, chlorthalidone or atenolol, as monotherapy, had little antihypertensive effect without dietary weight loss. Because of an increase in serum cholesterol in the chlorthalidone-treated group, calculated risk (Framingham criteria) actually increased. However, the group treated with a weight reduction program combined with atenolol had the greatest reduction in pressure and calculated decrease in risk.[2] There is no reason not to encourage weight reduction by safe means for overweight hypertensive persons; the challenge is for these patients to sustain their efforts to remain at a lower weight.

SALT RESTRICTION

Both experimental and clinical studies have shown that some hypertensive individuals (animals and humans) are salt sensitive (i.e., have an increased arterial pressure with increased dietary salt intake) and some are not. Apart from the rare cases in which an excess of a salt-retaining steroid is causing renal salt retention, the pathophysiology of salt sensitivity is not fully characterized. It has been suggested that salt sensitivity is a low renin or high volume state. If so, one might speculate that salt-sensitive hypertensive persons would be protected from development of cardiovascular disease.[9] Salt-sensitive hypertensive persons may have greater responsiveness to pressor substances than hypertensive patients who are salt resistant.[10] It has been suggested that salt-sensitive subjects are also insulin resistant.[11,12] While these observations are provocative from a mechanistic point of view, they do not provide a simple clinical test to distinguish salt-sensitive hypertensive individuals from salt-resistant ones. The only way to find out is by placing the patient on a low salt diet and determining whether the blood pressure falls or remains elevated.[13]

Meta-analyses suggest there is a trend toward a linear relationship between salt intake and the level of arterial pressure in Western-type cultures.[14,15] In a recent extensive international survey, INTERSALT, the most prominent relationship found was between the level of salt intake and the rate of increase in arterial pressure with age.[16] Whether salt intake alone accounts for the age-related increase in a population's average pressure is not yet certain.

The effect of reducing dietary salt intake on arterial pressure has been extensively studied. A meta-analysis of many such investigations suggests several conclusions: (1) the blood pressure lowering effect of reduced salt intake is greater in individuals with higher pressures, but still evident in normotensive persons, the range of reduction in systolic pressure being 5 to 7 mmHg and in diastolic pressure 3 to 5 mmHg; (2) a larger effect of salt restriction tends to be found in older patients; and (3) the relationship between salt intake and arterial pressure predicted by epidemiologic surveys[14,15] is fairly well duplicated in the few long-term studies of salt restriction, but not in short-term observations (less than 4 weeks).[17] However, only a fraction of those exposed to reduced salt intake have a clinically significant fall in pressure.[13] For a selected group of highly compliant subjects, an antihypertensive effect can be sustained for up to 1 year.[18] As with many interventions, most studies of salt restriction have relied on casual or clinic blood pressure measurements. When ambulatory blood pressure monitoring is used, the reduction in pressure is much less than that defined by clinic measurements.[19] Salt restriction has no known beneficial effects on nonhypertensive cardiovascular risk factors. Some subgroups may have small increases in serum lipid fractions during salt restriction[20] so that the long-term effects of reduction in dietary salt intake on cardiovascular disease rates is problematic. At this time, no evidence from clinical trials shows that a sustained reduction in salt intake actually causes reduction in either stroke or coronary heart disease rates, despite wishful extrapolation from the available data.[17]

POTASSIUM AND CALCIUM

Epidemiologic and experimental studies suggest that a potassium-deficient diet may increase blood pressure or the risk of stroke.[21] A recent meta-analysis has summarized the effect of potassium supplementation on blood pressure and concludes that a small, but significant, decrease in pressure may be associated with adding potassium to the diet.[22] It is not yet known whether potassium supplementation affects rate of stroke or ischemic heart disease.

The relationship between dietary calcium intake and hypertension has been a controversial subject.[23] From the perspective of meta-analysis, addition of calcium supplements to the diet appears to have little effect on arterial pressure in hypertensive subjects.[24]

ALCOHOL CONSUMPTION

Excessive alcohol intake is related to increased arterial pressure in epidemiologic surveys[25–27] and may contribute to stroke.[28] It is suggested, but not certain, that low level alcohol use (10 to 15 g/day) may decrease arterial pressure and/or reduce cardiovascular risk. In addition, it has recently been shown, in Australian beer drinking hypertensive subjects (with relatively high daily intake), that substitution of nonalcoholic beer reduces arterial pressure whether or not salt restriction is included in the program.[29] This is additional evidence for the view that hypertensive patients with high alcohol intake may indeed have "secondary hypertension," which is reversible when alcohol consumption is eliminated or reduced to a much lower level.

FISH OIL

Polyunsaturated fatty acid components of fish and vegetable oils have been thought to have beneficial effects with regard to prevention of atherosclerotic and thrombotic events, partly through their effects on prostaglandin metabolism.[30] Blood pressure lowering effects of fish oil ingestion had been shown in limited studies.[31] More recently, two studies with different and unbiased designs have demonstrated small but significant reductions in arterial pressure in subjects given fish oil diet supplements containing ω-3 fatty acids. Knapp and FitzGerald[32] showed that fish oil (at a dose of 50 ml/day) significantly reduced ambulatory arterial pressure by 7 mmHg systolic and 4 mmHg diastolic pressure. Neither a safflower oil control nor an oil mixture chosen to duplicate the average fat content of the American diet had an effect on ambulatory pressure. A population-based study comparing fish and corn oil supplements in a Norwegian community reported small but significant reductions in pressure only with the fish oil treatment. Patients with a high dietary fish intake had smaller changes in blood pressure during fish oil treatment than those who habitually ate less fish.[33]

Although it is tempting to endorse fish oil supplementation as a nondrug treatment for mild hypertension, a few warnings are in order. The daily amount needed for the modest antihypertensive effect achieved (30 to 50 ml/day) can add enough calories to the diet for weight to increase (or fail to decrease) in the overweight and sedentary. In addition, no long-term studies have been done to establish whether fish oil supplementation reduces cardiovascular morbidity or mortality when used as a treatment for hypertension in controlled trials. There is concern that the antithrombotic effect of fish oils might lead to an increased risk of hemorrhage in a hypertensive group if arterial pressure were not well controlled.

SMOKING CESSATION

In the past, cigarette smoking has not been well correlated with either the level of arterial pressure or the prevalence of hypertension in large-scale epidemiologic surveys. Despite this lack of correlation, the link between smoking and the risk of stroke or coronary heart disease is firmly established.[34,35] Cigarette smoking has, however, been linked to malignant hypertension[36,37] and to atherosclerotic renovascular hypertension.[38] Smoking cessation definitely reduces the risk of coronary heart disease[39] and thus can be firmly recommended on that basis alone. Hypertensive persons who do not stop smoking fail to gain maximal benefit from reduction of pressure by drug treatment.[40]

It is not surprising that cigarette smoking, an intermittent phenomenon, is not well correlated with casual or clinic blood pressures, as these pressures represent only a small sample of the pressure and its variation throughout an entire day. Ambulatory blood pressure monitoring has revealed that cigarette smokers tend to have either higher average pressures or transient elevations of daytime systolic pressures, probably related to the effect of smoking activity.[41,42]

Patients may be concerned about the weight gain that occurs with cessation of smoking.[43] The net benefit from discontinuing smoking far outweighs the independent risk of weight gain. However, whenever possible, patients should try to remain no more than 10 percent above their desirable weight for their height as reflected by their body mass index.

EXERCISE

Regular exercise has a protective effect for prevention of future cardiovascular disease.[44–46] This effect may be due to several mechanisms, including weight reduction and improvement in glucose tolerance and serum lipid patterns. However, lack of exercise has also been linked to increased arterial pressure.[25] When persons with mild hypertension engage in a pattern of regular aerobic exercise, a small but significant reduction in arterial pressure occurs.[47–49] Both resting and exercise pressures are decreased, as are levels of plasma norepinephrine.[47]

Sustained regular exercise increases maximal oxygen consumption, a beneficial training effect. In a direct comparison between a placebo and two β-blockers, treatment with the nonselective β-blocker propranolol prevented the training effect, whereas the selective β_1-antagonist metoprolol had no such action.[48] Little is known about the effects of other antihypertensive drugs on the training effect of regular exercise.

CONCLUSION

Several nonpharmacologic interventions may cause small, sustained reductions in arterial pressure and thus are treatments for hypertension. Table 14-1 provides a summary of the nonpharmacologic treatments discussed above.

Table 14-1. Summary of Nonpharmacologic or Life-Style Interventions for Treatment of Hypertension

Intervention	Change in Pressure	Comment
Weight reduction	Systolic 10–15 mmHg Diastolic 5–10 mmHg	Ideal treatment for overweight persons who are mildly hypertensive; may improve other risk factors and reduce insulin resistance
Salt restriction of 50–100 mmol/day	Related to level of pressure and age Systolic 5–7 mmHg Diastolic 3–5 mmHg	Individual variation in response; effects on other risk factors not defined; does not add to either weight reduction or decreased alcohol intake
Potassium supplementation	Small effects: diastolic reduction of 3–5 mmHg	May decrease likelihood of stroke
Calcium supplementation	Little overall effect documented	May have other benefits, such as prevention of osteoporosis in women
Fish oil supplementation	Small but uniform decrease: 4–5 mmHg diastolic	Changes in clotting mechanism; long-term effectiveness and safety not established
Cessation of smoking	No known effect on clinic pressures; may reduce transient surges in systolic pressure	Unequivocal benefit in reducing risk of coronary heart disease and stroke
Reduction of high alcohol intake	Definite but small reductions in pressure Systolic 5–10 mmHg Diastolic 3–6 mmHg	Potential benefit for noncardiovascular disease also; no long-term studies available
Increased regular aerobic exercise	Systolic decrease 5–10 mmHg Diastolic 3–5 mmHg	Appears to reduce long-term risk of coronary heart disease; may increase high-density lipoprotein cholesterol and decrease insulin resistance; assists in weight reduction
Meditation, relaxation and other stress-reduction techiques	Long-term effect on pressure not known	No known effects on rate of stroke or coronary heart disease; may be helpful as adjunct in secondary prevention of coronary heart disease[50]

Cessation of smoking is necessary, not so much for its effect on arterial pressure but because of its overall benefit in reducing the risk of atherosclerosis. Among the nonpharmacologic approaches for reducing arterial pressure, the most promising are weight reduction for the overweight; restriction of alcohol intake for those with excess intake; and increased regular aerobic exercise. Achieving compliance for these interventions is a formidable but not insurmountable problem. Lowering dietary salt intake may be beneficial in selected patients, but is less impressive than some investigators predicted. Potassium supplementation may cause small reductions in pressure and may confer a selective benefit against stroke. A high fish oil consumption may cause small reductions in pressure; long-term prevention of cardiovascular disease is not yet fully established. For patients with mild hypertension, nonpharmacologic intervention or favorable life-style changes may be all that is needed. When pressure is higher, combining nonpharmacologic treatment with antihypertensive medication is necessary for optimal prevention.

REFERENCES

1. Fuh MM-T, Shieh S-M, Wu D-A et al: Abnormalities of carbohydrate and lipid metabolism in patients with hypertension. Arch Intern Med 147:1035, 1987

2. Oberman A, Wassertheil-Smoller S, Langford HG et al: Pharmacologic and nutritional treatment of mild hypertension: changes in cardiovascular risk status. Ann Intern Med 112:89, 1990

3. Reisin E, Abel R, Modan M et al: Effect of weight loss without salt restriction on the blood pressure in overweight hypertensive patients. N Engl J Med 298:1, 1978

4. Tuck ML, Sowers J, Dornfeld L et al: The effect of weight reduction on blood pressure, plasma renin activity, and plasma aldosterone levels in obese patients. N Engl J Med 304:930, 1981

5. MacMahon SW, MacDonald GJ, Bernstein L et al: Comparison of weight reduction with metoprolol in treatment of hypertension in young overweight patients. Lancet 1:1233, 1985

6. MacMahon SW, Wilcken DEL, MacDonald GJ: The effect of weight reduction on left ventricular mass: a randomized controlled trial in young, overweight hypertensive patients. N Engl J Med 314:334, 1986

7. Rocchini AP, Key J, Bondie D et al: The effect of weight loss on the sensitivity of blood pressure to sodium in obese adolescents. N Engl J Med 321:580, 1989

8. Rocchini AP, Katch V, Kveselis D et al: Insulin and renal sodium retention in obese adolescents. Hypertension 14:367, 1989

9. Alderman MH, Madhavan S, Ooi WL et al: Association of the renin-sodium profile with the risk of myocardial infarction in patients with hypertension. N Engl J Med 324:1098, 1991

10. Campese VM, Karubian F, Chervu I et al: Pressor reactivity to norepinephrine and angiotensin in salt-sensitive hypertensive patients. Hypertension 21:301, 1993

11. Sharma AM, Ruland K, Spies K-P, Distler A: Salt sensitivity in young normotensive subjects is associated with a hyperinsulinemic response to oral glucose. J Hypertens 9:329, 1991

12. Sharma AM, Schorr U, Distler A: Insulin resistance in young salt sensitive nor-motensive subjects. Hypertension 21:273, 1993

13. Australian National Health and Medical Research Council Dietary Salt Study Management Committee: Fall in blood pressure with modest reduction in dietary salt intake in mild hypertension. Lancet 1:399, 1989

14. Law MR, Frost CD, Wald NJ: By how much does dietary salt reduction lower blood pressure? I—analysis of observational data among populations. BMJ 302:811, 1991

15. Frost CD, Law MR, Wald NJ: By how much does dietary salt reduction lower blood pressure? II—analysis of observational data within populations. BMJ 302:815, 1991

16. Intersalt Cooperative Research Group: Intersalt: an international study of elec-trolyte excretion and blood pressure. Results for 24 hour urinary sodium and potassium excretion. BMJ 297:319, 1988

17. Law MR, Frost CD, Wald NJ: By how much does dietary salt reduction lower blood pressure? III—analysis of data from trials of salt reduction. BMJ 302:819, 1991

18. MacGregor GA, Markandu ND, Sagnella GA et al: Double-blind study of three sodium intakes and long-term effects of sodium restriction in essential hyper-tension. Lancet 2:1244, 1989

19. Moore TJ, Maralick C, Olmedo A, Klein RC: Salt restriction lowers resting blood pressure, but not 24 H ambulatory blood pressure. Am J Hypertens 5:410, 1991

20. Egan BM, Weder AB, Petrin J, Hoffman RG: Neurohumoral and metabolic effects of short-term dietary NaCl restriction in men: relationship to salt-sen-sivity status. Am J Hypertens 4:416, 1991

21. Khaw K-T, Barrett-Connor E: Dietary potassium and stroke-associated mortali-ty. N Engl J Med 316:235, 1987

22. Cappucio FP, MacGregor GA: Does potassium supplementation lower blood pressure? A meta-analysis of published trials. J Hypertens 9:465, 1991

23. Kaplan NM: Non-drug treatment of hypertension. Ann Intern Med 102:359, 1985

24. Cappucio FP, Siani A, Strazullo P: Oral calcium supplementation and blood pressure: an overview of randomized clinical trials. J Hypertens 7:941, 1989

25. Beilin LJ: The fifth Sir George Pickering memorial lecture: epitaph to essential hypertension—a preventable disorder of known aetiology? J Hypertens 6:85, 1988

26. Stampfer MJ, Colditz GA, Willett WC et al: A prospective study of moderate alcohol consumption and the risk of coronary disease and stroke in women. N Engl J Med 319:267, 1988

27. Klatsky AL, Friedman GD, Siegelaub AB, Gerard MJ: Alcohol consumption and blood pressure: Kaiser-Permanente multiphasic health examination data. N Engl J Med 296:1194, 1977

28. Gill JS, Zezulka AV, Shipley MJ et al: Stroke and alcohol consumption. N Engl J Med 315:1041, 1986

29. Parker M, Puddey IB, Beilin LJ, Vandongen R: Two-way factorial study of alco-hol and salt restriction in treated hypertensive men. Hypertension 16:398, 1990

30. Leaf A, Weber PC: Cardiovascular effects of n-3 fatty acids. N Engl J Med 318:549, 1988

31. Singer P, Berger I, Luck K et al: Long-term effect of mackerel diet on blood pressure, serum lipids and thromboxane formation in patients with mild essential hypertension. Atherosclerosis 62:259, 1986

32. Knapp HR, FitzGerald GA: The antihypertensive effects of fish oil: a controlled study of polyunsaturated fatty acid supplements in essential hypertension. N Engl J Med 320:1037, 1989

33. Bonaa KH, Bjerve KS, Straume B et al: Effect of eicosapentaenoic and docosahexaenoic acids on blood pressure in hypertension. N Engl J Med 322:795, 1990

34. Manson JE, Tosteson H, Ridker PM et al: The primary prevention of myocardial infarction. N Engl J Med 326:1406, 1992

35. Willett WC, Green A, Stampfer MJ et al: Relative and absolute excess risks of coronary heart disease among women who smoke cigarettes. N Engl J Med 317:1303, 1987

36. Isles C, Brown JJ, Cumming AMM et al: Excess smoking in malignant-phase hypertension. BMJ 1:579, 1979

37. Bloxham CA, Beevers DG, Walker JM: Malignant hypertension and cigarette smoking. BMJ 1:581, 1979

38. Nicholson JP, Teichman SL, Alderman MH et al: Cigarette smoking and renovascular hypertension. Lancet 2:765, 1983

39. Rosenberg L, Kaufman DW, Helmrich SP, Shapiro S: The risk of myocardial infarction after quitting smoking in men under 55 years of age. N Engl J Med 313:1511, 1985

40. Heyden S, Schneider KA, Fodor JG: Smoking habits and antihypertensive treatment. Nephron, suppl. 1. 47:99, 1987

41. Mann SJ, James GD, Wang RS, Pickering TG: Elevation of ambulatory systolic blood pressure in hypertensive smokers. JAMA 265:2226, 1991

42. Groppelli A, Giorgi DMA, Omboni S et al: Persistent blood pressure increase induced by heavy smoking. J Hypertens 10:495, 1992

43. Williamson DF, Madans J, Anda RF et al: Smoking cessation and severity of weight gain in a national cohort. N Engl J Med 324:739, 1991

44. Paffenbarger RS Jr, Hyde RT, Wing AL, Hsieh C-C: Physical activity, all-cause mortality, and longevity of college alumni. N Engl J Med 314:605, 1986

45. Sandvik L, Erikssen J, Thaulow E et al: Physical fitness as a predictor of mortality among healthy middle-aged Norwegian men. N Engl J Med 328:533, 1993

46. Paffenbarger RS Jr, Hyde RT, Wing AL et al: The association of changes in physical-activity level and among other lifestyle characteristics with mortality among men. N Engl J Med 328:538, 1993

47. Nelson L, Jennings GL, Esler MD, Korner PI: Effect of changing levels of physical activity on blood-pressure and haemodynamics in essential hypertension. Lancet 2:473, 1986

48. Ades PA, Gunther PGS, Meacham CP et al: Hypertension, exercise, and beta-adrenergic blockade. Ann Intern Med 109:629, 1988

49. Arroll B, Beaglehole R: Does physical activity lower blood pressure: a critical review of the clinical trials. J Clin Epidemiol 45:439, 1992

50. Ornish D, Brown SE, Scherwitz LW et al: Can lifestyle changes reverse coronary heart disease? The Lifestyle Heart Trial. Lancet 336:129, 1990

15

DRUG TREATMENT

The antihypertensive drugs are accepted as the basis for effective control of elevated arterial pressure and prevention of cardiovascular disease, especially stroke, congestive heart failure, dissecting aneurism, progression of renal disease, and the malignant phase of hypertension. In addition, antihypertensive drug treatment may, to a limited extent, prevent ischemic or coronary heart disease. Current trends in clinical research are directed at improved therapy for primary prevention of coronary heart disease, regression of established left ventricular hypertrophy, and delayed progression of renal insufficiency in diabetes and chronic renal disease.

At present more than 50 individual agents are approved as antihypertensive drugs in the United States. Many combinations are also available for prescription. This imposes a burden on the treating physician's memory and the need to develop a systematic yet easily memorized classification system. It so happens that the first 4 letters of the alphabet, *A, B, C, D,* will suffice, as indicated in Table 15-1. Admittedly, this simple scheme overlaps the diverse pharmacologic actions within each major category, but it may prove useful as a practical start.

THE IDEAL ANTIHYPERTENSIVE DRUG

It is useful to compare existing medications or even proposed agents for the treatment of hypertension with theoretical drugs that would be the ideal. While no one therapeutic agent meets such criteria for all hypertensive patients, many individuals are so well controlled on one drug or another that their treatment seems to approach the optimum. Nonetheless, in the long run we should not settle for less than those characteristics given in Table 15-2.

Effectiveness

All antihypertensive drugs reduce arterial pressure in some patients or they would not be approved by regulatory agencies (the Food and Drug Administration [FDA] in the United States). However, the ability of antihypertensive agents to lower pressure in any one patient or the likelihood of effectiveness in a given subgroup of the hypertensive population (e.g., elderly diabetic patients compared with younger nondiabetic subjects) may not be well defined. When prescribing a particular drug, both physicians and patients would like a reasonable guarantee that the pressure will respond in a predictable manner. Assessment of response in many of the pertinent subgroups among the large hypertensive population is available for some agents and classes, but not necessarily for others.

Table 15-1. Alphabetic Classification of the Antihypertensive Drugs

Group	Drug names
A	Angiotensin converting enzyme inhibitors
	Antiadrenergic agents
	α-Receptor blockers
	Angiotensin receptor antagonists
B	β-Receptor blockers
C	Calcium channel entry blockers
	Central active agents
D	Diuretics
	Dilating agents: hydralazine-like, nitrate-like

Prolonged Duration of Action

Hypertension is, by and large, a symptomless disorder; effective treatment requires continuing commitment to taking the drugs each day—compliance. Several studies and abundant clinical experience suggest that the convenience of once a day dosing, by mouth, is most likely to achieve the high rate of compliance needed for sustained reduction of arterial pressure.[1] This requirement has been met through several mechanisms for nearly all the antihypertensive drug classes now widely used. Drugs have been developed that are well absorbed by the gastrointestinal tract and have slow rates of metabolism or elimination, thus favoring sustained action in relationship to well-preserved plasma levels or tissue delivery throughout the day. In addition, new delivery systems have appeared that release drugs with short half-lives over a prolonged span during their residence in the gut and thus convert short-acting agents to those with sustained antihypertensive effect. The latter strategy has been applied to several calcium channel blockers, such as verapamil, diltiazem, and nifedipine. One centrally acting drug, clonidine, has been placed in a transdermal delivery system (skin patch), which may be applied on a weekly basis. Thus, pharmaceutical development has responded to a growing consensus of physicians that the prolonged duration of action offered by those preparations that are effective when given once a day is necessary for optimal treatment.

Table 15-2. Characteristics of the Ideal Antihypertensive Drug

Effective in reducing systemic arterial pressure
Prolonged (24-hr) duration of action for once daily dosing
Absence of adverse reactions, including risk factor trade-off
Reversal of target organ damage (e.g., cardiovascular pathology)
Compatible with other necessary therapeutic agents
Affordable for the individual and the health care system

Absence of Adverse Reactions and Risk Trade-Off

The ideal drug will be free of adverse effects. These can be divided into four categories: (1) life-threatening reactions, (2) specific but minor diseases attributable to the drug (e.g., gout), (3) silent increases in risk (e.g., impaired glucose tolerance), and (4) decreases in quality of life.

Life-threatening actions attributable to the antihypertensive drugs are rare entities. However, several specific conditions led to the elimination of certain drugs. The β-blocker practolol was found to be the cause of blindness due to corneal ulceration secondary to a sicca syndrome also associated with a fibrous peritonitis (the oculomucocutaneous syndrome). A unique uricosuric diuretic, ticrynafen, was withdrawn from use in the United States shortly after approval because of its association with fatal hepatic necrosis and acute renal failure. Of the still available older therapies, reserpine has been associated with delayed appearance of severe depression; long-term use of methyldopa has been linked to chronic and severe hepatitis. Hydralazine has been associated with development of drug-induced systemic lupus erythematosus. Despite the apparent safety of nearly all currently used agents, there is, then, ample reason for concern that long-term safety requires continuing surveillance of more recently available drugs for rare, but severe, adverse effects.

A large number of specific and distinct, but infrequent drug-induced non-life-threatening disorders have been clearly related to antihypertensive drugs. Diuretic-induced gout, minor skin rashes, transient hepatitis, hypokalemia, distinct sleep disorders, transient depressive syndromes, retrograde ejaculation, Raynaud syndrome, pedal edema, and other entities may be seen as iatrogenic entities (i.e., diseases that usually require a change in medication). These are described in greater detail in relationship to the specific agents associated with them. Prescribing physicians should be familiar with these adverse effects. Inexpensive computer programs for identifying specific syndromes with their causative drugs are now available to aid the overtaxed memory. (The *Medical Letter* provides an excellent example.)

Of great concern to clinicians are the potential silent alterations in other cardiovascular risk factors that might offset the benefit of lowered arterial pressure—risk trade-off. There are several identifiable forms of risk trade-off caused by many of the antihypertensive drugs, as indicated in Table 15-3 (e.g., hemodynamic effects, the effects of hypovolemia, and metabolic actions).

The diuretics and older vasodilators, such as hydralazine and minoxidil, reduce blood pressure with activation of the sympathoadrenal and renin-angiotensin systems; heart rate, plasma catecholamines, and plasma renin activity may increase significantly. These mechanisms have the potential, based on experimental studies, to aggravate ischemic heart disease and may contribute to cardiac and vascular pathology due to the unopposed effects of the catecholamines and angiotensin II.

The well-documented adverse metabolic effects of the thiazide-type diuretics and, to some extent, the β-receptor blockers have been the subject of continuing debate and controversy. A report by Ames and Hill published

Table 15-3. Risk Trade-Off in Hypertensive Drug Treatment

Hemodynamic effects
    Baroreflex activation
        Activation of the sympathoadrenal system
        Increased heart rate
        Increased plasma catecholamines
        Activation of the renin system
Effects of hypovolemia
    Activation of the renin-angiotensin system
    Secondary aldosteronism, hypokalemia
    Increased blood viscosity due to higher hematocrit
Metabolic effects
    Adverse change in serum lipids
        Increased total and low-density lipoprotein cholesterol
        Reduced high-density lipoprotein cholesterol
    Impaired glucose tolerance
        Reduced insulin secretion
        Decreased sensitivity to insulin action: insulin resistance

in *Lancet* in 1976 first noted that diuretic-based therapy led to an increase in serum total cholesterol and glucose that, according to the Framingham risk calculations, could entirely offset the predicted benefit of decreased blood pressure. Since then, a large literature has accumulated essentially confirming, in short-term studies, that the thiazide-type diuretic drugs raise low-density lipoprotein (LDL) cholesterol and impair glucose tolerance. The latter is, in part, due to increased resistance to the action of insulin. β-Receptor antagonists have been shown to reduce high-density lipoprotein (HDL) cholesterol concentration by a small but statistically significant amount and to raise serum triglyceride concentration. Some of these untoward metabolic effects can be prevented or reversed by favorable changes in life-style behavior, namely, weight reduction, reduced intake of dietary cholesterol and saturated fat, and increased regular aerobic exercise. These behavioral changes may be beneficial by themselves and might be even more so if their effects were not required to overcome drug-induced alterations in metabolic patterns. Metabolic profiles, pertinent to known cardiovascular risk factors, are now well established for nearly all widely used antihypertensive agents. In choosing the most appropriate drug for each patient, these profiles should be considered to avoid or minimize risk trade-off during reduction of blood pressure.

Quality of life is a major issue for each patient and is the subject of several studies of antihypertensive therapy.[2–12] Extensive questionnaires have exposed some differences in the various categories included in quality of life indices. However, there is considerable heterogeneity in the response patterns noted. In reviewing such studies, it is surprising how many subjects do not have significant symptoms compared with placebo and how few are the differences between drugs. A recent report compared a placebo with the following: a diuretic (chlorthalidone), a β-blocker (acebutolol), an angiotensin converting enzyme (ACE) inhibitor (enalapril), a calcium channel blocker (amlodipine), and an α-receptor blocker (doxazosin). All were given at low doses and once daily.[13] No meaningful differences could be found for symptomatic adverse effects over the first year of the trial. Moreover, dropout rates due to symptoms related to medication were infrequent. This pattern is certainly not the case in all studies; when higher doses are used, subjects often display their lack of comfort on medication by removing themselves from the study. In a large-scale comparison of several drug classes conducted within the Veterans Administration (men only), trends indicated that the centrally acting agent clonidine and the α-receptor blocker prazosin produced more side effects than a diuretic, ACE inhibitor, calcium entry blocker, and β-receptor blocker.[14] In a within class comparison, quality of life indices seemed to improve in patients with captopril compared with little change observed for enalapril.[12] (I find this last study difficult to understand or explain, since the ACE inhibitors seem so similar in their basic mechanisms of action.)

For many patients, mild adverse symptomatic effects become a way of life that is acceptable when weighed against the risk of untreated hypertension. When patients have well-controlled arterial pressure and are compliant, yet indicate some degree of ongoing discomfort, the decision to change drug treatment becomes difficult and requires open discussion. Sometimes the symptoms mentioned bear no relationship to the known pattern of adverse effects reported for the drug in question. If the patient is willing, a double-blind trial (the n-of-1 approach[15]) comparing the drug with a placebo can be performed to establish both efficacy (i.e., whether there is a difference in arterial pressure) and relationship to the adverse effect in question. This may be time consuming, but is highly useful on occasion.

Reversal or Delay of Target Organ Pathology

Many hypertensive persons, either when first identified or during surveillance, have advanced target organ damage. The organ damage most likely to be detected includes (1) left ventricular hypertrophy, (2) microalbuminuria or proteinuria, or (3) mild renal insufficiency (creatinine clearance less than 80 ml/min). Evidence of atherosclerosis, vascular bruits, claudication, or ischemic changes on the electrocardiogram may also be found. Reversal of these abnormalities by reduction of arterial pressure alone is not yet established in all circumstances. However, it is well documented that regression of left ventricular hypertrophy can be achieved,[16] proteinuria can be reduced, and the progression of renal insufficiency (reduced creatinine clearance or glomerular filtration rate) can be delayed.[17] It is appropriate to consider the potential for such reversals or delays in the choice of drug therapy for patients with clinical evidence of target organ pathology.

Compatability With Other Agents

Use of other drugs for cardiovascular and other diseases is often necessary during the treatment of hypertension. This requirement is safer and easier when there is minimal or no risk of adverse drug interactions. Examples of such interactions are given in Table 15-4. The ideal drug for each patient should be chosen with the potential for negative drug interactions in mind.

Affordability

Since treatment of hypertension is a preventative measure, minimizing cost of therapy is imperative. Excessive cost to the patient will inhibit compliance and is a wasteful diversion of health care resources for society at large.[18] Relating cost of treatment to benefit is a problematic and somewhat theoretical exercise for which the therapy of hypertension has been an attractive model.[19–21] Apart from lives spared or strokes prevented, calculations of benefit versus harm or cost of therapy include consideration of adverse effects requiring additional medical care (such as a need for potassium supplements or treatment of a gout attack or drug-induced rash). Introduction of quality of life estimates for comparing various therapies might seem to settle some of the controversies generated by cost/benefit analysis alone in which the units are monetary. In cost-effective analysis, the calculation is made as dollar/quality adjusted years of life.[19] However, there are no simple ways to convert the indices used for such surveys to units of cost, dollars, or other currency.[22] Decisions to prescribe a specific hypertensive therapy instead of another one according to estimates of a better quality of life on the first treat-

Table 15-4. Drug Interactions Related to Antihypertensive Agents

Agents	Interaction
Nonselective β-blockers and insulin	Impaired compensatory response to hypoglycemia
Nonselective β-blockers and bronchodilators	Impaired bronchodilation by β_2-agonists prevents treatment of asthma
β-Blockers and verapamil	Additive negative inotropic effect may worsen cardiac contractility
ACE inhibitors and diuretics	Orthostatic hypotension, impaired renal function in bilateral renal artery stenosis
ACE inhibitors and nonsteroidal anti-inflammatory drugs	Reduced antihypertensive response due to reduction of prostaglandin synthesis
ACE inhibitors and potassium-sparing diuretics	Risk of hyperkalemia
Verapamil and digoxin	Increased plasma digoxin levels
Guanethidine or guanadrel (peripheral neuron depletors) and tricyclic antidepressants	Reduced antihypertensive effect due to blockade of neuron pump

ment need much additional study. At present it is not well known how physicians or their patients perceive what are the "best buys" in this regard.

In summary, the choice of one or more drugs for long-term treatment of hypertension represents one of the major preventative health interventions for adult medicine. These choices should be considered in relationship to optimal therapy, the ideal drug for each patient.

GOALS OF TREATMENT

The reason to treat with antihypertensive medication is reduction of arterial pressure as the basis for prevention of future cardiovascular disease. For all but the elderly (65 years of age or older) effectiveness is based only on the decrease in diastolic pressure in conformity with the clinical trials. By contrast, treatment of isolated systolic hypertension in the elderly appears to be beneficial. Drug treatment is started when the average pretreatment diastolic pressure is at least 95 mmHg when the patient is seated. Reasonable goals for treatment for most patients are to achieve an average diastolic pressure of less than 90 mmHg together with at least a 10-mmHg decrease below pretreatment pressure over a prolonged treatment period. However, excessive reduction of diastolic pressure during treatment—the J-curve effect—may be deleterious.[23,24] For those with mild to moderate hypertension, it is likely that the most appropriate target during drug treatment is a diastolic pressure of approximately 85 mmHg, with an absolute reduction from pretreatment pressure of 10 to 15 mmHg.

Since the demonstration that drug treatment of isolated systolic hypertension in the elderly is beneficial, it is reasonable to include this as a goal of treatment also. Whether a decrement of 15 to 20 mmHg in systolic pressure is a more acceptable goal than a specific level of pressure (e.g., 140 to 150 mmHg) remains unknown. Occasionally, young patients (those younger than 50 years old) have unexplained isolated systolic elevations. Whether these somewhat unique individuals have a better outlook on drug treatment is not yet established. My own approach is to be certain that such patients, if younger than 45 years old, do not have the "white coat syndrome" using 24-hour ambulatory blood pressure monitoring and a 6-month or longer observation period before considering drug treatment.

INITIAL DRUG SELECTION

All antihypertensive drugs reduce arterial pressure in some patients. For mild to moderate hypertensive persons, choice of a single drug (monotherapy) will often be effective. Table 15-5 summarizes the major factors to be considered in making the initial choice of drug treatment.

It is evident from examination of these factors that the choice of the initial drug may be easy in some patients and more difficult in others. It has been suggested by some consensus groups that initial therapy should be based on those drugs that have been shown to be effective in the large randomized

Table 15-5. Factors Determining the Choice of the Initial Antihypertensive Agent

Level of arterial pressure

Age of patient

Nonhypertensive risk status: glucose tolerance, lipids

Stage of cardiac, renal, neurologic, vascular disease

Allergies or other medical conditions (e.g., asthma or obstructive lung disease, depressive syndrome) likely to affect therapy

Clues to mechanism of hypertension, clinical signs of hyperadrenergic state (rapid heart rate), plasma renin activity, age or ethnic status suggestive of low renin status, and so forth

Cost to the patient (care system)

controlled trials, principally the thiazide-type diuretics and β-receptor antagonists.[25] This perspective limits consideration of the more recently available agents, ACE inhibitors and calcium entry blockers, since they have yet to be studied in long-term trials in which mortality and morbidity are the endpoints for primary prevention. Meta-analyses of the clinical trials[26] fail to demonstrate meaningful differences between diuretics and β-blockers for primary prevention, despite some differences in individual trials. With regard to the most consistent endpoint, stroke, it appears that reduction of pressure per se, regardless of the agent used, confers the benefit. For coronary heart disease, the issues are far more complex (see Ch. 5 for detailed discussion). There is no doubt that cost is an issue in the consensus groups' decision to emphasize the initial selection of the diuretics and β-blockers. This is not a trivial issue for either the patient, as payer, or the care system.[21]

The criteria indicated in Table 15-5 imply that cost-effective choices can be made if the patient is given due consideration. For example, an elderly mild hypertensive patient without either nonhypertensive risk factors or target organ damage apart from focal retinal arteriolar sclerosis might do just as well on a low dose of a diuretic drug as on a calcium entry blocker. The difference in cost is substantial. On the other hand, should such a patient develop hyperglycemia on the diuretic, transition to a calcium entry blocker might be entirely justified.

If there is little or no response to initial drug selection, the available options are to (1) increase the dose of the same drug, (2) add a suitable second agent, or (3) switch to a different class (sequential monotherapy). Individual considerations provide the basis for which strategy should be chosen for any one patient.

RATIONALE FOR THE NEXT AGENT

If the first drug chosen has a partial effect on pressure, choice of the next agent should take into account those compensatory mechanisms that may have been stimulated by the initial treatment and now prevent further reduction in pressure. Diuretics, vasodilators (hydralazine), or the dihydropyridine calcium channel blockers may stimulate the renin-angiotensin system. Thus, addition of a β-blocker (suppressing renin release) or an ACE inhibitor will often achieve a greater and, to some extent physiologic, decrease in pressure. Activation of the sympathetic nervous system by the volume-depleting action of diuretics or by the vasodilators may also prevent optimal treatment, providing another reason to select β-blockers and occasionally α-blockers. When β-blockers are chosen as the initial treatment, the hemodynamic effect is a predominant reduction in cardiac output with little change in systemic resistance. Addition of an α-receptor blocker or a dihydropyridine calcium channel blocker may be useful, as both of these drugs reduce systemic vascular resistance.

Addition of some drugs to each other has no additive effect or may be contraindicated for other reasons. β-Blockers suppress renin release; addition of an ACE inhibitor is rarely effective. Centrally acting adrenergic agents have little effect when peripheral α- and β-receptor blockers are already being taken. Both verapamil and β-blockers have negative cardiac chronotropic and inotropic actions; they should not be given together. When the addition of a second agent is fully effective in lowering pressure, cessation of the first may be considered. The patient then reverts to monotherapy. Thus, *sequential monotherapy* is achieved by either switching drugs or by adding a second with subsequent subtraction of the first.

The following section provides more detailed descriptions of the various classes and subclasses of the antihypertensive drugs. Details for individual drugs, including doses and duration of action, are given in Appendix 1.

CLASSIFICATION

Diuretics

Thiazide-Like Diuretics

Diuretic drugs, particularly the thiazide and thiazide-like agents, are effective in reducing blood pressure as monotherapy and in combination with antiadrenergic agents (especially the β-blockers) and ACE inhibitors. Diuretics have been the initial treatment in several randomized clinical trials of antihypertensive therapy. A large number of thiazide congeners and thiazide-like compounds (such as chlorthalidone) are available for use. All act at the distal renal tubule beyond the diluting segment and proximal to the aldosterone-sensitive site to cause net loss of sodium and water. Secondary increases in plasma renin activity cause elevation of aldosterone secretion and hypokalemia. Activation of the renin-angiotensin system limits reduction of arterial pressure because the action of angiotensin II is unopposed. The major action of diuretics in reducing pressure appears to be sustained loss of extracellular salt and water. Whether other mechanisms participate remains uncertain. The hemodynamic effects of sustained diuretic treatment are reduction in both cardiac output (probably secondary to reduced filling volumes) and systemic vascular resistance.

Common adverse effects of the thiazide-type diuretics include hypokalemia, increased serum uric acid, impaired glucose tolerance, and increased serum LDL and total cholesterol. Diuretic-induced hypokalemia and hyperlipidemia have been considered by some as a basis for increased risk opposed to the benefit (risk trade-off) of lowered arterial pressure.[27] Less common adverse effects are hypercalcemia and thrombocytopenia. The former may be due to unmasking of mild primary hyperparathyroidism.

Loop Diuretics

Furosemide, ethacrynic acid, and bumetanide are potent diuretics that act at the diluting segment of the thick ascending limb of the early distal renal tubule where chloride is actively reabsorbed. In general, these drugs have a brief duration of action. They may reduce arterial pressure by causing loss of salt and water, but activate the renin-angiotensin system like the thiazides. The loop diuretics appear to be more effective than thiazides in patients with renal insufficiency. Loop diuretics may be less likely to impair glucose tolerance in noninsulin-dependent diabetics. In specific contrast to the thiazides, the loop diuretics tend to enhance calcium excretion and may be used in the treatment of hypercalcemia.

Potassium-Sparing Agents

Potassium-sparing agents act to impair sodium reabsorption, but limit potassium excretion. Spironolactone is a specific antagonist for aldosterone receptors. Thus, its action is dependent on presence of a mineralocorticoid. By contrast, amiloride and triamterene prevent entry of sodium ion through specific sodium channels that are activated, in part, by mineralocorticoid action. All three drugs are useful in preventing or correcting hypokalemia due to the thiazide-type and loop active agents. It is perhaps important that successful clinical trials of drug treatment for elderly hypertensive patients employed amiloride in combination with hydrochlorothiazide as the active treatment.[28,29] The potassium-sparing agents have minimal antihypertensive effect as monotherapy. These drugs should ordinarily not be used in patients with renal insufficiency or given together with ACE inhibitors or potassium supplements because of the risk of hyperkalemia.

Central Antiadrenergic Agents

Drugs that reduce arterial pressure by an action within the central nervous system that diminishes sympathetic tone include reserpine, which depletes biogenic amines from intraneuronal stores; methyldopa, which has several effects; and the α_2-receptor agonists clonidine, guanabenz, and guanfacine. These agents may lower blood pressure as monotherapy or be additive to diuretics. All have significant sedative effects. Reserpine has been associated with severe depression, nasal congestion, and hyperacidity. The complex effects of methyldopa include inhibition of dopa decarboxylase, acting as a false transmitter after transformation to α-methyldopamine and as a central α_2-agonist, like clonidine. Methyldopa may cause an allergic hepatitis or positive Coombs reaction. The latter is rarely associated with frank hemolysis, possibly because of an impairment in reticuloendothelial function induced by the drug.[30]

The central α_2-agonists are associated with an "overshoot or rebound hypertension," which may occur if these medications are suddenly discontinued. The rapid rise in pressure is due to adrenergic excess with elevated plasma or urine catecholamine levels. Hypertensive crises and cerebrovascular accidents have occurred as a result of α_2-agonist rebound hypertension.

The adverse symptoms and reactions caused by the central adrenergic drugs make them less desirable than more recently developed medications.[2] However, these agents may still be useful when other drugs are unsuitable or ineffective. Methyldopa is still considered useful for hypertension during pregnancy because of its substantial safety record.[31]

Peripheral Antiadrenergic Drugs

Neuron Depletors

Neuron depletor antihypertensive agents include those that reduce sympathetic action outside the central nervous system. Guanethidine, guanadrel, and bethanidine deplete peripheral adrenergic neurons of norepinephrine. All three agents may cause orthostatic hypotension, but differ in that guanadrel and bethamidine have a shorter duration of action. To be effective, these agents enter the adrenergic neuron by an active uptake. This uptake system is inhibited by tricyclic antidepressants (such as imipramine), which can reverse the antihypertensive effect of the peripheral neuron depletors.

β-Receptor Blockers

β-Adrenergic receptor antagonists are effective antihypertensive drugs. They reduce sympathetic effect by selective competitive inhibition of agonist binding to β-receptors in the heart and juxtaglomerular apparatus. β-Blockers lower pressure by diminishing cardiac output and renin secretion. These drugs may have central effects, including reduction of baroreflex activity.

The effects of β-receptor blockade on cardiac function and hemodynamics depend on whether they have intrinsic sympathomimetic action (ISA).[32] β-Blockers *without ISA* (such as propranolol) initially decrease cardiac output due to a fall in heart rate; systemic vascular resistance increases. Subsequently, systemic vascular resistance tends to decrease, perhaps due to autoregulatory changes or to resetting of baroreflex pathways. β-Blockers without ISA reduce both resting and exercise heart rate. By contrast, β-blockers *with ISA* (such as pindolol) increase resting heart rate and cardiac output, but reduce exercise-induced changes. Partial agonist effects of β-blockers with ISA on β_2-vascular receptors may reduce systemic vascular resistance as an initial and as a sustained effect.

As monotherapy, β-blockers appear to be most effective in younger and nonblack patients. A wider spectrum of efficacy is found when β-blockers are added to either a diuretic agent or a dihydropyridine calcium channel blocker for treatment of moderate hypertension.

All β-blockers may be effective for treatment of hypertension. There are, however, differences that may be important in their selection. $β_1$-Selective agents (atenolol, metoprolol, or betaxolol) are less likely to cause pulmonary airway obstruction (a $β_2$-effect). However, $β_1$-selectivity is dose dependent, being less apparent at higher doses. β-Blockers with ISA (e.g., pindolol, acebutolol, or carteolol) have less bradycardia effect than those without ISA (e.g., propranolol, among others). However, the β-blockers with ISA tend to increase heart rate during sleep. Another difference between β-blockers is duration of action; atenolol, nadolol, and betaxolol have prolonged half-lives and are suitable for once a day administration at even small doses. The shorter acting β-blockers (e.g., propranolol) are more lipid soluble and thus may penetrate the blood-brain barrier more easily than the more water-soluble agents. It has been suggested that this difference accounts for a greater frequency of central nervous system side effects (depressive symptoms and sleep disorders) reported with the shorter acting agents.

The most common symptomatic adverse reactions of the β-blockers are fatigue, reduced exercise tolerance, and cold fingers and toes. These are best explained by the primary reduction in cardiac output observed during treatment. Other potential adverse effects are worsening of asthma or obstructive pulmonary disease, impotence, depressive symptoms, and sleep disorders. Symptoms of insulin-induced hypoglycemia may be masked by β-blockers, particularly with the nonselective agents that block $β_2$-receptors and impair the counter-regulatory effect of epinephrine-induced glycogenolysis. Intermittent claudication may be worsened by β-blockers. These drugs may precipitate congestive heart failure in patients with borderline left ventricular systolic function. A silent effect of β-blockers (without ISA) is a small but significant reduction in serum HDL cholesterol; the long-term effect of this change is uncertain.

Despite the spectrum of adverse effects associated with β-blocker therapy, their effectiveness for secondary prevention of coronary heart disease is well established. This applies to β-blockers without ISA, but has yet to be shown for those with ISA. It has been suggested that treatment of mild to moderate hypertension with β-blockers may confer primary prevention of coronary or ischemic heart disease.[33–35] This remains a controversial issue because of conflicting studies.[36]

α-Receptor Blockers

$α_1$-Postsynaptic antagonists (prazosin, terazosin, and doxazosin) reduce peripheral resistance at the arteriolar level due to their inhibition of action of neuronally released norepinephrine. The primary hemodynamic effect of the $α_1$-antagonists is to reduce systemic vascular resistance. The major difference between the various $α_1$-blockers is duration of action. Prazosin has the shortest half-life and must be given two to three times a day. Terazosin is effective when given twice a day, and doxazosin may be prescribed as a once a day agent. All three $α_1$-antagonists have a favorable effect on serum lipids by reducing LDL cholesterol and increasing HDL cholesterol. The changes are small, but significant.[13]

The most common adverse effect of α_1-receptor blockade is orthostatic hypotension, which may be particularly bothersome after the first dose. Adaptation to this effect occurs rapidly; patients are often told to take the first dose (on starting or during upward titration) at bedtime to avoid the orthostatic effect that is likely to occur within an hour or two after dosing.

Phentolamine and phenoxybenzamine are nonspecific α-receptor blockers that act on both postsynaptic and vascular α-receptors. They are indicated only for management of pheochromocytoma where massive circulating catecholamine excess may occur.

Combined α_1- and β-receptor antagonism is effective in a single agent (labetalol) or as a combination of two specific agents. Labetalol is available as a tablet for oral administration and as an intravenous preparation for hypertensive emergencies.

Primary Vasodilators

Nitrates reduce arterial pressure through arterial and venodilation and have a short-term effect. The primary indication for these agents is cardiac ischemia reflected by anginal pain or electrocardiographic evidence of ischemia. Reduction in pressure concurrent with relief of pain is often observed. The long-acting nitrates (isosorbide) have not been shown to be effective sustained antihypertensive drugs.

Intravenous nitroprusside is a rapid, highly effective agent, reducing venous and arteriolar tone. It is useful in hypertensive emergencies where it is given in medical intensive care units. Nitroprusside is highly toxic; the parent compound is converted to thiocyanate. Free cyanide ion may accumulate with long-term use.

Hydralazine and minoxidil are potent arteriolar vasodilators with a similar hemodynamic action—reduction in systemic vascular resistance. However, their administration causes reflex tachycardia, increases cardiac output, and may precipitate angina and ischemic cardiac disease. Fluid retention, due in part to activation of the renin-angiotensin-aldosterone system, often occurs. For these reasons, these agents are often given with diuretics and β-receptor antagonists as "triple therapy" for severe hypertension. These nonspecific vasodilators have mostly been replaced by newer agents for treatment of severe hypertension, particularly ACE inhibitors, the dihydropyridine calcium channel blockers, and α_1-receptor blockers. In addition to tachycardia and fluid retention, well-known adverse effects of hydralazine and minoxidil are a lupus-like syndrome and peripheral neuropathy (hydralazine); and hirsutism, pericardial effusion, and pulmonary hypertension (minoxidil).

Diazoxide is a nonspecific vasodilator with hemodynamic actions like those of hydralazine. Intravenous injections of diazoxide have been effective in hypertensive emergencies. The uncertainty of its effect and risk of substantial hypotension have led to selection of other agents for this purpose in recent years. Prolonged use of diazoxide causes hyperglycemia, which may require insulin therapy.

Renin System Antagonists

Angiotensin Converting Enzyme Inhibitors

The ACE inhibitors are effective antihypertensive agents[37] that interrupt the renin-angiotensin system by preventing conversion of angiotensin I to angiotensin II. This effect reduces arteriolar constriction and aldosterone secretion. ACE inhibitors may also enhance action of the kallikrein-kinin system and stimulate release of vasodilating prostaglandins. While ACE inhibitors may be most effective in high renin states, significant reduction in pressure has been observed in those with normal or even low plasma renin levels. This may be due to potentiation of kinins (converting enzyme also inactivates bradykinin) and stimulation of vasodilatory prostaglandins by kinins. Enhanced sensitivity to angiotensin II may be present in some hypertensive persons, whose pressure is elevated by an excessive action of angiotensin II maintained by a normal or even low renin level. Thus, while the immediate hypotensive effect of ACE inhibitors is correlated with plasma renin activity, long-term antihypertensive effects of these agents are not.

As monotherapy, ACE inhibition is most effective in high renin states, which may occur in younger patients and in whites. However, when combined with diuretics, ACE inhibitors are as effective in black as in white patients. Diuretics activate the renin system, which then prevents further reduction in pressure. Addition of ACE inhibition to diuretic administration is highly effective for control of pressure; the reduction in aldosterone secretion caused by ACE inhibition then limits potassium loss of diuretic treatment.

ACE inhibitors have, in short-term studies, been shown to cause regression of left ventricular hypertrophy in hypertensive patients.[38,39] Their effectiveness in management of congestive heart failure is well established.[40-42] ACE inhibitors may also be valuable for long-term treatment of those with mild left ventricular dysfunction, often found in those with hypertension and ischemic heart disease.[43-45] Experimental studies provide a rationale for the hope that ACE inhibitors will prevent progression of renal insufficiency. Clinical trials have been conducted to test this hypothesis, particularly in those with diabetic nephropathy, the most commonly found cause of renal insufficiency in most populations.[17,46]

Patients with *unilateral renal artery stenosis* may be effectively treated with ACE inhibitors as monotherapy. However, in *bilateral renal artery stenosis* or *stenosis of the artery to a solitary kidney* (as after renal transplantation), reduction of arterial pressure by ACE inhibition may be associated with development of reversible renal insufficiency.[47,48] This effect is due both to the decrease in systemic arterial pressure (reducing renal perfusion) and to loss of constriction by efferent (postglomerular) arterioles, which is needed to maintain intraglomerular filtration pressure when preglomerular stenosis is present.

Adverse effects of ACE inhibitors are infrequent. The most common symptom is a dry, persistent cough, which occurs in 2 to 5 percent of patients taking ACE inhibitors and varies from a minimal irritation to a disabling one. Angioneurotic edema of the tongue or pharynx is a rare but serious adverse effect. Skin rash, loss of taste, leukopenia, and proteinuria were originally reported during captopril treatment when doses used tended to be high and patients with multisystem disease were first studied. It was once suggested that these adverse effects may be more frequent with captopril, because of its sulfhydryl group, than with the nonsulfhydryl agents enalapril and lisinopril. In recent years, the ACE inhibitors, as a class, have been found to be remarkably safe, with little or no clear-cut differences observed for the various agents now available. On balance, ACE inhibitors are well tolerated, causing few of the symptoms associated with diuretic agents, central adrenergic agents, or β-receptor blockers. A direct comparison of captopril, methyldopa, and propranolol demonstrated that the ACE inhibitor resulted in significantly fewer adverse effects that would diminish quality of life.[2] Another potentially positive effect of ACE inhibition is a small but significant reduction in resistance to insulin action, which has been shown for captopril[49] in comparison with hydrochlorothiazide.

ACE inhibitors may be useful for initial therapy of mild to moderate hypertension. If additional antihypertensive effect is desired, combining the ACE inhibitor with low dose diuretics or a calcium channel blocker may reach the therapeutic goal.

New Renin System Inhibitors

Two new subclasses that interrupt the renin-angiotensin system have been developed for experimental exploration and preliminary clinical investigation: the nonpeptide, orally absorbable angiotensin receptor antagonists and the direct renin inhibitors. Losartan (formerly DuP 753) is a nonpeptide, orally active angiotensin II receptor antagonist that has been studied in a small number of hypertensive patients.[50-52] Initial studies reveal, using 24-hour ambulatory blood pressure monitoring, that this agent significantly decreases both systolic and diastolic pressures without changing heart rate. During treatment, plasma renin activity increased without a change in plasma aldosterone, potassium, or creatinine. A small reduction in serum uric acid occurred.[50] Should additional investigations confirm the efficacy of these drugs and provide evidence of adequate safety, the angiotensin antagonists may prove to be useful, particularly for those patients who cannot tolerate the adverse effects (mainly cough) of the ACE inhibitors. The role of specific angiotensin antagonists in congestive heart failure will likely be a subject of considerable future research.

Calcium Channel Entry Blockers

Reduction of arterial pressure in hypertensive patients has been observed with the following calcium channel blockers[53]: the negative chronotropic, inotropic agents verapamil and diltiazem and the dihydropyridines, nifedipine, nicardipine, isradipine, felodipine, and amlodipine, which are primary vasodilators. Verapamil and diltiazem act on cardiac tissue, reducing cardiac contractility, sinus node conduction, and atrioventricular conduction, but are also arterial vasodilators. By contrast, the dihydropyridines decrease pressure primarily by reduction of peripheral resistance.[54] The initial effects of the dihydropyridines are to reduce arterial pressure and increase cardiac output and heart rate. The latter actions may be transient, with heart rate and output returning toward pretreatment levels while pressure (resistance) remains reduced. Calcium channel blockers may cause a mild diuresis in some patients as an additional hypotensive action; weight is slightly decreased. Calcium channel blockers have been shown to cause regression of left ventricular hypertrophy.[55,56] Verapamil[55] and nifedipine (in the GITS formulation[57]) may improve left ventricular diastolic dysfunction during treatment. It is not yet established whether calcium channel blockers prevent progression of renal insufficiency during treatment of those with renal disease. A recent report, however, suggests that calcium channel blockers may prevent the impairment of glomerular filtration rate associated with cyclosporine following renal transplantation.[58]

Calcium channel blockers may be effective as monotherapy in mild to moderate hypertensive persons. They may have special benefit in patients with ischemic heart disease because of the coronary artery vasodilating effect. It has been reported that these blockers are most effective in older patients and equally effective in white and black patients.[59] It has been suggested that calcium channel blockers have no additive action when combined with diuretic drugs or a low salt diet.[60] This remains a controversial issue. Calcium channel blockers have little effect on renin secretion or sympathetic function as long-term therapy; hence, they may be effectively combined with β-blockers or ACE inhibitors. The exception is verapamil, which has the most negative chronotropic and inotropic actions. It should not be used with β-blockers.

Adverse effects associated with calcium channel blockers are headache, flushing of the face, palpitations, and edema of the feet and ankles. The edema is not due to salt and water retention, but to local changes in vascular permeability. It is not associated with weight gain. Flushing, headache, and palpitations seem to be more frequently observed with the shorter acting calcium channel blocker preparations and are less frequently reported with sustained release or controlled release delivery systems. Verapamil and, to a lesser extent, diltiazem may impair cardiac conduction, resulting in atrioventricular conduction abnormalities. As previously mentioned, verapamil is a negative inotropic agent and should be avoided in patients with systolic ventricular dysfunction.

REFERENCES

1. Greenberg RN: Overview of patient compliance with medication dosing: a review of the literature. Clin Ther 6:592, 1984
2. Croog SH, Levine S, Testa MA et al: The effects of antihypertensive therapy on the quality of life. N Engl J Med 314:1657, 1986
3. Jachuck SJ, Brierly H, Jachuck S, Willcox PM: The effect of hypotensive drugs on the quality of life. J R Coll Gen Pract 32:103, 1982
4. Doing better, feeling worse. Lancet 336:1037, 1990

5. Bulpitt CJ, Fletcher AE: The measurement of quality of life in hypertensive patients: a practical approach. Br J Clin Pharmacol 30:353, 1990

6. Fletcher AE, Chester PC, Hawkins CMA et al: The effects of verapamil and propranolol on quality of life in hypertension. J Hum Hypertens 3:125, 1989

7. Fletcher AE, Bulpitt CJ, Hawkins CM et al: Quality of life on anti-hypertensive therapy: a randomized double-blind controlled trial on captopril and atenolol. J Hypertens 8:463, 1990

8. Palmer A, Fletcher A, Hamilton G et al: A comparison of verapamil and nifedipine on quality of life. Br J Clin Pharmacol 30:365, 1990

9. Applegate WB, Phillips HL, Schnaper H et al: A randomized controlled trial of the effects of three antihypertensive agents on blood pressure control and quality of life in older women. Arch Intern Med 151:1817, 1991

10. Skinner MH, Futterman A, Morrisette D et al: Atenolol compared with nifedipine: effect on cognitive function and mood in elderly patients. Ann Intern Med 116:615, 1992

11. Fletcher AE, Bulpitt CJ, Chase DM et al: Quality of life with three antihypertensive treatments: cilazapril, atenolol, nifedipine. Hypertension 19:499, 1992

12. Testa MA, Anderson RB, Nackley JF et al: Hypertension Study Group. Quality of life and antihypertensive therapy in men: a comparison study of captopril and enalapril. N Engl J Med 328:907, 1993

13. Treatment of Mild Hypertension Research Group: The Treatment of Mild Hypertension Study: a randomized, placebo-controlled trial of a nutritional-hygienic regimen along with various drug monotherapies. Arch Intern Med 151:1413, 1991

14. Materson BJ, Reda DJ, Cushman WC et al: Single-drug therapy for hypertension in men: a comparision of six antihypertensive agents with placebo. N Engl J Med 328:914, 1993

15. Guyatt GH, Keller JL, Jaeschke R et al: The n-of-1 randomized controlled trial: clinical usefulness. Ann Intern Med 112:293, 1990

16. Dahlof B, Pennert K, Hansson L: Reversal of left ventricular hypertrophy in hypertensive patients: a metaanalysis of 109 treatment studies. Am J Hypertens 5:95, 1992

17. Kasiske BL, Kalil RSN, Ma JZ et al: Effect of antihypertensive therapy on the kidney in patients with diabetes: a meta-regression analysis. Ann Intern Med 118:129, 1993

18. Fletcher A: Pressure to treat and pressure to cost: a review of cost-effectiveness analysis. J Hypertens 9:193, 1991

19. Weinstein MC, Stason WB: Hypertension: A Policy Perspective. Harvard University Press, Cambridge, 1976

20. Edelson JT, Weinstein MC, Tosteson ANA et al: Long-term cost effectiveness of various initial monotherapies for mild to moderate hypertension. JAMA 263:408, 1990

21. Kawachi I, Malcolm LA: The cost-effectiveness of treating mild to moderate hypertension: reappraisal. J Hypertens 9:199, 1991

22. Scheiner LB, Melmon KL: The utility function of antihypertensive therapy. Ann NY Acad Sci 304:112, 1978

23. Alderman MH, Ooi WL, Madhavan S, Cohen H: Treatment-induced blood pressure reduction and the risk of myocardial infarction. JAMA 262:920, 1989

24. Farnett L, Mulrow CD, Linn WD et al: The J-curve phenomenon and the treatment of hypertension. Is there a point beyond which pressure reduction is dangerous? JAMA 265:489, 1991

25. Joint National Committee on Detection and Treatment of Hypertension: The 5th Report of the Joint National Committee on Detection, Evaluation and Treatment of High Blood Pressure (JNC V). Arch Intern Med 153:154, 1993

26. Collins R, Peto R, MacMahon S et al: Blood pressure, stroke, and coronary heart disease. Part 2. Short-term reductions in blood pressure: overview of randomized drug trials in their epidemiological context. Lancet 335:827, 1990

27. Grimm RH, Leon AS, Hunninghake DB et al: Effects of thiazide diuretics on plasma lipids and lipoproteins in mildly hypertensive patients: a double blind controlled trial. Ann Intern Med 94:7, 1981

28. Dahlof B, Lindholm LH, Hansson L et al: Morbidity and mortality in the Swedish Trial in Old Patients with hypertension (STOP-Hypertension). Lancet 338:1281, 1991

29. Medical Research Council Working Party: Medical Research Council trial of treatment of hypertension in older adults: principal results. BMJ 304:405, 1992

30. Kelton JG: Impaired reticuloendothelial function in patients treated with methyldopa. N Engl J Med 313:596, 1985

31. Cunningham FG, Lindheimer MD: Current concepts: hypertension in pregnancy. N Engl J Med 326:927, 1992

32. van den Meiraker AH, Man in't Veld AJ, van Eck RHJ et al: Hemodynamic and hormonal adaptations to beta-adrenoceptor blockade. Circulation 78:957, 1988

33. IPPPSH Collaborative Group: Cardiovascular risk and risk factors in a randomized trial of treatment based on the beta-blocker oxprenolol: the International Prospective Primary Prevention Study in Hypertension (IPPPSH). J Hypertens 3:379, 1985

34. Wikstrand J, Warnold I, Olsson G et al: Primary prevention with metoprolol in patients with hypertension: mortality results from the MAPHY study. JAMA 259:1976, 1988

35. Psaty BM, Koepsell TD, LoGerfo JP et al: Beta-blockers and primary prevention of coronary heart disease in patients with hypertension. JAMA 261:2087, 1989

36. Wilhelmsen L, Berglund G, Elmfeldt D et al: Beta-blockers versus diuretics in hypertensive men: main results from the HAPPHY trial. J Hypertens 5:561, 1987

37. Williams GH: Converting-enzyme inhibitors in the treatment of hypertension. N Engl J Med 319:1517, 1988

38. Nakashima Y, Fouad FM, Tarazi RC: Regression of left ventricular hypertrophy from systemic hypertension by enalapril. Am J Cardiol 53:1044, 1984

39. Asmar RB, Pannier B, Santoni JP et al: Reversion of cardiac hypertrophy and reduced arterial compliance after converting enzyme inhibition in essential hypertension. Circulation 78:941, 1988

40. CONSENSUS Trial Study Group: Effects of enalapril on mortality in severe congestive heart failure: results of the Cooperative North Scandinavian Enalapril Survival Study (CONSENSUS). N Engl J Med 316:1429, 1987

41. SOLVD Investigators: Effect of enalapril on survival in patients with reduced left ventricular ejection fractions and congestive heart failure. N Engl J Med 325:293, 1991

42. Cohn JN, Johnson G, Ziesche S et al: A comparison of enalapril with hydralazine-isosorbide dinitrate in the treatment of chronic congestive heart failure. N Engl J Med 325:303, 1991

43. SOLVD Investigators: Effect of enalapril on mortality and the development of heart failure in asymptomatic patients with reduced left ventricular ejection fractions. N Engl J Med 327:685, 1992

44. Yusuf S, Pepine CJ, Garces C et al: Effect of enalapril on myocardial infarction and unstable angina in patients with low ejection fractions. Lancet 340:1173, 1992

45. Pfeffer MA, Braunwald E, Moye LA et al: Effect of captopril on mortality and morbidity in patients with left ventricular dysfunction after myocardial infarction: results of the survival and ventricular enlargement trial. N Engl J Med 327:669, 1992

46. Keane WF, Anderson S, Aurell M et al: Angiotensin converting enzyme inhibitors and progressive renal insufficiency. Ann Intern Med 111:503, 1990

47. Hricik DE, Browning PJ, Kopelman R et al: Captopril-induced functional renal insufficiency in patients with bilateral renal-artery stenoses or renal-artery stenosis in a solitary kidney. N Engl J Med 308:373, 1983

48. Curtis JJ, Luke RG, Whelchel JD et al: Inhibition of angiotensin-converting enzyme in renal-transplant recipients with hypertension. N Engl J Med 308:377, 1983

49. Pollare T, Lithell H, Berne C: A comparison of the effects of hydrochlorothiazide and captopril on glucose and lipid metabolism in patients with hypertension. N Engl J Med 321:868, 1989

50. Tsunoda K, Abe K, Hagino T et al: Hypotensive effect of losartan, a nonpeptide angiotensin II receptor antagonist, in essential hypertension. Am J Hypertens 6:28, 1993

51. Weber MA: Clinical experience with the angiotensin II receptor antagonist losartan. A preliminary report. Am J Hypertens 5:247S, 1992

52. Munafo A, Christen Y, Nussberger J et al: Drug concentration response relationships in normal volunteers after oral administration of losartan, an angiotensin II receptor antagonist. Clin Pharmacol Ther 51:513, 1992

53. Kaplan NM: Calcium entry blockers in the treatment of hypertension. JAMA 262:817, 1989

54. Andersson OK, Persson B, Hedner T et al: Blood pressure control and haemodynamic adaptation with the dihydropyridine calcium antagonist isradipine: a controlled study in middle-aged hypertensive men. J Hypertens 7:465, 1989

55. Schulman SP, Weiss JL, Becher LC et al: The effects of antihypertensive therapy on left ventricular mass in elderly patients. N Engl J Med 322:1350, 1990

56. Geizhals M, Phillips RA, Ardeljan M, Krakoff LR: Sustained calcium channel blockade in the treatment of severe hypertension. Am J Hypertens 3:313S, 1990

57. Phillips RA, Ardeljan M, Shimabukuro S et al: Normalization of left ventricular mass and associated changes in neurohormones and atrial natriuretic peptide after 1 year of sustained nifedipine therapy for severe hypertension. J Am Coll Cardiol 17:1595, 1991

58. Hauser AC, Derfler K, Stockenhuber F et al: Effect of calcium-channel blockers on renal function in renal-graft recipients treated with cyclosporine. N Engl J Med 324:1517, 1991

59. Cubeddu LX, Aranda J, Singh B et al: Comparison of verapamil and propranolol for the initial treatment of hypertension: racial differences in response. JAMA 256:2214, 1986

60. Nicholson JP, Resnick LM, Laragh JH: The antihypertensive effect of verapamil at extremes of dietary sodium intake. Ann Intern Med 107:319, 1987

16

EMERGENCIES

Hypertensive emergencies are a group of disorders characterized by both markedly elevated arterial pressure and clinical evidence that a life-threatening event is present or nearly at hand. With these disorders the pressure is sufficiently elevated that its reduction is immediately necessary.

A hypertensive emergency is defined both by the level of arterial pressure (usually a diastolic pressure of 130 mmHg or more in adults)—evidence that the pressure has increased suddenly and recently—and symptoms, signs, and findings of a serious life-threatening condition. The success of programs for indentification and treatment of hypertension has markedly reduced the incidence of hypertensive emergencies during the past several decades. Nonetheless, these problems still occur and should be anticipated, especially in the emergency departments of urban centers.[1] In addition to well-described diagnostic entities, several new syndromes causing hypertensive emergencies may be encountered.

Table 16-1 lists those conditions for which immediate reduction of arterial pressure is advisable, usually through the use of intravenous agents. Patients with these conditions should be managed in a medical intensive care unit or equivalent facility with experienced nursing personnel and the availability of specialized services to provide optimum support.

PATHOPHYSIOLOGY AND DIAGNOSIS

The hypertensive emergencies comprise diseases that have in common markedly elevated arterial pressure, but differ, to some extent, from each other in the specific mechanisms that have caused the elevation. For some of these disorders, more than one cause may be participating. The initial evaluation of a patient with a hypertensive emergency will be brief and focused on the most obvious urgent problems. However, unless the patient is in full-blown ("flash") pulmonary edema or is unconscious, a rapid pertinent history can usually be obtained. The physical examination should quickly include evaluation of the retinae, and the pulmonary, cardiac, and neurologic status. There is time to listen for cervical and abdominal bruits and evaluate the extremities for pulsation and edema. Chest or upper abdominal pain requires an electrocardiogram and chest radiograph as minimal measures to distinguish between myocardial ischemia and aortic dissection. Subsequent use of echocardiography (transthoracic or transesophageal in selected cases)

Table 16-1. Hypertensive Emergencies

Hypertensive encephalopathy
Dissecting aortic aneurism
Intracerebral or subarachnoid hemorrhage
Acute pulmonary edema
Syndrome of malignant hypertension
    Due to essential hypertension
    Due to secondary hypertension: scleroderma renal crisis, renal artery stenosis,
        pheochromocytoma, other causes
Unstable angina or acute myocardial infarction with hypertension
Acute cerebral infarction or ischemia with hypertension
Toxemia of pregnancy
Hypertensive drug reactions: amphetamine, hallucinogens, cocaine,
    over-the-counter diet pills, monoamine oxidase inhibitor/tyramine syndrome, α_2-
    agonist withdrawal syndrome, alcohol withdrawal syndrome

or computed tomography (CT) scanning may be necessary if dissection is strongly suspected. Neurologic abnormalities may be due to hypertensive encephalopathy or to focal intracranial disease—hemorrhage or infarction. Appropriate use of modern neurologic imaging (CT scan or magnetic resonance imaging [MRI]) may be helpful for determining optimal management. Ordinarily, antihypertensive therapy should be started promptly and maintained during completion of the diagnostic assessments.

The routine laboratory studies are rarely decisive for the initial management of hypertensive emergencies, but the blood count, urinalysis, and determination of serum electrolyte, urea nitrogen, and creatinine levels offer useful information for subsequent consideration. Microangiopathic hemolysis (schistocytes, burr, and helmet cells) on the peripheral blood smear point to malignant hypertension. Hypokalemia suggests secondary aldosteronsim due to a high renin state, as in renal artery stenosis or scleroderma renal crisis (and some patients with the malignant phase of essential hypertension). Evidence of chronic renal disease in the form of proteinura with casts may be revealed by the urinalysis. Renal function is quantified by measurement of the serum urea nitrogen and creatinine levels.

Familiarity with the various specific hypertensive emergencies is crucial for informed management. The following sections briefly summarize the most pertinent mechanisms and diagnostic features. Implications for therapy are noted where pertinent. The most often used drugs for hypertensive emergencies are listed in Table 16-2.

HYPERTENSIVE ENCEPHALOPATHY

Any patient with a history of a sudden increase in arterial pressure to very high levels in association with an alteration in neurologic status may be considered to have hypertensive encephalopathy. Most often, severe heachache, blurred vision, nausea, vomiting, confusion, seizures, and minor focal abnormalities will be present, along with papilledema and retinal hemorrhages and exudates. In general, major focal deficits will be absent, as will signs of meningeal irritation. This disorder must be distinguished from cerebral trauma, intracranial hemorrhage, brain tumor, pseudotumor, and even encephalitis. Appropriate use of the CT scan and examination of cerebrospinal fluid by lumbar puncture is necessary.

The mechanism of hypertensive encephalopathy is a breakthrough of autoregulation of cerebral blood flow due to the abrupt increase in perfusion pressure.[1] This leads to capillary hyperfiltration, focal cerebral edema, and neurologic dysfunction. Prompt and controlled reduction in arterial pressure is necessary, but within the limits of autoregulation. In most hypertensive persons, the autoregulatory range is moved upward compared with normal. Thus, during treatment of hypertensive encephalopathy, the initial reduction of pressure should be kept to a 20- to 30-mmHg decrease in diastolic pressure (to 90 to 110 mmHg). Otherwise, cerebral ischemia may occur if perfusion pressure falls below the autoregulatory range. Lowering the arterial pressure by any appropriate drug leads to clearing of the neurologic picture, which may take days to weeks for full recovery.

DISSECTING AORTIC ANEURYSM

The initial clues to aortic dissection are usually severe "ripping" pain with hypertension, variably unequal pulses, a new murmur of aortic valve insufficiency, and a widened mediastinal shadow on chest radiograph. The diagno-

Table 16-2. Drugs That Are Effective for Management of Hypertensive Emergencies

Drug	Type
Intravenous agents	
Nitroprusside	Arteriolar and venodilator
Labetolol	α- and β-Receptor blocker
Trimethaphan	Ganglionic blocking agent
Enalapril	Angiotensin converting enzyme inhibitor
Phentolamine	α-Receptor blocker
Nitroglycerine	Venous, arterial, and coronary vasodilator
Hydralazine, diazoxide	Arteriolar vasodilator
Propranolol, metoprolol, esmolol	β-Blockers
Nicardipine	Vasodilator calcium entry blocker
Methyldopa	Central antiadrenergic agent
Furosemide, bumetanide	Rapid "loop" site diuretics
Oral agents	
Nifedipine, bite and swallow	Vasodilator calcium entry blocker
Clonidine	α_2-Receptor agonist
Captopril	Angiotensin converting enzyme inhibitor
Nitroglycerine, sublingual	Nitrate vasodilator, coronary dilator

sis may be suspected or confirmed by ultrasound (echo). Transesophageal methods may be more sensitive than transthoracic assessment. CT scans or MRI are often definitive.

Severe hypertension often, but not always, precedes aortic dissection. Marfan syndrome or a solitary congenital or acquired abnormality of the aorta alone should be suspected. The degree of hypertension present when the patient is seen with the dissection represents both the previous status and the elevation due to pain, hence an adrenergic component. Both the mean distending pressure and the rate of rise in aortic pressure are thought to contribute to the aortic tear and its propagation. Treatment is directed toward the prompt and controlled reduction of arterial pressure and of the rate of rise in aortic pressure. The administration of intravenous nitroprusside in combination with a β-blocker is clearly indicated. The intravenous ganglionic blocking agent trimethaphan can sometimes be useful as a substitute.

INTRACEREBRAL OR SUBARACHNOID HEMORRHAGE

Severe hypertension of any cause is a risk factor for intracerebral or subarachnoid hemorrhage. However, when these catastrophes occur, additional elevations in pressure may be due to activation of sympathoadrenal mechanisms triggered by neurologic pathways. Intravenous labetalol can be useful, but reduction in arterial pressure should be cautious and controlled. In addition, spasm of meningeal or cerebral vessels may contribute to deterioration. Use of nimodipine, a calcium entry blocker that crosses the blood-brain barrier, may be beneficial for preventing or reversing vasospasm in subarachnoid hemorrhage.[2] Nimodipine can also reduce arterial pressure to a variable extent. Once the clinical condition is stable, imaging studies are necessary for accurate anatomic diagnosis and subsequent decisions regarding management. Neurosurgical evacuation of an intracranial hematoma may be necessary.

ACUTE PULMONARY EDEMA

Sudden occurrence of severe dyspnea with cough productive of frothy pink sputum and associated severe hypertension has acquired the term *flash pulmonary edema*. This condition is caused by abrupt congestion of the pulmonary circulation due to the increased afterload impeding left ventricular ejection and impaired diastolic filling of the left ventricle.[3] Tachycardia is often present, reducing the diastolic filling interval. Increased venous return and right ventricular pumping of returned blood to the lungs augments preload. Acute pulmonary edema may complicate essential or secondary hypertension. It may be a specific complication of bilateral renal artery stenosis in elderly patients due to excessive vasoconstriction by an activated renin system and impaired renal excretion of extracellular fluid overload at even high arterial pressures.[4]

Treatment of acute pulmonary edema due to hypertension includes reduction of arterial pressure and diuresis. Sedation with morphine and oxygen by mask are necessary. Intravenous furosemide is often effective, having an initial venodilating effect and a subsequent diuresis. Decreased arterial pressure may be achieved by nitroprusside, nitroglycerine, and/or intravenous enalapril. The nitrate vasodilators have the advantage of reducing preload by a venodilator effect, as well as decreasing afterload. Direct arteriolar vasodilation by agents with little or no negative cardiac inotropic effect (dihydropyridine calcium channel blockers, hydralazine, diazoxide) may be beneficial. β-Blockers and verapamil (negative inotropic agents) are usually contraindicated because of the threat of impaired cardiac systolic function. If the dominant cardiac abnormality is impaired diastolic function (which is worsened by rapid heart rate), *cautious* use of these agents may be attempted. Increasingly, use of echocardiography is helpful in distinguishing between impaired systolic and diastolic function in the pathogenesis of severe pulmonary congestion.[3] In severe pulmonary edema, face mask oxygen delivered at positive pressure can be life saving and can reduce the need for tracheal intubation when compared with oxygen delivered by mask at ambient pressures.[5] However, endotracheal intubation is sometimes required for adequate ventilation.

MALIGNANT HYPERTENSION

When patients are seen with severe hypertension and grade III (retinal hemorrhages and exudates) or grade IV (papilledema) retinopathy, the diagnosis of malignant hypertension is established. Variable degrees of pulmonary congestion due to left ventricular decompensation and renal pathology may be present. Signs of left ventricular hypertrophy and strain are often found on the electrocardiogram. The cause of this clinical constellation may be uncontrolled essential hypertension or an identifiable form of secondary hypertension. The need to decrease arterial pressure, however, precludes an extensive diagnostic assessment before starting treatment. In our experience, the most common forms of associated secondary hypertension are (1) renal artery stenosis and (2) scleroderma renal crisis. Various chronic renal diseases may be present. Pheochromocytoma should be, at least briefly, considered. If encephalopathy is prominent and arterial pressure is not elevated above 130 mmHg diastolic pressure, a primary intracranial disease (e.g., subdural hematoma, brain tumor) should be kept in mind.

The various causes of the the syndrome of malignant hypertension imply different therapies. An activated renin-angiotensin system accounts for scleroderma renal crisis and malignant hypertension due to renal artery stenosis. Intravenous enalapril or captopril by mouth are the most rapid and appropriate means for decreasing pressure. Where there is evidence that fluid volume retention is a dominant mechanism, as in chronic renal disease or essential hypertension complicated by advanced nephrosclerosis, intravenous furosemide may be effective or hemodialysis may be necessary. Malignant hypertension due to uncontrolled essential hypertension is a complex entity in which vasoconstriction due to the renin system or local vascular mechanisms may be prominent. Weight gain and edema, if present, imply that volume retention is also a factor in pathogenesis. Selection of drug treatment should take these mechanisms into account. Combining an angiotensin converting enzyme inhibitor with a dihydropyridine calcium channel blocker may be highly effective. Addition of a diuretic will depend on evidence of volume retention. Finally, if suggestive evidence of a hyperadrenergic syndrome (such as pheochromocytoma) is present, intravenous phentolamine or labetolol is appropriate.

HYPERTENSION WITH UNSTABLE ANGINA OR ACUTE MYOCARDIAL INFARCTION

Patients with acute chest pain due to unstable angina or evolving myocardial infarction may have elevated arterial pressure. Reflex mechanisms may account for this finding. Treatment directed at the underlying cause may be effective, especially intravenous nitroglycerine or selective administration of β-receptor blockers and/or calcium channel entry blocking agents. The role of antithrombotic or thrombolytic agents in *hypertensive* patients who have acute ischemic cardiac syndromes is not certain due to the suspected greater risk of deleterious hemorrhage in these patients. Patients with hypertension at entry usually have been excluded from the trials of antithrombotic or thrombolytic agents. Caution in their use is strongly advised.

HYPERTENSION DUE TO ACUTE CEREBRAL ISCHEMIA

Hypertensive episodes may occur during the course of ischemic cerebral events that are either self-limited (transient ischemic attacks or reversible ischemic neurologic deficits) or evolve to complete infarctions. Presumably such episodes are due to sympathoadrenal activation as a result of ischemia or irritation at hypothalamic or brain stem sites. It has been suggested that the increased pressure is a compensatory mechanism for preserving cerebral perfusion and that reduction in pressure may be harmful, in contrast to the consensus that reduced arterial pressure is beneficial for prevention of stroke. No clinical trials have yet resolved this issue. Nimodipine, a calcium channel blocker that crosses the blood-brain barrier and that can reduce arterial pressure, has been assessed in acute ischemic stroke, with conflicting results in two studies.[6,7]

TOXEMIA OF PREGNANCY

An increase in arterial pressure to higher than 90 mmHg diastolic during the third trimester of pregnancy that is associated with proteinuria, edema, and altered neurologic status (most often seizures) defines eclampsia of pregnancy. A variant that includes *h*emolysis, elevated *l*iver enzymes, *l*ow *p*latelets (thrombocytopenia) is called the HELLP syndrome; renal failure may also occur. Upper abdominal pain may be a clue to this entity. In severe toxemia or eclampsia of pregnancy, both the patient and the fetus are at risk. The hemodynamic status of such patients is due to vasoconstriction with reduced blood volume; hence, diuretic agents are generally avoided. Appropriate antihypertensive agents are intravenous or intramuscular hydralazine, diazoxide (given by intermittent boluses intravenously), or methyldopa. Nitroprusside and the intravenous ganglionic blocker trimethaphan are contraindicated because of risk to the fetus.[1] Angiotensin converting enzyme inhibitors may cause impaired renal development and function in the fetus during the third trimester and thus are also contraindicated.[8] There has been controversy about the role of β-receptor blockers in pregnancy because of concern about the potential of propranol to cross the placental barrier and cause fetal bradycardia. Atenolol, however, has been shown to be beneficial for pregnancy-induced hypertension.[9] Nifedipine, a calcium entry blocker, may also be effective.[10] There is general agreement that expedient delivery of the fetus reverses eclampsia. Hypertension that persists 4 to 6 weeks beyond the end of pregnancy should be considered a chronic condition; evaluation for reversible causes and long-term treatment is indicated.

HYPERTENSIVE DRUG REACTIONS

Hypertensive episodes are associated with headache, anxiety or agitation, and tachycardia in the presence of a variety of licit and illicit drugs: amphetamines, diet pills (phenylpropanolamine), cocaine, hallucinogens, monoamine oxidase inhibitor with tyramine-containing foods, α_2-agonist withdrawal, or even alcohol withdrawal. In general, these reactions are due to activation of the sympathoadrenal nervous system. In one case report, it was suggested that concurrent use of a nonsteroidal anti-inflammatory drug (inhibiting vasodilatory prostaglandin synthesis) potentiated the effect of diet pill overdose. The evidence that all these disorders share a common mechanism—excessive stimulation of either the sympathetic system directly or its α- and β-receptors—provides the therapeutic rationale for adrenergic receptor blockade. Either intravenous phentolamine with or without a parenteral β-receptor blocker or intravenous labetolol may be beneficial. In α_2-agonist withdrawal or alcohol withdrawal syndromes, oral clonidine may be the most effective approach, since there is evidence that the sympathetic excess is due to central activation that is suppressible by central α_2-receptor stimulaton.

HYPERTENSIVE URGENCIES

Patients with severe hypertension (diastolic pressure of 115 mmHg or higher) that is untreated or previously treated often appear at emergency departments because of minor complaints, not necessarily related to their blood pressure and without signs of the hypertensive emergencies described in the previous sections. While such patients are at high risk of future cardiovascular disease, their *immediate* risk is low. Some patients can be restarted on their previous treatment if they have simply run out of their pills. Intravenous drugs, labetolol, and nicardipine (a calcium channel blocker of the dihydropyridine type) have been studied in such patients.[11] However, effective treatment can be achieved by administration of rapidly acting oral agents such as clonidine, captopril, or nifedipine. The advantage of the latter two agents is that they do not sedate the patient by altering the function of the central nervous system, as does clonidine. The risk of rapid blood pressure reduction in such patients is that of acute myocardial ischemia, which has been observed with several vasodilators and nifedipine.[12] If patients are properly screened, however, this risk is quite low. Minor reversible T-wave abnormalities without chest pain during a rapid decrease in pressure may be due to transient repolarization abnormalities unrelated to ischemia.[13]

There is no evidence that these severely hypertensive patients will incur any benefit from a brief reduction in their pressure,[14] unless the pressure is kept under control by entry and maintainence in a long-term management program where *sustained treatment* of arterial pressure will prevent future cardiovascular disease.[15,16]

AFTER THE EMERGENCY IS OVER

Once the patient's blood pressure is controlled and the acute emergency situation is past, diagnostic reassessment should be undertaken to search for causes of reversible hypertension. If a patient is sick enough to be hospitalized for hypertension, it is reasonable to believe that failure to detect and eliminate one of the correctable forms of secondary hypertension will not fully address the patient's disorder. I recommend that all patients admitted for hypertensive emergencies be re-evaluated for likely reversible disease: pheochromocytoma and renal artery stenosis are often overlooked, especially in elderly patients.[17–19] Should a curable cause of hypertension not be found, every effort should be made to convice the patient to remain compliant with antihypertensive therapy,

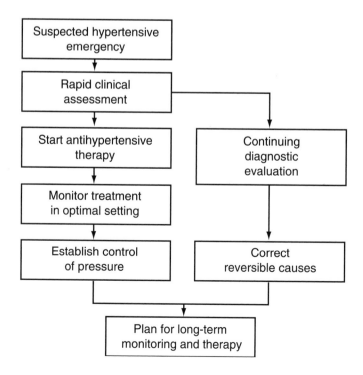

because that is the most likely method to prevent future cardiovascular disease. Development of simplified drug regimens relying on once-a-day, long-acting agents will definitely be helpful in minimizing noncompliance.[20]

REFERENCES

1. Calhoun DA, Oparil S: Current concepts—treatment of hypertensive crisis. N Engl J Med 323:1177, 1990

2. Allen GS, Ahn HS, Preziosi T et al: Cerebral arterial spasm: a controlled trial of nimodipine in patients with subarachnoid hemorrhage. N Engl J Med 308:619, 1983

3. Topol EJ, Traill GV, Fortuin NJ: Hypertensive cardiomyopathy of the elderly. N Engl J Med 312:277, 1985

4. Pickering TG, Herman L, Devereux RB et al: Recurrent pulmonary oedema in hypertension due to bilateral renal artery stenosis: treatment by angioplasty or surgical revascularization. Lancet 2:551, 1988

5. Berstein AD, Holt AW, Vedig AE et al: Treatment of severe cardiogenic pulmonary edema with continuous positive airway pressure delivered by face mask. N Engl J Med 325:1825, 1991

6. Gelmers HJ, Gorter K, De Weerdt CJ, Wiezer HJA: A controlled trial of nimodipine in acute ischemic stroke. N Engl J Med 318:203, 1988

7. Trust Study Group: Randomised double-blind, placebo controlled trial of nimodipine in acute stroke. Lancet 336:1205, 1990

8. Hanssens M, Keirse MJ, Vankelecom F, Van Assche FA: Fetal and neonatal effects of treatment with angiotensin-converting enzyme inhibitors in pregnancy. Obstet Gynecol 78:128, 1991

9. Lowe SA, Rubin PC: The pharmacological management of hypertension in pregnancy. J Hypertens 10:201, 1992

10. Fenakel K, Fenakel G, Appelman Z et al: Nifedipine in the treatment of severe preeclampsia. Obstet Gynecol 77:331, 1991

11. Wallin JD: Intravenous nicardipine hydrochloride: treatment of patients with severe hypertension. Am Heart J 119:434, 1990

12. O'Mailia JJ, Sander GE, Giles TD: Nifedipine-associated myocardial ischemia or infarction in the treatment of hypertensive urgencies. Ann Intern Med 107:185, 1987

13. Phillips RA, Goldman ME, Ardeljan M et al: Isolated T-wave abnormalities and evaluation of left ventricular wall motion after nifedipine for severe hypertension. Am J Hypertens 4:432, 1991

14. Fagan TC: Acute reduction of blood pressure in asymptomatic patients with severe hypertension: an idea whose time has come—and gone. Arch Intern Med 149:2169, 1989

15. Veterans Administration Cooperative Study Group on Antihypertensive Agents: Effects of treatment on morbidity in hypertension: results in patients with diastolic blood pressures averaging 115 through 129 mm Hg. JAMA 202:1028, 1967

16. Veterans Administration Cooperative Study Group on Antihypertensive Agents: Effects of treatment on morbidity in hypertension. II. Results in patients with diastolic blood pressure averaging 90 through 114 mm Hg. JAMA 213:1143, 1970

17. Cooper ME, Goodman D, Frauman A et al: Pheochromocytoma in the elderly: a poorly recognized entity? BMJ 293:1474, 1986

18. Vidt DG: Geriatric hypertension of renal origin: diagnosis and management. Geriatrics 42:59, 1987

19. Messina LM, Zelenock GB, Yao KA, Stanley JC: Renal revascularization for recurrent pulmonary edema in patients with poorly controlled hypertension and renal insufficiency: a distinct subgroup of patients with arteriosclerotic renal artery occlusive disease. J Vasc Surg 15:73, 1992

Section IV

SPECIAL PROBLEMS

17

ELDERLY PATIENTS

Nearly all physicians, caring for adults, have a large and increasing fraction of older (defined here as greater than 65 years of age) patients in their practices. This trend, in part, reflects the increased survival of patients who in prior decades would have died of various causes. In this regard, the most important change over the past 20 years has been the reduction in death due to cardiovascular disease, stroke, and coronary heart disease. The individuals who are living longer as a result of this reduction are not free of cardiovascular risk or disease. Indeed, they are equally or more likely to have future cardiovascular morbidity or mortality, but at a later age.

Compared with those less than 65 years of age, an older population presents with an array or spectrum of signs and symptoms that require clinical management. These signs and symptoms have two major components: (1) those related to the aging process itself and (2) the disease burden that accrues with the years of exposure to risk factors and other causative processes. These separate characteristics are summarized in Table 17-1. They form the rationale for shifts in emphasis for both diagnosis and treatment of elderly patients.

DIAGNOSTIC CONSIDERATIONS

Figure 17-1 displays, as a simplified diagram, the increased likelihood that an older hypertensive patient will have more target organ damage (cardiovascular and renal disease) than a younger one, but is less likely to have secondary hypertension. The specific forms of either secondary hypertension or target organ damage that may occur in the elderly are somewhat predictable and should be assessed first during initial appraisals, as described in the following sections.

Arterial Pressure

Typically, the older hypertensive patient will have a relatively high systolic pressure with the same diastolic pressure as a younger one (i.e., 180/100 mmHg for the 70-year-old compared with 150/100 mmHg for the 50-year-old). In addition, the older patient will more often have an orthostatic decrease (greater than 10 mmHg) in systolic pressure (with or without symptoms) and may also have other sources of variability in pressure, such as postprandial hypotension. A small fraction of the elderly will have isolated systolic hypertension (pressure above 160 mmHg systolic and below 90 mmHg dias-

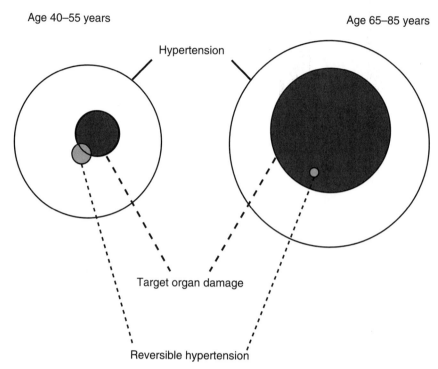

Fig. 17-1. Relationship between age and likelihood of reversible secondary hypertension or target organ damage in hypertensive patients. Estimates were obtained and pooled from several studies.

tolic), a condition that warrants consideration for treatment. In addition, because of impaired baroreflex function, blood pressure is more variable in the elderly, giving a firm basis for the necessity of repeated measurements to yield an adequate baseline before therapy. Supplemental blood pressure determinations from home measurements by the patient, companion, or caretaker or ambulatory blood pressure monitoring can be useful in completing the assessment.[1,2]

Nonhypertensive Risk Factors

Evaluation of nonhypertensive risk factors follows the principles that apply to younger patients, but with each decade above the age of 60 patterns shift and strategy becomes less certain. Persons with multiple risk factors tend to die before age 75 so that those who do reach 80 years of age and beyond, with good overall health, but having either hyperlipidemia or uncomplicated non-insulin-dependent diabetes have, in a sense, adapted to their risk status by beating the odds. There is, moreover, little or no evidence from controlled trials that aggressive reduction of these risk factors in those older than 75 years of age favorably affects outcome. This is especially so for cholesterol, and I avoid prescribing cholesterol-lowering medications in these patients. Cessation of smoking is desirable at any age. However, when an older patient

Table 17-1. Characteristics of Elderly Hypertensive Patients

Age-related

Reduced cardiac β-receptor–mediated responsiveness: tendency for slow heart rate and decreased heart rate response to exercise and demand; resting and exercise cardiac output maintained more by stroke volume

Tendency to left ventricular hypertrophy, independent of hypertension

Reduced rate of left ventricular early diastolic filling; in presence of left ventricular hypertrophy, may increase pulmonary capillary pressure with tendency to chronic congestion

Increased stiffness (reduced compliance) of large arteries, augmented by diabetes, smoking, and hyperlipidemia

Delayed excretion of salt/volume load and possibly impaired ability to maintain intravascular volume when salt/volume depleted

Tendency to lower plasma renin activity and aldosterone concentrations, both unstimulated and stimulated; may account for limited ability to maintain normal fluid volumes, greater likelihood of salt depletion, and dehydration

Disease-related

Greater prevalence of ischemic cardiac disease, myocardial infarction, impaired left ventricular systolic dysfunction, and tendency to arrhythmias

Greater prevalence of atherosclerotic occlusive arterial disease of coronary, cerebrovascular, renal, and peripheral arteries; greater prevalence of abdominal aortic aneurysm

Higher incidence and prevalence of diabetes mellitus (usually noninsulin dependent) and cardiovascular complications of earlier diabetes

Presence of other diseases and organ impairment: obstructive pulmonary disease, depression, neoplasms, and so forth

Less likelihood of most forms of secondary (reversible) hypertension, but greater likelihood of atherosclerotic renal artery disease

stops smoking, it may be as beneficial for those younger family members and friends who are less exposed via passive smoking as it is for the patient.

Target Organ Damage

Figure 17-1 and Table 17-1 clearly show that a major difference between younger and older hypertensive patients is the far greater prevalence of target organ damage or an advanced stage of cardiovascular disease in the latter group. Abnormalities in cardiac function, cerebral vasculature, renal function, peripheral arterial perfusion, and the abdominal aorta (e.g., aneurysm) imply greater absolute risk of future disease and mortality. The presence of such pathology needs to be acknowledged in therapeutic decisions. Table 17-2 lists target organ damage or dysfunction often found in elderly hypertensive persons if appropriate tests are performed.

SECONDARY HYPERTENSION

Most forms of reversible secondary hypertension are less likely to be found in older hypertensive patients. Some forms, such as oral contraceptive hypertension and congenital coarctation of the aorta, should be entirely absent.

Table 17-2. Target Organ Abnormalities Most Often Detected in Elderly Hypertensive Patients

Abnormality	Comment
Retinal arterial sclerosis: focal or diffuse, "copper" or "silver wire" changes	While often found and the only direct evidence of arteriolosclerosis, these have little prognostic or therapeutic significance
Asymptomatic carotid bruit	Indicative of atherosclerotic disease elsewhere; increased risk of stroke *and* coronary heart disease
S-4 sound on cardiac examination	Consistent with left ventricular diastolic filling abnormality requiring increased left atrial contraction; correlates with left atrial enlargement on the electrocardiogram and/or mild left ventricular hypertrophy on echocardiography; consider the patient at higher risk than if not present
Systolic cardiac murmur	Often found in older hypertensive persons; may be due to nonobstructive aortic valve sclerosis or mitral valve regurgitation; echocardiography may be needed for clarification
Irregular cardiac rhythm	Increased frequency of atrial premature beats often found with left atrial hypertrophy, as precurser of atrial fibrillation; increased frequency of ventricular premature beats suggests left ventricular hypertrophy or ischemia; low serum potassium may be the cause
Systolic abdominal bruit	Renal artery stenosis is possible, but not certain; may be due to stenosis of other arteries or aortic atherosclerosis
Prominent abdominal aortic pulsation	Possibility of aortic aneurysm is raised; sonography is needed for greater sensitivity in detection
Signs of peripheral arterial disease: ankle/arm systolic pressure ratio <0.9, femoral artery bruit, claudication, reduced pedal pulses	Symptomatic peripheral arterial disease needs treatment, but may alter choice of antihypertensive drug (avoid β-blockers); conveys higher risk of mortality and cerebrovascular or cardiac morbidity
Electrocardiographic abnormalities	Increased voltage, ST-T wave changes of left ventricular enlargement; signs of ischemia: old myocardial infarction, left axis deviation, left bundle branch block, atrioventricular conduction defects, ectopic atrial or ventricular beats, arrhythmias; any or all increase risk; several imply specific or altered therapy
Chest radiograph: cardiac enlargement, uncoiled and calcified aorta	Often found; convey greater risk, but have no therapeutic significance in the absence of pulmonary congestion

(Continues)

Table 17-2. *(Continued)*

Abnormality	Comment
Echocardiographic abnormalities: left ventricular hypertrophy (LVH) or diastolic filling abnormalities	Often found; LVH conveys higher risk and can be reduced by treatment; diastolic filling can be improved by some agents (significance not yet certain); may reduce pulmonary capillary pressure and likelihood for congestion
Impaired left ventricular systolic function by echocardiography (fractional shortening) or nuclear technique (ejection fraction); either global or regional abnormalites of contraction	Findings indicate high risk; patient is close to congestive heart failure; therapeutic value of angiotensin converting enzymes inhibitors have been established in several studies
Microalbuminuria or proteinuria	Implies renal disease, but not specific in older patients; consider renal artery stenosis, nephrosclerosis, urinary tract infection
Increased serum urea nitrogen and creatinine	Definitely add to risk; may be reversible if due to excessive diuresis, congestive heart failure, urinary tract abnormality (i.e., obstruction of bladder of ureters), or infection
Neurologic dysfunction: transient ischemic episodes, completed stroke with fixed deficits, dementia	All too frequent in older hypertensive persons; consider embolism from heart, aorta, or carotids; ultrasound assessment of arteries and cardiac chambers may be needed; consider value of antithrombotic/anticoagulant therapy

The important exception to this rule is atherosclerotic renal artery stenosis, now becoming a more prominent problem in this age group.[3,4] The typical elderly patient with renal artery stenosis will have signs of atherosclerotic disease elsewhere in carotid, coronary, and/or peripheral arteries. There will usually be a background of multiple risk factors for atherosclerosis as the substrate. Renal function is often subnormal due either to nephrosclerosis or bilateral renal artery narrowing. Frequently, the older patient with renal artery stenosis will have a history of hypertension, once well controlled but now progressively worsening despite more medication. An abdominal systolic bruit may often be heard, but is not specific, since it may be due to aortic, mesenteric, or ileofemoral arterial stenosis. Ordinary laboratory tests in elderly patients with renal artery stenosis will reveal a moderately elevated serum creatinine level. Serum potassium may actually be reduced due to secondary aldosteronism. Plasma renin activity will be inappropriately elevated for the patient's age. Repeated episodes of pulmonary congestion in such patients reflect impaired left ventricular function due to increased afterload and increased preload caused by the volume-retaining effects of multiple renal vascular lesions. Once the diagnosis of renal artery stenosis is established (see Ch. 10), aggressive interventional therapy with angioplasty or vascular surgery may be necessary to correct the hemodynamic burden and prevent progression of renal insufficiency to end-stage disease requiring dialysis.

Occasional cases of pheochromocytoma, primary aldosteronism, or Cushing syndrome (more often due to adrenal neoplasms or adrenocorticotropic hormone producing carcinomas than pituitary adenomas) are reported in older patients.[5] While rare, their occurrence serves notice that these forms of secondary hypertension cannot be entirely ignored in older subjects.

THERAPY

Nonpharmacologic Treatment

The available information from the published clinical trials is sufficient to support the value of antihypertensive therapy for older patients up to age 85 (see Ch. 5). Beyond that, however, we are left to our own devices in deciding whether or how to reduce pressure in octo- and nonagenerians. For patients with minimal elevations in pressure, the nondrug approach (see Ch. 14) may be effective. However, salt restriction should, in my view, be considered with caution and related to overall nutritional and therapeutic goals for each patient. Excessively high or low salt intake may harm the older patient who has reduced cardiac performance and limited salt/volume-conserving renal and endocrine mechanisms. A target level of 2 to 3 g sodium (85 to 130 mmol/day) seems reasonable for most patients. If the older patient is obese, weight reduction is desirable. However, as in younger patients, this should be coupled with increased daily activity and attention to appropriate nutrition. The value of low-fat diets to prevent atherosclerosis in older patients remains to be explored. Where hyperlipidemia is clearly present, available guidelines for diet therapy of elevated cholesterol should be (gently) imposed.

Drug Treatment

The successful therapeutic trials for older patients have used a variety of antihypertensive drugs. Most prominent, however, have been low-dose diuretic drugs often with a potassium-sparing component such as 25 mg hydrochlorthizide with 2.5 mg amiloride. Several β-blockers, at low doses, have been added for control in various studies. In the Systolic Hypertension in the Elderly Program (SHEP) trial of isolated systolic hypertension, chlorthalidone alone (at a starting dose of 12.5 mg/day), or with atenolol (starting dose, 25 mg/day) as the β-blocker, proved effective.

Other studies, however, address several of the target organ pathologies so often found in older patients. It is now evident that angiotensin converting enzyme (ACE) inhibitors offer benefit when left ventricular systolic dysfunction is present with or without the symptoms of pulmonary congestion. Both ACE inhibitors and calcium entry blockers can reduce left ventricular hypertrophy. Regression of left ventricular hypertrophy may or may not be accompanied by improvement in left ventricular diastolic filling abnormalities.

Older patients may have pulmonary congestion due to diastolic dysfunction alone because of severe hypertrophy, but with well-preserved systolic function. It has been suggested that such patients are best treated with drugs that reduce heart rate (if bradycardia is not present), as well as improve filling abnormalities, thereby lengthening the diastolic filling interval. β-Blockers or verapamil have value for this approach. However, regression of hypertrophy alone, as produced by ACE inhibitors and the dihydropyridine calcium channel entry blockers, may also improve diastolic filling and reduce the likelihood of pulmonary congestion.

When ischemic coronary heart disease is present, the potential value of calcium entry blockers increases because of their selective dilation of the coronary arteries. It is not yet certain whether any drugs reverse the structural changes in larger arteries that account for their increased stiffness with age and the predominance of systolic pressure elevation. Several studies are in progress to determine whether calcium entry blockers may be effective in this regard. I have observed that calcium channel blockers (nifedipine) are remarkably effective in reducing systolic pressure in the elderly, often at relatively low and well-tolerated doses.

Choices of antihypertensive drug therapy in the elderly should be made with full consideration of the patient's overall picture, including the likely physiology of the patient and the pharmacology of the drug to be chosen. There is less margin for error with elderly than with younger patients, who have more normal baroreflexes and cardiac and renal status. Experience

Table 17-3. Frequently Encountered Problems in Elderly Hypertensive Patients

Condition	Effect on Management
Orthostatic hypotension (fall in systolic pressure >20 mmHg from sitting to standing) with or without symptoms	Avoid excessive diuresis or use of α-blockers; evaluate other medications (i.e., antidepressants)
Bradycardia	May be due to reduced sinus rate or to heart block; electrocardiogram needed; caution regarding use of β-blockers or verapamil
Obstructive pulmonary disease	Avoid β-blockers, if possible; for angina, lowest possible use of $β_1$-selective agents, if needed
Men with symptoms of prostatic obstruction	Optimal situation for trial of $α_1$-receptor antagonists; evaluate for urinary tract obstruction; monitor for orthostatic hypotension
Claudication	Minimize use of nonselective β-blockers; theoretically, vasodilating calcium channel blockers (dihydropyridines) or $α_1$-receptor antagonists should be valuable, but not enough studies available

(Continues)

Table 17-3. *(Continued)*

Condition	Effect on Management
Depression	Avoid use of centrally acting agents and β-blockers; shift to ACE inhibitors and dihydropyridine-type calcium channel blockers; be aware of all drugs; avoid drug interactions; monitor for orthostatic hypotension
Exertional dyspnea	May be due either to left ventricular or pulmonary dysfunction; careful assessment of each needed
Foot and leg edema	Consider congestive failure, renal salt retention, venous disease, hypoalbuminemia; but if no weight gain, often due to calcium channel entry blockers
Need for antithrombotic agents (aspirin or ticlopidine) or anticoagulants	When indicated, likelihood of hemorrhagic events (especially cerebrovascular hemorrhage) is related to level of arterial pressure; safety may increase if pressure is *well*-controlled; anticoagulation level must be strictly maintained at optimum level; ticlopidine treatment requires serial determination of the blood count (leukopenia has been reported during the first few months of therapy)
Bone and joint pain; symptomatic arthritis, usually osteoarthritis or due to osteoporosis	Often found in older patients; use of nonsteroidal agents is all too common; these drugs may increase pressure, reducing effectiveness of antihypertensive agents; they may also cause renal impairment and gastritis; the latter is a special risk for those on antithrombotic or anticoagulant drugs

leads me to select a few of the more common situations that have altered strategy. These are listed in Table 17-3.

ADVERSE EFFECTS AND QUALITY OF LIFE

As most patients age they tend to focus more on their present than their future. Symptomatic adverse effects of medication become especially troublesome and less well tolerated. Such symptoms may be difficult to distinguish from those of an underlying disease. Withdrawal rates from treatment, in part because of adverse effects, have been as high as 20 to 30 percent in some studies. However, the adverse effect rate in the SHEP trial, which recruited from a very healthy older group and generally used low doses, was less than 10 percent.

In the follow-up assessment of older hypertensive patients on antihypertensive medication, enough time should be taken at each visit for a thorough reconsideration of the value and possible harm of treatment, as well as whether there has been any change in overall function and well being. As a general guide, I look for reasons to reduce the total drug burden, sometimes the most reversible step one can provide for the patient's improvement. For those over 80 years of age, symptoms are the best guide and numbers become less and less pertinent to therapeutic decisions.

REFERENCES

1. Ruddy MC, Bialy GB, Malka ES et al: The relationship of plasma renin activity to clinic and ambulatory blood pressure in elderly people with isolated systolic hypertension. J Hypertens 6:S412, 1988

2. Thijs L, Amery A, Clement D et al: Ambulatory blood pressure monitoring in elderly patients with isolated systolic hypertension. J Hypertens 10:693, 1992

3. Vidt DG: Geriatric hypertension of renal origin: diagnosis and management. Geriatrics 42:59, 1987

4. Olin JW, Vidt DG, Gifford RW Jr, Novick AC: Renovascular disease in the elderly: an analysis of 50 patients. J Am Coll Cardiol 5:1232, 1985

5. Cooper ME, Goodman D, Frauman A et al: Pheochromocytoma in the elderly: a poorly recognized entity? BMJ 293:1474, 1986

18

DIABETIC PATIENTS

In previous chapters, diabetes mellitus in its various forms, including the precursor states of insulin resistance and intermediate glucose tolerance, were described during the assessment of overall risk (see Ch. 6) and, to a limited extent, as affecting choice of treatment (see Chs. 14 and 15). However, the combination of hypertension and diabetes is highly lethal and has many implications that merit additional consideration for management. Thus, this chapter focuses on the various strategies that should be considered when confronting the hypertensive diabetic patient.

Several series suggest that 6 to 7 percent of the adult hypertensive population has diabetes mellitus, defined by a fasting blood glucose above 140 mg/dl, or is receiving antidiabetic treatment. Only a small proportion of patients with diabetes and hypertension will have insulin-dependent diabetes (IDDM), either resulting from early or juvenile onset or because the diabetes cannot be controlled by diet and oral agents. Most hypertensive diabetics will have noninsulin-dependent diabetes (NIDDM). While the clinical spectrum of IDDM and NIDDM overlaps within the hypertensive population, there are sound reasons for separating these two entities with regard to an approach to antihypertensive management.

INSULIN-DEPENDENT DIABETES MELLITUS

In the initial and early phases (1 to 5 years) of IDDM, blood pressure is usually normal. After 5 to 10 years of the disorder, several events occur that are associated with increased arterial pressure. These are the appearance of retinopathy and nephropathy. The latter is often preceded by microalbuminuria before obvious diabetic proteinuric nephropathy is evident. The tendency to increased blood pressure concurrent with diabetic nephropathy is not uniform. It has been suggested that those with a prior tendency to become hypertensive, possibly related to a membrane transport defect reflected by altered red cell sodium/lithium countertransport, are also more likely to develop diabetic nephropathy.[1,2] Whereas all patients with IDDM lack adequate insulin production, it has also been noted that those with nephropathy tend to have insulin resistance as well.[3] Many clinical and experimental studies suggest that prior to the development of proteinuric diabetic nephropathy there is a phase of increased glomerular perfusion and hyperfiltration. This phase is possibly related to excessive constriction of postglomerular (i.e. efferent) arterioles by the intrarenal renin angiotensin system. This mechanism persists even after proteinuria has become present.

217

The supposition that the intrarenal renin system participates in the pathogenesis of diabetic proteinuric nephropathy and its relentless progression to renal failure, which then requires renal replacement therapy, has led to clinical trials of the angiotensin converting enzyme (ACE) inhibitors as a strategy for reducing diabetic proteinuria and preventing the progression of renal insufficiency. Initial short-term studies demonstrated that ACE inhibitor therapy could reduce the proteinuria of diabetic nephropathy.[4] Some calcium channel blockers (verapamil and diltiazem) have also been shown to decrease diabetic proteinuria.[5] The dihydropyridine calcium channel blocker nifedipine may worsen proteinuria in diabetic nephropathy.[6] The crucial question has been: Can ACE inhibitors reduce the progression of nephropathy in IDDM patients in a clinically significant manner? This question has now been answered definitively (Fig. 18-1).

Captopril has been compared to placebo in a large randomized trial with the result that the ACE inhibitor treated group had significantly decreased progression as assessed by either changes in serum creatinine or need for renal replacement therapy.[7] The benefit of ACE inhibitor treatment was not clearly related to changes in arterial pressure. In fact, the pressures at baseline and during treatment were not markedly elevated. These considerations provide a rationale for the view that the major goal of drug therapy for IDDM (of the juvenile-onset type) is the preservation of renal function, which may, in younger patients, even supersede the need to prevent stroke or coronary heart disease.

When IDDM patients become frankly hypertensive, after many years of their disease, autonomic neuropathy may be present in addition to varying degrees of renal insufficiency. Impaired autonomic function may explain why some of these patients have a lack of or reversal in the circadian pattern of blood pressure (see Fig. 6-5). Their supine, nighttime, or sleep pressures may be well into the hypertensive range, while daytime and upright (standing) pressures are lower, to the point that symptomatic orthostatic hypotension is present. Twenty-four hour average pressures may be markedly elevated in such patients, yet even minimal doses of antihypertensive medication worsen symptoms of the orthostatic decrease in pressure. Since the calcium channel entry blockers have a minimal effect on cardiovascular reflexes, cautious attempts to reduce pressure, beginning at very low doses, may be considered. Certainly, volume-depleting diuretic drugs and α_1-receptor blockers should be avoided for management of hypertensive diabetics with signs of autonomic neuropathy. β-Receptor blockers (especially those that are nonselective and inhibit β_2-receptors) are also unsuitable for therapy for IDDM patients. This warning is due to the increased risk of asymptomatic hypoglycemia as a result of blocking the epinephrine-mediated counterregulatory mechanism of glycogenolysis when β_2-receptors are antagonized.

In my view, patients with IDDM should receive ACE inhibitor therapy when microalbuminuria or proteinuria appears and as an initial management for elevated blood pressure. Should pressure not be adequately controlled on ACE-inhibitor monotherapy, addition of a calcium channel entry blocker as the next step is suggested. Whether verapamil and diltiazem are preferable to the dihydropyridines when combined with ACE inhibitors in the management of hypertensive patients with IDDM is not yet established. These patients must be monitored at each visit for orthostatic hypotension. Adjustment of medication to avoid syncope yet maintain adequate control of average pressure may be a difficult challenge in those with advanced neuropathy.

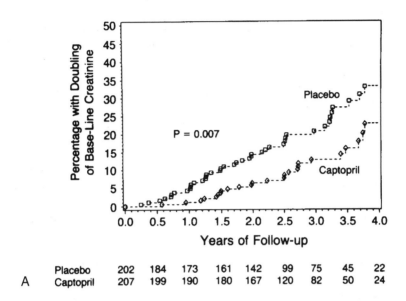

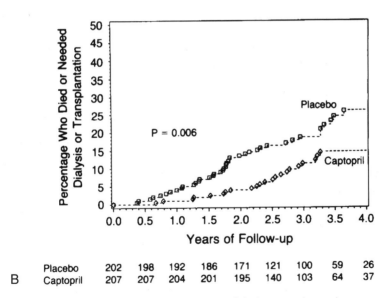

Fig. 18-1. Effect of ACE inhibitor on course of diabetic nephropathy in patients with IDDM. **(A)** Fraction treated with either placebo or captopril, having a doubling of baseline serum creatinine. **(B)** Fraction in each treatment group proceeding to renal replacement therapy, either dialysis or transplantation. (From Lewis et al.,[7] with permission.)

NONINSULIN-DEPENDENT DIABETES MELLITUS

There is no doubt among either clinicians or cardiovascular epidemiologists that the combination of hypertension and NIDDM (H-NIDDM) is a high-risk situation for development of cerebrovascular, coronary artery, and peripheral vascular disease. This cluster, usually but not limited to obese individuals, accounts for 6 to 10 percent of most adult hypertensive groups. Many H-NIDDM patients also have serum lipid patterns that add to their risk of future cardiovascular disease, namely, increased low-density lipoprotein cholesterol, and/or reduced high-density lipoprotein fractions in association with raised serum triglyceride concentration. Despite the high-risk state of H-NIDDM, randomized clinical trials of antihypertensive therapy have either excluded known diabetics or have not recruited enough subjects for subgroup analysis to compare active drug treatment with a nontreated group. The only study that attempted such a comparison, the HDFP trial, yielded equivocal results when the special care and referred care groups were compared. Nonetheless, nearly all physicians (I among them) consider effective and safe antihypertensive therapy to be necessary for all H-NIDDM patients.

For optimal safety and a coordinated attack on the usual risk factors present in most H-NIDDM patients, blood pressure reduction should ordinarily begin with nonpharmacologic steps or life-style interventions: weight reduction, increased aerobic exercise, and a diet appropriate for their glucose intolerance and serum lipid disorder. While this approach is potentially effective, I surmise that nearly all clinicians reading this advice will immediately raise their collective brows in skepticism; nonpharmacologic therapy is very difficult to achieve on a sustained basis. To be realistic, most patients with H-NIDDM are destined for antihypertensive drug treatment in conjunction with diet and/or use of oral antidiabetic agents.

Which agents should then be chosen for initial and subsequent treatment of H-NIDDM? Should the same approach be used as for hypertension without diabetes, or are there compelling reasons to shift the spectrum of antihypertensive drug choices for hypertensive patients with NIDDM? Since the randomized clinical trials fail to yield definitive answers to this question, such decisions should, to me, be based on the natural history and pathophysiology of H-NIDDM and the clinical pharmacology of currently available drugs.

In contrast to IDDM, H-NIDDM is, for the most part, a disorder affecting the same age spectrum as that of essential hypertension (i.e., middle-aged and elderly subjects). The most likely causes of cardiovascular morbidity and mortality in H-NIDDM are stroke and ischemic or coronary heart disease, as is the situation for hypertension in patients without NIDDM. Furthermore, H-NIDDM patients are more likely to develop these diseases than are those without diabetes. H-NIDDM persons may also develop microalbuminuria that can be reduced by ACE inhibitor treatment in association with a delayed increase in serum creatinine.[8] However, it is not yet known whether end-stage renal disease, requiring renal replacement therapy, can be prevented in H-NIDDM patients by antihypertensive therapy in general or ACE inhibitors in particular. These considerations prompt me to conclude that the primary goals of therapy for patients with H-NIDDM should be similar to those for hypertensive patients without NIDDM, prevention of stroke and coronary heart disease with less certainty that prevention of renal insufficiency can be obtained in the same way as for younger insulin-dependent diabetics. In other words, there is less reason to rely on ACE inhibitors as the cornerstone of management of H-NIDDM than of IDDM with microalbuminuria or proteinuric nephropathy, unless the arterial pressure is decreased. Instead, those agents that significantly reduce arterial pressure with either improvement or, at least, no deterioration of the patient's overall metabolic status should be favored. For some, this may indeed be the ACE inhibitors. For others, β-receptor blockers, calcium channel entry blockers, or α_1-receptor antagonists as monotherapy or in appropriate combination may be desirable. For example, when there is evidence of symptomatic coronary heart disease, angina, the value of β-receptor blockers and calcium entry blockers should not be overlooked. On the other hand, if a patient with H-NIDDM has impaired left ventricular systolic function, ACE inhibitors offer special benefit.

This leads to a strategy for initiating and adjusting antihypertensive drug therapy in H-NIDDM patients. First, thiazide-type diuretic agents are to be avoided. Many studies amply demonstrate that these agents worsen glucose tolerance through several mechanisms, including increased resistance to insulin action. In addition, the well-established potential for the increased serum low-density lipoprotein cholesterol and the reduction of serum potassium attendant on the use of this class of diuretics are a cause of concern for patients in whom metabolic risk factors are so prominent. Some clinicians have also expressed concern about the use of β-blockers in H-NIDDM, despite the benefit related to these agents in the randomized trials of antihypertensive therapy and for secondary prevention of coronary heart disease. Those skeptical about the use of β-blockers emphasize studies that show that β-blockers without intrinsic sympathomimetic activity (e.g., propranolol, metoprolol, atenolol) cause a small, but consistent reduction in serum high-density lipoprotein cholesterol and increase in serum triglyceride concentration. Other studies suggest that β-blockers may (in association with thiazide diuretics) worsen glucose tolerance or increase insulin resistance. Whether these adverse effects of β-blockade, small in magnitude as they are, offset the benefit of this drug class in H-NIDDM remains unknown. However, therapeutic alternatives are now available.

From the perspective of metabolic change, the more recently developed antihypertensive agents offer promise for reduction of blood pressure in H-NIDDM with either a neutral or favorable change in insulin resistance, glucose tolerance, and serum lipid profile. Table 18-1 summarizes the effects of ACE inhibitors, α_1-blockers, and calcium channel entry blockers on pertinent metabolic effects or risk factors likely to be found in H-NIDDM.

As a strategy, I prefer to initiate antihypertensive drug therapy in H-NIDDM patients with an ACE inhibitor, especially if either microalbuminuria or proteinuria is present. When coronary heart disease is evident as revealed by angina or a recent myocardial infarction, monotherapy with either a cal-

Table 18-1. Comparison of Antihypertensive Drug Classes for Metabolic Effects

Drug Class	Carbohydrate Metabolism	Serum Lipids
Thiazide-type diuretics	Worsen glucose tolerance, increase insulin resistance	Increase serum total and low-density lipoprotein cholesterol
β-Blockers without ISA	May worsen glucose tolerance; possible synergy with thiazide diuretics	Increase serum triglycerides, decrease high-density cholesterol (15–20%)
β-Blockers with ISA	In small studies had little effect	Few long-term studies
α_1-Blockers	May improve glucose tolerance and insulin resistance	Reduce total and low-density lipoprotein cholesterol; increase high-density lipoprotein fraction
ACE inhibitors	Decrease insulin resistance	No effect
Calcium entry blockers	No effect in most studies; tendency for decreased insulin resistance in a few	No effect in nearly all studies

Abbreviation: ISA, intrinsic sympathomimetic activity.

cium channel entry blocker of the verapamil or diltiazem type or a selective β_1-receptor blocker is a reasonable option. When monotherapy with an ACE inhibitor fails to normalize pressure, addition of either a calcium channel entry blocker or an α_1-receptor blocker is suggested. Conversely, failure to normalize pressure with a calcium entry blocker calls for addition of an ACE inhibitor. The combination of a dihydropyridine calcium channel blocker with low doses of β-blockers may be especially useful to correct the tachycardia that sometimes is the result of monotherapy using a dihydropyridine. These selections permit control of pressure in most H-NIDDM patients without the need for thiazide-type diuretic exposure.

Occasionally, blood pressure remains above the desired therapeutic range despite the combinations mentioned in the previous discussion. Adding small doses of the diuretics (e.g., 12.5 to 25 mg hydrochlorothiazide or chlorthalidone daily) may permit better control. It has been suggested that low doses of the loop diuretics (e.g., furosemide 20 to 40 mg/day) may be as effective and less likely to impair glucose tolerance further. Reduced serum potassium is to be avoided in these patients as it may impair glucose metabolism. Potassium-sparing agents, such as amiloride 5 mg/day, may be added to correct hypokalemia. Serial measurement of blood glucose, glycohemoglobin, and serum lipids is then needed to adjust for the metabolic effects that may occur. The long-term goal remains effective control of blood pressure with normalization or improvement in the metabolic status of each patient with H-NIDDM. Until and unless clinical trials provide a better rationale, a high degree of individualization is warranted in selection of antihypertensive agents for this high-risk population.

REFERENCES

1. Krowlewski AS, Canessa M, Warram JH et al: Predisposition to hypertension and susceptibility to renal disease in insulin-dependent diabetes mellitus. N Engl J Med 318:140, 1988

2. Mangili R, Bending JJ, Scott G et al: Increased sodium-lithium countertransport activity in red cells of patients with insulin-dependent diabetes and nephropathy. N Engl J Med 318:146, 1988

3. Yip J, Mattock MB, Morocutti A et al: Insulin resistance in insulin-dependent diabetic patients with microalbuminuria. Lancet 342:883, 1993

4. Bakris GL: Angiotensin-converting enzyme inhibitors and progression of diabetic nephropathy. Ann Intern Med 118:643, 1993

5. Bakris GL: Effects of diltiazem or lisinopril on massive proteinuria associated with diabetes mellitus. Ann Intern Med 112:701, 1990

6. Demarie BK, Bakris GL: Effects of different calcium antagonists on proteinuria associated with diabetes mellitus. Ann Intern Med 113:987, 1991

7. Lewis EJ, Hunsicker LG, Bain RP for the Collaborative Study Group: The effect of angiotensin-converting-enzyme inhibition on diabetic nephropathy. N Engl J Med 329:1456, 1993

8. Ravid M, Savin H, Jutrin I et al: Long-term stabilizing effect of angiotensin-converting enzyme inhibition on plasma creatinine and on proteinuria in normtensive type II diabetic patients. Ann Intern Med 118:577, 1993

19

REFRACTORY HYPERTENSION

Some patients do not seem to respond to well-intentioned and appropriate antihypertensive therapy. What does this mean? The answer must be related to the goals of treatment. For hypertension, the goal is prevention of future cardiovascular disease via reduction of arterial pressure. However, this goal is portrayed in different ways. For some, it is a specific decrease in pressure (e.g., -10 mmHg systolic and/or -5 mmHg diastolic pressures. In other studies, the percentage of reduction is considered a target. Guideline statements often refer to a fixed level or range of pressure (e.g., below 140 mmHg systolic and/or below 90 mmHg diastolic pressure), considered to represent a minimum or low risk state.

The term *refractory hypertension* as found in recent literature is used in a vague way, but implies that the patient's pressure has not fallen as expected after whatever therapy was started. In reviewing various studies, it seems likely that a fall of 10 mmHg or more in seated diastolic pressure, measured carefully, can be taken as a response to drug treatment. For mild-to-moderate hypertension, many physicians aim for this as a minimum response and would like to reduce clinic pressures to below 140 mmHg systolic and 90 mmHg diastolic as an optimal target. If so, then *refractory* hypertension implies either that the pressure has decreased less than 10 mmHg or has failed to reach 140/90 mmHg. I prefer the former approach and begin to consider the pressure refractory or resistant to treatment when the decrease in clinic diastolic pressure is less than 10 mmHg. If isolated systolic hypertension is being treated, a reduction of at least 15 mmHg is considered a response. Use of ambulatory blood pressure monitoring provides different criteria, since this method can define average daily pressures more precisely. A decrement of 5 to 6 mmHg in daytime diastolic pressure as measured by ambulatory pressure recording is usually significant.

Most patients treated do indeed respond to treatment. It is assumed here that during the initial evaluation and phases of treatment some time will be spent with the patient, by the physician or other professional, explaining the rationale for treatment to elicit cooperation. Attention to patient education with ample opportunity to ask questions can be valuable in hopes of preventing lack of compliance due to misunderstanding. Additional information and reminders provided by community or work-site programs can assist in gaining a patient's cooperation for treatment. Refractory hypertension has become associated with some specific features that can be characterized and evaluated. These are listed in Table 19-1.

Table 19-1. Factors To Be Considered for Refractory Hypertension

Lack of patient compliance or adherence to treatment
Lack of patient compliance or adherence to treatment
Lack of patient compliance or adherence to treatment
Ineffective intervention (e.g., incorrect drug[s])
Drug interactions
Excessive "white coat" effect in clinic or office
Unrecognized secondary hypertension
Progression of disease

COMPLIANCE/ADHERENCE

It is the firm belief of many treating physicians that when a patient's blood pressure does not fall after reasonable patient education, life-style changes have been advised, and/or a prescription has been given, it must be because the patient has not kept their part of the (implied) contract (i.e., the patient is noncompliant or nonadherent). In many cases, this may well be true. The first three items in Table 19-1 reflect this prevailing view; the repetition is intended to make the point. What then might contribute to the compliance/adherence dilemma? Surprisingly, there have been few studies that shed light on the problem of patient noncompliance. Experience and clinical impressions provide what little guidance there is (Table 19-2).

In formal studies of drug treatment, compliance or adherence is usually defined by such measures as pill counts or missed visits. However, the analysis of which patients are noncompliant and their specific characteristics remains largely unaddressed, as these patients are often initially excluded or removed from the trial. It is impractical (and time consuming) to do pill counts on a routine clinic visit. Compliance is far easier to assess for the life-style changes or nonpharmacologic interventions. Very simply, weight and 24-hour urine sodium or chloride levels are the numerical indices that document whether the patient has implemented the request to lose weight or reduce salt intake. Measurement of blood or serum level of an antihypertensive agent is not ordinarily available for the antihypertensive drugs. Indirect assessments can be made, however, such as the response of serum potassium to a thiazide diuretic or a reduction in heart rate after a β-blocker has been prescribed. The presence of an adverse effect (cough caused by an angiotensin converting enzyme [ACE] inhibitor, edema caused by a calcium channel blocker) may be used as a guide that patients are indeed taking the drug, but absence of these manifestations does not imply that they are nonadherent.

What then are the useful clinical clues to detect the noncompliant patient? First, one suspects that patients with a pattern of erratic visits are probably no more committed to taking medication than they are to keeping appointments. This may not always be the case. The availability of clinic or office facilities to those with domestic and/or work responsibilities must be considered.

Table 19-2. Possible Causes of Poor Patient Compliance

Lack of patient education/motivation
Excessively complex or inconvenient regimen (too many pills, too often)
"Negative reinforcement" of adverse effects, phobia to medication
Excessive cost of medication relative to patient's resources
High risk or denying behavior pattern with unwillingness to accept
   long-term preventive care

Work-site treatment programs have been successful and overcome the difficulty some have with keeping appointments elsewhere. It has been suggested that the use of home blood pressure measurements taken by the patient or companion may be helpful. Blood pressures can be phoned in and evaluated, reducing the need for office visits. Patient education can be performed over the phone and does not always need a face to face encounter. Next, look at the drug list. Can the regimen be simplified to one or two pills once a day, with a shift to the long-acting agents? Reassessment of adverse effects may be helpful. Patients with a history of several bothersome side effects may lose confidence that any medication can be effective and not annoying. A few patients become almost phobic about taking medication and become convinced that no medicine is safe or tolerable. Cost of medication could be an issue for some; a gentle, but open approach to this issue is advisable. Last, behaviors that could diminish compliance, particularly substance or alcohol abuse, should be considered apart from the metabolic effect of the behavior on blood pressure, itself, or drug metabolism. In the absence of a history of excessive alcohol intake, detection of hepatomegaly or abnormal hepatic enzyme patterns unexplained by other causes of hepatic disease may suggest furtive alcohol excess. Other kinds of substance abuse may be difficult to assess unless they are admitted by the patient or they are detected by chemical screening tests.

Some patients, seen once or twice, give the impression that their overall life choices are of the high-risk type. They may simply deny the likelihood that their future can be altered and refuse treatment or, after consideration, choose to accept the long odds that they will not incur disease. Current medical ethics stress patient autonomy along with informed consent; choices made by rational patients are to be respected. However, those who initially choose to refrain from drug treatment may reconsider their odds and risks later on. Whenever possible we try to keep such patients under medical surveillance and schedule re-visits at regular intervals, if only for additional education and counseling.

INEFFECTIVE THERAPY

Some treatments work in some patients; few are effective in all. The heterogeneity of pathophysiologic mechanisms at work in hypertensive patients ensures that the response to any single treatment modality will vary from patient to patient. Only the salt sensitive (20 to 30 percent) will respond to reduced salt intake or, by analogy, to diuretics. Several studies confirm that older patients and those of African origin are more likely to respond to diuretics or calcium channel entry blockers and less likely to respond to β-blockers or ACE inhibitors, whereas younger patients and those of European or Hispanic origin have better responses to these drugs.[1] There are, however, exceptions to such generalizations. Most often, the reason that a drug combination does not work is because it does not include agents that work together in an additive manner. For example, there is little basis for combining a centrally acting agent (all of which act via reduction of sympathetic tone) with peripheral α- and/or β-adrenergic receptor antagonists. Another example, the β-receptor blockers, reduce pressure in part by diminishing renin secretion. Measurement of plasma renin activity on treatment with a β-blocker will define the extent to which the β-blocker has worked in this respect. An ACE inhibitor may have little additive effect if renin release has already been reduced to a very low level by the β-blocker. However, patients on the combination of a diuretic and a β-blocker may not achieve full suppression of plasma renin activity; addition of an ACE inhibitor can then be effective.

A few recent studies suggest that there is little additive effect with thiazide diuretics and calcium channel entry blockers. By contrast, combinations that do have additive or even synergistic action for decreasing pressure (as described in Ch. 15) include β-blocker or ACE inhibitor with a diuretic, α- and β-blockers, and β-blocker and dihydropyridine calcium channel blocker. Each of these drug classes has a long-acting, once-a-day agent to maximize convenience for the patient.

DRUG INTERACTIONS IMPAIRING ANTIHYPERTENSIVE TREATMENT

When well-controlled pressure becomes elevated with no other explanation, the answer can sometimes be found in a re-examination of *all medications* that the patient now takes. Several drug classes should be considered: the tricyclic antidepressants, the nonsteroidal anti-inflammatory drugs (NSAIDs), and the steroids themselves. Tricyclic antidepressants have a specific action, blocking the neuron pump of the adrenergic terminal. Guanethidine and its analogs are taken up by this pump. Tricyclics then reverse the antihypertensive action of these peripheral neuron depletors. The NSAIDs, by antagonizing cyclo-oxygenase, prevent formation of vasodilating prostaglandins. This may diminish the effect of the ACE inhibitors, specifically, and perhaps that of other antihypertensive agents. Use of glucocorticoids such as prednisone may increase arterial pressure through a variety of mechanisms and may account for an unexpected loss of antihypertensive control. Now that cyclosporine is being used more widely, it should also be on the list of suspect drugs for increased arterial pressure. In brief, patients with refractory hypertension need a careful history to assess the possibility that drugs prescribed for other illnesses may account for resistance to blood pressure lowering medication.

THE "WHITE COAT" COMPONENT

All who have studied ambulatory blood pressure monitoring have quickly recognized the frequent disparity between clinic pressure and average ambulatory blood pressure. For patients whose clinic pressure is consistently higher than their ambulatory pressure, the "white coat" factor becomes a particularly difficult problem at the time of initial diagnosis, as described in Chapter 6. Unless a "white coat" component is identified before treatment is started, there may be misinterpretation of clinic pressures as failing to respond when, in fact, they only represent the patient's recurring response to the clinic setting. The transient elevation of pressure due to brief stress (i.e., of a clinic visit) can override the effect of treatment. As a result, more medication is prescribed, adverse effects may occur, and a frustrating situation for both patient and physician results. Once a patient is suspected of having an excessive white coat component, the only diagnostic step that will confirm that suspicion is ambulatory blood pressure monitoring. This then will provide the needed baseline for consideration of any change in treatment. Usually those with the white coat pattern are taking medication unnecessarily. This is supported by Figure 19-1, taken from a sequential study of ambulatory blood pressure measurements at baseline and during treatment with either lisinopril or isradipine. The authors have concluded that only those with daytime average pressures of 135/85 mmHg or higher are likely to respond to drug treatment.[2] This is a reasonable guideline that I can agree with until better information becomes available.

UNRECOGNIZED SECONDARY HYPERTENSION

Most older textbooks carry the statement that resistant or refractory hypertension should suggest secondary, potentially reversible hypertension. Surprisingly, apart from anecdotes, there is little documentation for this opinion. With the current availability of new and potent antihypertensive drugs that can act at diverse sites in the cardiovascular system, it is likely that nearly all forms of secondary hypertension can be controlled with drug treatment. Therefore, failure to respond to drug treatment may not be either sensitive or specific for predicting the presence or absence of a reversible condition. The following are some examples. Primary aldosteronism can be well controlled with potassium-sparing diuretics, particularly spironolactone. Arterial pressure levels and fluctuations in pheochromocytoma can be modified by α- and β-blockade, sometimes with addition of ACE inhibitors. The renin-dependent hypertension of unilateral renal artery stenosis can often be controlled by ACE inhibitor monotherapy. Patients with bilateral stenosis respond to calcium channel entry blockers. It is easy to see that secondary hypertension might escape detection if response to drug treatment was the only basis for diagnosis.

It is likely that individuals with refractory or resistant hypertension have received more diagnostic attention than the responders, and thus a selection bias has led to more accurate diagnosis in these patients. In fact, it has been argued in the past (and may still be valid) that only those not responding to

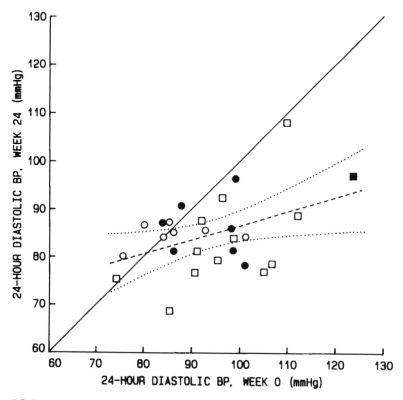

Fig. 19-1. Comparison between baseline and on-treatment diastolic pressures measured by ambulatory blood pressure monitoring. The line of identity is shown. Open squares indicate lisinopril monotherapy; open circles, isradipine monotherapy; closed symbols, hydrochlorothiazide added to either lisinopril (squares) or isradipine (circles). (From Fagard et al.,[2] with permission.)

drug treatment should be evaluated for renal artery stenosis. This is based on cost-effectiveness and lack of evidence that interventional treatment is superior to drug therapy for those who are compliant and do respond to medication without adverse effects.

My own strategy is to recognize that those with secondary hypertension may escape detection during their initial evaluations and to remind myself to reconsider the possibility during follow-up after a few years, irrespective of their response to treatment. A thorough review of the chart and available laboratory values can be helpful. A borderline low serum potassium level might have been missed, and primary or secondary aldosteronism remain unrecognized. A repeat physical examination with the clues to secondary hypertension in mind is in order. It is easy, in a busy practice, to overlook that the second or third careful look for patients in treatment over many years can still correct false-negative initial findings.

PROGRESSION OF DISEASE

A time-trend look at the patient's pressure over several years may indicate a period of stable control and good compliance, with little change in medication, followed by a slow upward drift in systolic and diastolic pressure. Two mechanisms should be considered that represent evolution of the patient's natural history: deterioration in renal function and/or progression of atherosclerosis.

It is my impression that those patients with evidence of renal disease initially or who acquire it during the course of observation (not limited to diabetic nephropathy, the most often found) often follow the course described above: a period of good control gradually merging into higher pressures on the same treatment. This pattern might be explained by insidious progression of renal insufficiency with diminution of glomerular filtration rate. Small gains in weight in these patients might reflect retention of salt and water; effectiveness of thiazide diuretics may be diminished. Instead, the use of the loop active agents, such as furosemide, may achieve natriuresis and reduce volume and arterial pressure. In some instances progressive focal renal ischemia may cause increased renin secretion; addition of an ACE inhibitor may be effective. Often ACE inhibitors can be safe in patients with moderate renal insufficiency. However, serum potassium, urea nitrogen, and creatinine should be monitored frequently, as hyperkalemia and worsening renal function may occur. If the latter is evident, evaluation for bilateral renal artery stenosis (or stenosis of the artery to a renal transplant) is indicated (see Ch. 10).

As hypertensive patients age, their arteries slowly become less compliant; a disproportionate increase in systolic arterial pressure then takes place. It has been suggested that several drug classes, the ACE inhibitors and calcium channel entry blockers, may increase large artery compliance. Substituting or adding one of these to the treatment might reduce systolic pressure. Experience from the SHEP trial suggests that low-dose diuretics and the β_1-selective antagonists (e.g., atenolol, as used in this study) may be effective in those with isolated systolic hypertension.

SUMMARY

Widespread education, conducted by a variety of agencies, has taught much of the public about the risk of untreated hypertension and the preventive benefit of its treatment. The increased awareness of this problem and greater acceptance of therapeutic interventions, life-style change, and drug prescription are documented in recent trends. These favorable changes coupled with advances in antihypertensive drugs imply that the problem of refractory hypertension due to lack of patient information will diminish. To achieve an even higher response rate in those patients who truly need drug treatment, better patient selection to eliminate the "white coat" hypertensive patient is suggested, and more widespread use of ambulatory blood pressure monitoring could be useful. Careful attention to all drugs taken by the patient is necessary surveillance; some drugs may account for a resistant pattern. Finally, during long-term follow-up, close attention to trends in blood pressure, weight, and renal function (perhaps made more efficient by computerization of records so that these changes will be more apparent) may unmask progression of disease that requires an alteration in therapy.

REFERENCES

1. Materson BJ, Reda DJ, Cushman WC et al: Single-drug therapy for hypertension in men: a comparision of six antihypertensive agents with placebo. N Engl J Med 328:914, 1993

2. Fagard R, Bielen E, Staessen J et al: Response of ambulatory blood pressure to antihypertensive therapy guided by clinic pressure. Am J Hypertens 6:648, 1993

20

NONDIABETIC CHRONIC RENAL DISEASE

Chapter 11 provides a survey of the various forms of irreversible renal diseases associated with hypertension. This chapter focuses to a greater extent on the rationale for antihypertensive therapy in chronic renal diseases. It is based on recently concluded clinical trials that are relevant to an overall approach to patients with stable chronic nondiabetic renal diseases, particularly the glomerular diseases, polycystic renal disease, and nephrosclerosis whose course tends to be somewhat predictable. By contrast, the connective tissue diseases cannot be included because their courses are too variable and dependent on the changing vicissitudes of their pathology and its treatment.

Hypertension and chronic renal disease have been intertwined since Bright described the association of albuminuria and the *hard pulse* during life with the shrunken kidneys and enlarged heart at autopsy characteristic of those who died of uremia. Subsequently, the various forms of chronic progressive glomerular diseases, polycystic renal disease, and nephrosclerosis secondary to elevated arterial pressure itself have become defined through many correlative studies of many renal disorders. It was once thought that hypertension might be a necessary compensating mechanism for impaired renal blood flow and/or glomerular perfusion and filtration in patients with the chronic renal diseases or even nephrosclerosis. On that basis, reduction of systemic arterial pressure would inevitably make matters worse by further reduction in renal perfusion and glomerular filtration rate, hastening the advance of renal failure. As modern antihypertensive therapy became recognized for its effectiveness in preventing stroke, ischemic heart disease, and heart failure, clinicians began to suspect that progression of several forms of chronic renal disease might be delayed by the same treatment.

Experimental models of hypertension have demonstrated that afferent arteriolar nephrosclerosis is due to elevated arterial pressure and is preventable by several interventions that include lowered systemic pressure. A hemodynamic basis for the relationship between arteriolar pressure and progressive glomerular injury in animals with reduced nephron populations has become recognized. In brief, this set of hypotheses, based on a large literature, suggests that when the effective nephron population is reduced, the remaining glomeruli are perfused at high pressure, in part due to transmission of high systemic pressure through afferent arterioles that are only partially constricted and in part by efferent arteriolar constriction, largely maintained by an active intrarenal renin angiotensin system. The resultant intraglomerular "hypertension" provides the substrate for progressive glomerular obsolescence, in parallel with the underlying primary pathology (i.e., immunologically mediated glomerulopathies, polycystic renal disease, interstitial inflammation, fibrosis). These mechanisms imply that reduction of systemic arterial pressure may be beneficial by reducing the glomerulus' afferent pressure load. In addition, those drugs that decrease the action of the intrarenal renin system (i.e., angiotensin converting enzyme [ACE] inhibitors and angiotensin II receptor blockers, and perhaps even β-blockers) may be especially effective in preventing progression of chronic renal disease, independent of their effect on systemic pressure.[1]

Observations made during the clinical trials of antihypertensive therapy suggested that reduction of arterial pressure may have prevented a tendency for increased serum creatinine (as an estimate of glomerular filtration) that occurred in untreated subjects.

This trend was noted in the earliest observations of the most severely hypertensive patients included in Veterans Affairs Clinical Trials. However, some disturbing exceptions have also been noted. Observations during antihypertensive therapy of black American hypertensive persons have suggested that the rate of increase in serum creatinine was unaffected by treatment designed to bring blood pressure to a level usually considered beneficial for prevention of stroke or ischemic heart disease.[2,3] By contrast, non-black Americans tended to have a decrease in serum creatinine when treated conventionally. These reports have led to the suggestion that the goal blood pressure to be reached during treatment of susceptible groups (e.g., black American hypertensive patients) with slightly elevated baseline serum creatinine (1.2 to 2.0 mg/dl) or moderately reduced creatinine clearance (40 to 80 ml/hr) should be as low as 92 mmHg mean arterial pressure (MAP) compared with the usual or conventional goal of less than 107 mmHg.[4] MAP is calculated from measured systolic (S) and diastolic (D) pressures by the formula: MAP = (S + 2D)/3 (see Ch. 1). Table 20-1 displays the various systolic and diastolic pressures that would give equivalent MAPs of 107 and 92 mmHg.

While the older antihypertensive agents have been used to treat hypertension in the chronic renal diseases and have been effective for blood pressure reduction, the rationale for drugs such as the antiadrenergic agents (e.g., methyldopa, clonidine, and so forth) has never been certain. The loop active diuretics (e.g., furosemide) have often been employed on the basis that excessive volume, salt, and water, retained by impaired filtration was part of the pathophysiology of these disorders. That may still be so. However, the recognition of the role of the intrarenal renin system and the effectiveness of the ACE inhibitors in experimental models has clearly been influential in shifting attention to these agents. By contrast, the newer calcium channel

Table 20-1. Paired Systolic and Diastolic Pressures Equivalent to Goals for Mean Arterial Pressure (MAP) Used in Trials of Chronic Renal Disease[a]

MAP = 107 mmHg		MAP = 92 mmHg	
Systolic	Diastolic	Systolic	Diastolic
120	101	100	88
125	98	105	86
130	96	110	83
135	93	115	81
140	91	120	78
145	88	125	76
150	86	130	73
155	83	135	71
160	81	140	68

[a]MAP ≤107 mmHg is considered "usual"; MAP ≤92 mmHg is considered "low pressure." (From Klahr,[4] with permission)

entry blockers and α_1-receptor blockers, although effective for reduction of pressure, dilate afferent arterioles. If perfusion pressure (arterial pressure) is substantially decreased, they might also decrease intraglomerular pressure and prevent progression. By contrast, if afferent resistance was reduced *without a sufficient fall in systemic pressure,* glomeruli would still be hyperperfused and progression might continue. A summary of the effects of these newer antihypertensive agents is given in Table 20-2.

CHRONIC NONEND-STAGE RENAL DISEASE

One large clinical trial, the Modification of Diet in Renal Disease (MDRD) study,[5] has been completed that addresses the issues raised above regarding the effect of antihypertensive drug treatment on progression of renal disease. This trial studied patient with many types of renal disease: chronic glomerular diseases, polycystic renal disease, and hypertensive nephrosclerosis, and patients with noninsulin-dependent diabetes with nephropathy. Other large trials are, as this is written, either in progress or being planned to provide much needed information beyond the scope of the MDRD study.

As the title of the study suggests, the role of reduced dietary protein is also a subject of study because of its possible value in preventing progression of the chronic renal diseases. In the MDRD study, interventions included both reduced diet protein and antihypertensive drug therapy to achieve either the conventional level of control (MAP of lower than 107 mmHg) or very low pressure (MAP of 92 mmHg or lower). This study was composed of two parts. In the first part, subjects with moderate reduction in renal function (glomerular filtration rate 24 to 55 ml/min) were treated with either usual or

Table 20-2. Drug Selection of Newer Agents in Chronic Renal Disease

Renal Disease	Drug	Comment
Chronic glomerular pathology	ACE inhibitors	Variable effect on arterial pressure, may prevent progression through intrarenal effect; consider as first or second choice
	α_1-Receptor blockers	May be effective; value for prevention of progression is unknown
	Calcium channel blockers	Valuable primarily as antihypertensive drug
Adult polycystic renal disease	ACE inhibitors	First choice agents; very likely to be effective
	Calcium channel entry blockers	Beneficial only for reduction of arterial pressure
	α_1-Receptor blockers	May be effective; value for prevention of progression is unknown
Hypertensive nephrosclerosis	All agents	It is not known whether any drugs are specifically beneficial for prevention of nephrosclerosis

low protein intake or usual or low blood pressure control (i.e., four groups). The second part of the study evaluated a sicker group of patients, those with a glomerular filtration rate of 13 to 24 ml/min, who were placed on low or very low protein intakes and either usual or low pressure control. Blood pressure control was to be achieved by both nonpharmacologic measures and drug treatment. ACE inhibitors were recommended, but not required. These interventions were "open" and not blinded to either investigators or patients.

The overall effect of either intervention—reduced diet protein or blood pressure control to low levels—was disappointingly ineffective in the MDRD study. The rates of progression to either death or renal replacement therapy (dialysis) in those with more advanced disease (part 2 of the study) was nearly identical irrespective of the therapy, as shown in Figure 20-1. Of note, patients with higher baseline proteinuria and polycystic renal disease, and who were black tended to have more rapid progression. However, subgroup analysis gives some reason for optimism. Irrespective of the initial level of the glomerular filtration rate, aggressive blood pressure reduction was most effective for delaying progression in those with urine protein excretion of 1 g/24 hr or more, as shown in Figure 20-2.

The potential benefit of antihypertensive therapy in individuals with a chronic renal disease is not limited to preventing progression of renal insufficiency. There is no reason to consider that these individuals are exempt

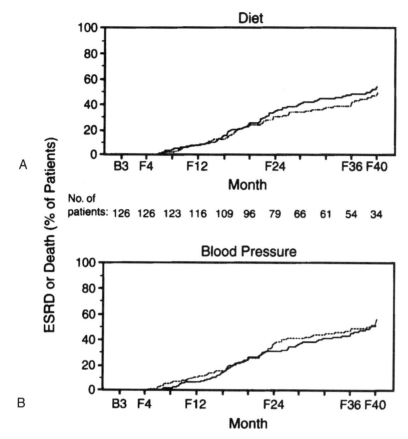

Fig. 20-1. Lack of effect of **(A)** very low protein diet or **(B)** low blood pressure on progression of chronic renal disease in the more severely affected subjects (study 2) in the MDRD study. There was no significant effect of the more aggressive interventions on either mortality or end-stage renal disease (ESRD), defined by the need for dialysis or transplant. Abscissa, month of followup; ordinate, percentage of death or ESRD. Fig. A: Solid line, low protein diet: dash/dot line, very low protein diet. Fig. B: solid line, low pressure group; dashed line, usual pressure group.

from the risk of stroke and cardiac disease that hypertension confers. For those with familial adult polycystic renal disease, there may be an even greater risk of intracranial hemorrhage, should blood pressure be uncontrolled. Effective antihypertensive therapy becomes especially important for those with reduced renal function, whatever the cause of their renal disease. Two issues remain unresolved. First, what should be the treatment goal for blood pressure reduction? The lower level of pressure sought in the MDRD study was not well tolerated by some patients. Perhaps some middle ground is needed. My own preference is to lower the diastolic pressure to within the 80 to 85 mmHg range and the systolic pressure to within 130 to 140 mmHg, resulting in an MAP of about 95 to 100 mmHg. Second, whether the ACE inhibitors (or, when available, the angiotensin II receptor

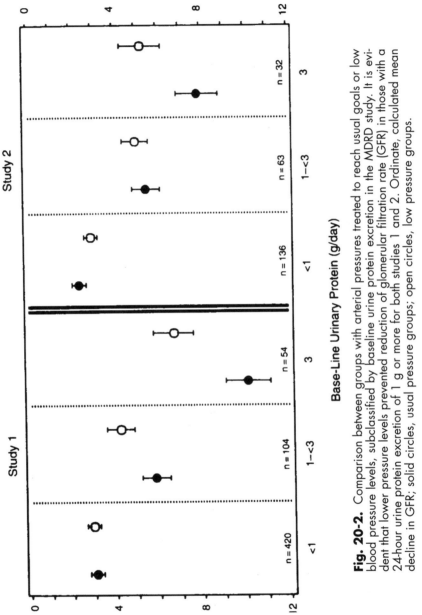

Fig. 20-2. Comparison between groups with arterial pressures treated to reach usual goals or low blood pressure levels, subclassified by baseline urine protein excretion in the MDRD study. It is evident that lower pressure levels prevented reduction of glomerular filtration rate (GFR) in those with a 24-hour urine protein excretion of 1 g or more for both studies 1 and 2. Ordinate, calculated mean decline in GFR; solid circles, usual pressure groups; open circles, low pressure groups.

antagonists) convey additional value, because of their intrarenal effect in reducing efferent arteriolar constriction, remains an unproven (in clinical trials) yet attractive hypothesis. At present the ACE inhibitors seem especially effective in adult polycystic renal disease and, perhaps, in other renal diseases with microalbuminuria or proteinuria. As with other hypertensive persons, attention to the other risk factors remains necessary. Finally, is there a J-curve for on-treatment blood pressure with regard to progression of renal insufficiency? In other words, is there some lower limit below which renal prefusion is not optimally maintained? Time and good clinical research will (one hopes) prevail.

REFERENCES

1. Keane WF, Anderson S, Aurell M et al: Angiotensin converting enzyme inhibitors and progressive renal insufficiency. Ann Intern Med 111:503, 1990

2. Rostand SG, Brown G, Kirk KA et al: Renal insufficiency in treated essential hypertension. N Engl J Med 320:684, 1989

3. Walker GW, Neaton JD, Cutler JA et al: Renal function change in hypertensive members of the Multiple Risk Factor Intervention trial: racial and treatment effects. JAMA 268:3085, 1992

4. Klahr S: The modification of diet in renal disease study. N Engl J Med 320:864, 1989

5. Klahr S, Levey AS, Beck GJ et al: The effects of dietary protein restriction and blood-pressure control on the progression of chronic renal disease. N Engl J Med 330:877, 1994

21

PREGNANCY IN HYPERTENSIVE WOMEN

This chapter is devoted to management of those hypertensive women who are considering the possibility of becoming pregnant or become pregnant after the diagnosis of hypertension has been made. Most of these patients are already being cared for by primary care internists or family practitioners. Increasingly, if the patient has a medical disease, such as *chronic hypertension* (the term used in the obstetrics literature), the later stages of pregnancy and the period surrounding delivery are managed by those within the field of obstetrics who deal with high-risk pregnancies as a subspecialty. For optimal management and continuity of care, a close cooperative relationship between these two is suggested. Pregnancy-induced hypertension (i.e., hypertension that occurs only during gestation and ceases after delivery or the end of pregnancy) has received much attention as a distinct entity with its own pathophysiology.[1] The syndrome of pre-eclampsia includes hypertension, but with other features, notably proteinuria, and represents a high-risk state that can develop into a hypertensive emergency (see Ch. 16).

Ideally, young women should be screened and identified as having hypertension before they begin to consider having children. Several questions are more important at this point than for older patients or men. Is there any likelihood of reversible hypertension that can be cured before the occurrence of pregnancy? The risk of undetected reversible secondary hypertension, particularly pheochromocytoma or renal artery stenosis, during pregnancy fully justifies the search for these disorders well before child bearing is contemplated. Likewise it is important to identify other medical illnesses in which hypertension may occur, such as the connective tissue diseases or diabetic nephropathy, in order to anticipate problems that may arise. The methods for detection of these disorders are described in Section II.

It is most important to establish whether the young woman is, in fact, hypertensive or has the "white coat" syndrome, which is more frequent in younger women compared with men.[2,3] When a young woman has office or clinic measurements in the mild hypertensive range, 140/85 to 160/100 mmHg, with no other abnormalities, I question whether hypertension is present at all. If there is no clinical evidence of either secondary hypertension or target organ damage, such patients should be carefully evaluated using ambulatory blood pressure monitoring before deciding whether the pressure is high enough to initiate antihypertensive drug treatment.[4] These steps may prevent some of the complex decisions that come when a drug-treated hypertensive woman becomes pregnant.

It is not unusual to be asked by a woman who has been advised to take antihypertensive medication and is contemplating bearing children whether her medications will be safe, with regard to fetal development, during her gestation. Implicit in this question is the relative risk of untreated high blood pressure to her and the fetus, particularly during the first 6 months of gestation, compared with the risk of the drugs. When the patient has moderate or severe hypertension with other risk factors or target organ damage, such as renal insufficiency or left ventricular hypertrophy, the value of continuing antihypertensive treatment is assumed to be fully established. For uncomplicated mild hypertension without other risk factors, there are too few studies for an unequivocal set of conclusions. Most of the recently developed antihypertensive agents have not been well studied for their safety vis á vis human fetal development during the initial phases of pregnancy. Blood pressure during this period rarely increases and is often lower than during the nonpregnant state. The available evidence suggests that antihypertensive drug therapy has no demonstrated value in this setting.[5–7]

If antihypertensive drug therapy is required during the initial phases of pregnancy, which drugs are effective and safe for the mother-to-be and for the fetus? Concern about fetal development and the risk to its proceeding without defect have been weighed by those concerned with this issue against the risk to the mother of uncontrolled severe hypertension that may occur if therapy is discontinued. Many of the recently available antihypertensive drugs have not been studied in human pregnancy due to concern that they might cause fetal abnormality on the basis of experimental studies in animal models. Thus, our knowledge of the potential for benefit versus harm for use during pregnancy is severely limited. The available consensus suggests that the older drugs—methyldopa and hydralazine—are considered the safest agents throughout pregnancy with regard to the fetus.[6,8] There is concern about the β-blockers and calcium channel blockers in early pregnancy and universal agreement that the ACE inhibitors are contraindicated throughout pregnancy.

In contrast to the views just stated with regard to the use of β-blockers and calcium channel entry blockers early in pregnancy, there is much more acceptance of these agents during pregnancy-induced hypertension or the increase in pressure occurring in the second half of gestation in patients with "chronic" hypertension. In this setting some of the newer agents have been used and appear to be affective for control of maternal pressure without fetal harm. Table 21-1 summarizes these agents.

Control of blood pressure during the second half of pregnancy by antihypertensive drugs may be beneficial, but does this effectiveness prevent the more serious complications associated with pre-eclampsia? Studies have shown that reduction of pressure does not necessarily prevent this complication.[6,9] Recent reports provide evidence that aspirin (60 mg/day) can prevent

Table 21-1. Efficacy and Safety of Antihypertensive Drugs During Pregnancy

Agent	First Half of Pregnancy (1–25 weeks)	Second Half of Pregnancy (≥25 weeks)
Methyldopa	Considered safe and effective	Safe and effective
Hydralazine	Considered safe and effective	Safe and variably effective
β-Blockers	Concern about safety of the fetus	Generally considered safe and effective, especially atenolol[8]
Labetalol	No information	Effective; reports suggest reasonable safety[9,11]
Nifedipine	Concern about safety of the fetus	Effective, more so than hydralazine[12]
Nicardipine	No studies	Effective for pressure, probably safe, few reports[13]
Other calcium blockers	No studies found	Few small studies
ACE inhibitors	Contraindicated	Contraindicated

pre-eclampsia, particularly in those with higher pressures. In a large randomized clinical trial, 11.6 percent of the women with systolic pressures at entry of 120 to 135 mmHg and given a placebo developed pre-eclampsia, compared with 5.6 percent in the aspirin-treated group, a reduction by aspirin of nearly 50 percent in the appearance of pre-eclampsia.[10] A higher rate of placental bleeding did occur in the aspirin-treated subjects, but the overall benefit seemed to favor aspirin use for patients with higher pressure.

After delivery, antihypertensive medication will need adjustment. For patients with pure pregnancy-induced hypertension, tapering and cessation of drug treatment is in order. For patients with persistent hypertension, a change to the previous medications or to those best suited for optimal control is desirable. To repeat once more, if there is doubt about whether the patient is, in fact, hypertensive following pregnancy, I recommend consideration of withdrawal of all medication and redefining the baseline using the supplemental methods, preferably ambulatory blood pressure monitoring.

REFERENCES

1. Cunningham FG, Lindheimer MD: Current concepts: hypertension in pregnancy. N Engl J Med 326:927, 1992
2. Pickering TG, James GD, Boddie C et al: How common is white coat hypertension? JAMA 259:225, 1988
3. Eison H, Phillips RA, Ardeljan M, Krakoff LR: Differences in ambulatory blood pressure between men and women with mild hypertension. J Hum Hypertens 4:400, 1990

4. Rayburn WF, Zuspan FP: Portable blood pressure monitoring for borderline or mild hypertension during pregnancy. Clin Obstet Gynecol 35:395, 1992

5. Sibai BM: Hypertension in pregnancy. Obstet Gynecol Clin North Am 19:615, 1992

6. Kyle PM, Redman CW: Comparative risk-benefit assessment of drugs used in the management of hypertension in pregnancy. Drug Safety 7:223, 1992

7. Hjertberg R, Belfrage P, Hanson U: Conservative treatment of mild and moderate hypertension in pregnancy. Acta Obstet Gynecol Scand 71:439, 1992

8. Lowe SA, Rubin PC: The pharmacological management of hypertension in pregnancy, editorial. J Hypertens 10:201, 1992

9. Cruickshank DJ, Robertson AA, Campbell DM, MacGillivray I: Does labetalol influence the development of proteinuria in pregnancy hypertension? A randomised controlled study. Eur J Obstet Gynecol Reprod Biol 45:47, 1992

10. Sibai BM, Caritis SN, Thom E et al: Prevention of preeclampsia with low-dose aspirin in healthy, nulliparous pregnant women. N Engl J Med 329:1213, 1993

11. Mahmoud TZ, Bjornsson S, Calder AA: Labetalol therapy in pregnancy induced hypertension: the effects on fetoplacental circulation and fetal outcome. Eur J Obstet Gynecol Reprod Biol 50:109, 1993

12. Fenakel K, Fenakel G, Appelman Z et al: Nifedipine in the treatment of severe preeclampsia. Obstet Gynecol 77:331, 1991

13. Carbonne B, Jannet D, Touboul C et al: Nicardipine treatment of hypertension during pregnancy. Obstet Gynecol 81:908, 1993

22

HYPERTENSION AND SURGERY

Before the era of effective antihypertensive therapy (since 1970), the hypertension of those patients who needed surgery was often uncontrolled, which, no doubt, added to their intra- and postoperative risks of cardiovascular morbidity, stroke, myocardial infarction, and acute pulmonary congestion. Advances in treatment of moderate and severe hypertension plus improvement in anesthetic care and postoperative monitoring have markedly improved this picture.[1] The recent development of less invasive or "minimal access" surgery (i.e., laparoscopy) may also be of benefit by reducing the risk as compared with more invasive procedures. In this chapter, the pertinent considerations for hypertensive patients requiring noncardiac surgery are divided into three sections: preoperative, intraoperative, and postoperative phases.

PREOPERATIVE MANAGEMENT

The hypertensive patient who is to undergo a surgical procedure should be reassessed with regard to overall status, including control of arterial pressure and target organ damage. Most pertinent is the presence of a recent myocardial infarction or stroke. Past experience and recent studies tend to agree that such events occurring within the previous 6 months increase the risk of intraoperative and postoperative cardiovascular morbidity and mortality. Now that most hypertensive patients can have their pressure well controlled prior to surgery, a history of hypertension, itself, is less of a risk than once was the case.[1,2]

How then should the patient be managed immediately before surgery? There are several important issues in this regard. First, communication between the physician providing continuing care and the anesthesiologist is necessary. A summary of the patient's medical status, current medications, and pertinent recent test results should be made available for review. In general, patients should continue taking their antihypertensive medications through the day of surgery. There is no basis for discontinuing medications, and there is a risk of a sudden increase in pressure if clonidine-like agents (α_2-agonists) are suddenly stopped. For those with ischemic heart disease, β-blockers and probably calcium channel entry blockers must be continued.

Several long-acting preparations are available for 24- to 48-hour control. When these agents are used daily and given on the morning of surgery, they will last throughout the operative and immediate postoperative period, almost until oral intake is re-established. Oral medications can be given safely with small amounts of water a few hours before anesthesia. For those on α_2-blockers, the clonidine patch (TTS-system) is a clever way to deliver this drug continuously during periods when the patient cannot take medication by mouth.[3] Overshoot hypertension due to withdrawal of α_2-agonists can thus be avoided.

INTRAOPERATIVE MANAGEMENT

Strictly speaking, intraoperative management of blood pressure is within the control of the anesthesiologist. However, a few suggestions are in order. To me, the intraoperative period begins with the onset of anesthesia and ends when the patient enters the recovery room. If monitored carefully, arterial pressure fluctuates considerably during this interval. Often blood pressure falls during anesthesia and surgery. There are a few times, however, when increases in pressure are predictable. These are during endotracheal intubation, skin incision, and pain perception if anesthesia is too "light." Whether such brief elevations in pressure are deleterious remains uncertain. However, attention has been given to these transient episodes. These pressure "spikes" can be blunted or prevented by either increased anesthesia or increased rapidly acting antihypertensive agents.[4,5] The overall pattern of pressure during surgery will reflect fluid shifts, hemorrhage, fluid replacement, and the effects of anesthetic agents and use of vasoactive substances. Unexpected or unpredicted blood pressure elevations should raise the possibility of hitherto unsuspected pheochromocytoma. Immediate use of phentolamine or nitroprusside is necessary; if possible, surgery should be terminated until pheochromocytoma is either detected or excluded.

POSTOPERATIVE MANAGEMENT

After surgery, when the effect of anesthesia dissipates and the fluid balance reaches the resultant of losses, infusions, and shifts, blood pressure may become elevated, particularly in patients with a prior history of moderate or severe hypertension. Such elevations may be due to uncontrolled pain; appropriate analgesia is needed. Next, fluid volume status needs assessment; if excess fluid has been given and results in high cardiac filling pressures, cardiac output may increase and raise pressure if peripheral resistance remains normal or elevated (as may be the case for patients with established hypertension). This is the setting in which pulmonary congestion may occur. An intravenous diuretic drug (furosemide or bumetanide) can correct this abnormality. For those patients with postoperative hypertension, unexplained by the preceding causes, control of arterial pressure can be provided by several rapidly acting intravenous agents, summarized in Table 22-1.

Table 22-1. Intravenous Agents Suitable for Postoperative Hypertension

Agent	Advantage	Disadvantage
Nitroglycerine	Coronary vasodilator, may reduce preload and afterload	Some tendency for tolerance, reduced effect on pressure
Sodium nitroprusside	Rapid control of pressure as vasodilatory	Cyanide toxicity if use is prolonged
Trimethaphan	Ganglionic blocking agent, antiadrenergic effects	May cause cholinergic blockade, intestinal ileus, urine retention; tolerance can develop
Enalapril	Intravenous ACE inhibitor	Little experience
Labetalol	Combined α/β-receptor antagonist	Predominantly β-blocker; may cause bronchoconstriction; avoid in bronchospasm
Phentolamine	Nonselective α-receptor	Tachycardia; indicated for massive catecholamine excess as in pheochromocytoma
Nicardipine	Dihydropyridine calcium channel blocker; arteriolar and coronary vasodilator	May cause reflex adrenergic activation; can be countered by β-receptor blockade
Esmolol	β-Receptor antagonist	Caution in obstructive pulmonary disease, bronchospasm
Furosemide, bumetanide, ethacrynic acid	Rapid, loop-site diuretics	Volume depletion, potassium depletion, contraction alkalosis

Optimal control of arterial pressure during the immediate postoperative period, before the patients can resume their oral regimen, is now possible due to the variety of agents currently available and the technology for their delivery at controlled rates. Close, minute-to-minute surveillance of arterial pressure is now also possible and standard using intra-arterial monitoring or reasonably accurate automatic noninvasive devices. It is not yet fully established, however, whether tight control of arterial pressure in the postoperative period confers benefit. Perhaps most important is the avoidance of intra- and postoperative myocardial ischemia through a variety of measures: adequate oxygenation, restoration of normal circulating hemoglobin levels, and avoidance of hypotension.

Once the patient can take medication by mouth, the patient's usual antihypertensive medications may be slowly resumed, albeit with close observation to avoid hypotension in those with altered fluid balance and, perhaps, sluggish baroreflexes. It is often observed that hypertensive patients have much lower pressures, *without any antihypertensive medication*, following surgery. As they begin to become active and return to their usual activities, pressure often increases to levels that require reinstitution of active treatment. If prior hypertension was mild, it may take weeks or months for the blood pressure to reach the hypertensive range. On occasion, weight loss following surgery seems to explain why blood pressure remains much lower than it was in the past. When previously hypertensive patients are discharged on no medication, my habit is to see them within 1 month to determine whether resumption of antihypertensive medication is necessary. It may take up to 1 year for their pressures to require drug treatment. If there is any previous history of ischemic heart disease, an electrocardiogram during the postoperative phase may, occasionally, reveal a silent myocardial infarction that accounts for a lowered pressure but worsens the overall risk/target organ profile of the patient.

REFERENCES

1. Mangano DT: Risk assessment for noncardiac surgery. p. 447. In Kapoor AS, Singh BN (eds): Prognosis and Risk Assessment in Cardiovascular Disease. Churchill Livingstone, New York, 1993

2. Ashton CM, Peterson NJ, Wray NP et al: The incidence of perioperative myocardial infarction in men undergoing noncardiac surgery. Ann Intern Med 118:504, 1993

3. Segal IS, Jarvis DJ, Duncan SR et al: Clinical efficacy of oral transdermal clonidine combinations during the perioperative period. Anesthesiology 74:220, 1991

4. Goto F, Kato S, Sudo I: Treatment of intraoperative hypertension with enflurane, nicardipine, or human atrial natriuretic peptide: haemodynamic and renal effects. Can J Anaesth 39:932, 1992

5. Omote K, Kirita A, Namiki A, Iwasaki H: Effects of nicardipine on the circulatory responses to tracheal intubation in normotensive and hypertensive patients. Anaesthesia 47:24, 1992

23

OTHER MEDICAL PROBLEMS

PERIPHERAL VASCULAR DISEASE

Presence of symptomatic peripheral vascular disease (i.e., intermittent claudication) indicates that the patient has an atherosclerotic burden involving the aorta, iliac, femoral, and distal arteries. Usually the patient is at least 55 years old and has a history of nonhypertensive risk factors, especially smoking, with hyperlipidemia and noninsulin-dependent diabetes mellitus as well. Clinical evidence of carotid arterial narrowing and/or coronary artery disease are commonly found. Even before symptoms appear, the examination may reveal signs of peripheral arterial disease such as an ankle/arm systolic pressure ratio of less than 0.9 and lower abdominal or groin bruits. Those patients with chronic obstructive pulmonary disease (evidence of their prior smoking habits) often have silent or symptomatic peripheral vascular disease. Noninvasive assessment of the lower leg perfusion at rest and exercise using Doppler ultrasound can provide quantitative assessment of the patient's status for baseline and serial observation.

The experience with antihypertensive medications in patients with peripheral vascular disease is summarized in Table 23-1. Since peripheral arterial blood flow, particularly during exercise, is related to the level of cardiac output, there has been suspicion that use of the β-receptor blockers (in particular the nonselective β-blockers that reduce β_2-receptor–mediated vasodilation) might worsen symptoms of peripheral arterial occlusive disease. The well-known adverse effects of β-blocker treatment—cold digits and Raynaud-like symptoms—support the suspicion. Worsening of peripheral vascular disease during treatment with β-blockers has been found in some, but not all, studies.[1,2] It had been suggested that those β-blockers that are nonselective and without intrinsic sympathomimetic activity (ISA) should be more likely to aggravate peripheral vascular disease compared with the β_1-selective agents with ISA. However, the available studies fail to confirm uniformly that (1) β-blockers invariably worsen symptoms of peripheral vascular disease1 or (2) that β-blockers with ISA or α-blockade (labetalol) are superior to those without ISA or α-blockade.[2-4] When ischemic coronary heart disease is present, the cardiac active calcium channel blockers verapamil and diltiazem would appear theoretically preferable to β-blockers, as the former tend to have less reduction of resting and exertional cardiac output than the latter.

Table 23-1. Effect of Antihypertensive Drugs on Peripheral Vascular Disease

Drug Class	Effect
Diuretics	No effect reported
β-Blockers	Inconsistent; some evidence of increased symptoms, reduced walking distance; other studies report no effect
Calcium channel blockers	No effect or change in symptoms or walking distance
Angiotensin converting enzyme inhibitors	No change in symptoms or walking distance
α_1-Receptor blockers	No effect on walking distance or symptoms

Other matters being equal, drugs with vasodilator effects should be more effective for treating hypertensive patients with peripheral vascular disease. Agents with theoretical value would be the dihydropyridine calcium channel blockers (such as nifedipine) and the α_1-receptor blockers. As yet, however, neither the calcium entry blockers[5,6] nor the α_1-receptor antagonists[7] have been shown to be significantly effective for symptomatic improvement. One report indicates that neither atenolol nor nifedipine had an effect on symptoms (walking distance) when used as monotherapy; however, the combination worsened symptoms.[5]

Circulating angiotensin II can certainly cause peripheral vasoconstriction; several studies suggest that captopril may increase calf blood flow in peripheral vascular disease with variable effect on exercise symptoms.[2,8,9] In one study, neither captopril nor nifedipine caused a change in walking distance.[2]

Antihypertensive drug therapy in patients with peripheral vascular disease will often be combined with measures to reduce the other risk factors and concurrent disorders that are present. The resultant drug burden for many such patients is a large one and thus requires counseling and reassessment of the patient's compliance to avoid the potential for over and under dosing due to confusion about the drug schedule. The potential for adverse drug interactions is increased when many agents are simultaneously prescribed. Particular attention is necessary for patients taking anticoagulants; close monitoring of the prothrombin time when drugs are started or stopped or doses are changed is required.

The rate of progress of peripheral vascular disease in hypertensive persons seems to be similar to patients with normal blood pressure. Emphasis on the concurrent value of positive life-style changes, diet, and regular exercise may delay the need for arteriography and invasive therapy.

ASTHMA AND CHRONIC OBSTRUCTIVE PULMONARY DISEASE

Occasionally a young hypertensive patient will also have asthma of the usual type. More often chronic obstructive pulmonary disease (COPD) and high blood pressure coexist and share the nonhypertensive risk factor, many years of cigarette smoking, as a substrate. As noted earlier, peripheral vascular disease will often be found in such patients if carefully searched for. Few studies have singled out the subgroup of hypertensive persons with either asthma or COPD for special analysis of either long-term risk or natural history or for the results of treatment in randomized trials. For this reason, management of such patients depends on knowledge of the mechanisms involved rather than an established data base for guidance.

There is no compelling reason not to attempt blood pressure reduction in those with asthma or COPD, as the risk of future stroke or cardiac disease must be at least that of patients without pulmonary disease and may well be higher. Considerations regarding antihypertensive medication are given in Table 23-2. The primary lung dysfunction is airway obstruction, which is ordinarily treated with β_2-receptor agonists. It is also possible that airway resistance is, to some extent, kept lower by endogenous circulating epinephrine, the natural β_2-receptor agonist. These considerations imply that antagonism of β_2-receptors by the nonselective β-blockers often used to treat hypertension (e.g., propranolol or timolol) may impair pulmonary function in those with asthma or COPD. Even the β_1-selective receptor antagonists (e.g., metoprolol or atenolol) become less selective at higher doses and antagonize β_2-receptors and, thus, should be avoided whenever possible. Whether those β-blockers with ISA might be safer or more suitable for use in patients with asthma or COPD remains uncertain, as these β-blockers inhibit the heart rate response to exercise. On occasion, a patient with chronic obstructive airway disease, hypertension, and angina may benefit from a low dose of a β_1-selective blocker through a reduction in heart rate. In general, however, I prefer to avoid use of the β-blockers for treatment of the hypertensive patients with asthma or COPD.

Many of the other antihypertensive agents have received little formal evaluation in either asthmatics or patients with COPD. Diuretics may be

Table 23-2. Effect of Antihypertensive Drugs on Asthma or Chronic Obstructive Pulmonary Disease

Drug Class	Effect
Diuretics	Theoretic disadvantage resulting from hypokalemia, excessive volume loss
β-Receptor blockers	Can increase airway resistance and antagonize β_2-receptor agonists
Calcium channel entry blockers	Seem to have little effect; theoretically beneficial, based on experimental studies; alternative to β-blockers for angina
Angiotensin converting enzyme inhibitors	Theoretical disadvantage due to potentiation of kinins; clinical studies suggest no deleterious effect on airway resistance; cough can be a problem

effective, but hypokalemia should be avoided due to its potential for cardiac arrhythmias given the setting of β_2-agonist treatment and resultant tachycardia that often occurs in these patients. Excessive diuresis is to be avoided, as it may increase blood viscosity in those already hypoxic and who perhaps have secondary polycythemia. The thickening effect of dehydration on pulmonary secretions is also to be avoided.

Since the calcium entry blockers relax smooth muscle, there is a theoretical basis for their being useful in asthma. Experimental studies suggest that verapamil inhibits agonist-induced bronchoconstriction.[10–12] In clinical evaluations, however, oral verapamil has no effect on airway function in patients with asthma or chronic obstructive airway disease.[13,14] In one comparison, neither verapamil nor the angiotensin converting enzyme (ACE) inhibitor captopril altered pulmonary function in asthmatic patients; no cough occurred in those given captopril.[13]

The kinins have been implicated as bronchoconstricting agents, which might participate in asthma. Converting enzyme is a kininase; inhibition of this enzyme by ACE inhibitors then potentiates kinin action. Indeed, it is this effect of the ACE inhibitors that has been suggested as the mechanism for the nonproductive cough that is the most common adverse effect of these drugs. However, in clinical use the ACE inhibitors fail to increase airway reactivity significantly in patients selected for hyperreactivity. In general, these agents have no deleterious effect on airway resistance.[15] Patients with asthma who become hypertensive during or after steroid use may have increased renin levels. Their blood pressure responds well to ACE inhibition without deleterious effect on their airway disease.[16] The occasional nonproductive cough induced by ACE inhibitors may occur more often in those with pulmonary disease, but has no known effect on outcome. However, the appearance of a new cough complicates the clinical picture, since it may be due to medication or progression of the pulmonary disease. Appropriate diagnostic steps are necessary, including withdrawal of the ACE inhibitor if this drug is the likely culprit.

A search of current literature reveals no information on the value of α_1-receptor blockers for patients with either asthma or chronic obstructive airway disease. In summary, those with the combination of obstructive pulmonary disease and hypertension can be effectively treated with either the calcium channel blockers or the ACE inhibitors. Diuretics should be used with caution and extra attention to the risk of hypokalemia. β-Receptor blockers of all types should be avoided. In unusual circumstances, low doses of the β_1-selective antagonists may be given with careful assessment for changes in airway function.

HYPERLIPIDEMIA

The risk cluster of hypertension with one of the hyperlipidemias is a common problem. In part, this combination is related to the high prevalence of obesity in the population of those with high blood pressure. This short section does not address the management of the hyperlipidemic patient, per se,

Table 23-3. Effect of Lipid Lowering Agents on Blood Pressure

Agent	Effect on Blood Pressure or Antihypertensive Response
Fish oils	Small reduction (~5 mmHg) in pressure; may be additive to antihypertensive medication
Cholestyramine	Unknown effects
Lovastatin	No effect on response to treatment
Simvastin	No effect on response to treatment
Privastatin	Unknown
Niacin	Unknown
Probucol	Unknown
Fibric acid derivatives (clofibrate and gemfibrizol)	Unknown

but instead summarizes the effects of lipid lowering drugs on the treatment of hypertension. The most commonly used lipid or lipoprotein lowering agents are listed in Table 23-3. Most of these drugs have not been systematically evaluated for their effects either on the blood pressure itself or on the response to antihypertensive therapy. Lovastatin is the exception. Two studies agree that this HMG coenzyme A reductase inhibitor, when used for reduction of low-density lipoprotein cholesterol, had no discernible effect on control of hypertension in patients treated with a variety of antihypertensive agents, including diuretics and β-blockers.[17,18] Another report indicates that the antihypertensive effect of either lisinopril or nifedipine was unaltered by lovastatin therapy.[19] Looking at the other side of this issue, in the few studies available, antihypertensive medications (thiazide diuretics, β-blockers, lisinopril, nifedipine) have no apparent effect on cholesterol reduction by the HMG coenzyme A reductase inhibitors lovastatin or simvastin or the fibric acid derivative gemfibrizol.

My own view is that those hypertensive patients who have hyperlipidemias that persist after weight reduction and diet therapy have been tried should be treated with lipid lowering drugs on the same basis as normotensive persons. Patients with evidence of atherosclerotic disease of the coronary, carotid, renal, or peripheral arteries are to be treated aggressively with the minimum goal being to reduce the total serum cholesterol to below 200 mg/dl and the low-density lipoprotein cholesterol to below 130 mg/dl.

HYPERURICEMIA AND/OR GOUT

Increased serum uric acid levels that are a mild degree (1 to 2 mg/dl) above the upper limit of normal are often found in untreated hypertensive patients. This may occur in patients with normal glomerular filtration rates, as reflected by serum urea nitrogen, but is more likely to occur with reduced glomerular filtration. While elevated serum uric acid concentrations have been associated with increased cardiovascular morbidity and mortality (mainly due to coronary heart disease), no pathogenetic or causal relationship has been demonstrated; hyperuricemia is merely an association.

Twenty years ago the most common cause of hyperuricemia in hypertensive patients was diuretic therapy. For example, the usual doses of hydrochlorothiazide prescribed at that time (50 to 100 mg/day) caused serum uric acid to increase by 1 to 3 mg/dl. Most patients with diuretic-induced hyperuricemia never developed gout. During the past 10 years, there has been an overall reduction in the frequency of high-dose diuretic treatment; the usual daily dose of hydrochlorothiazide is 25 mg/day. Several studies have used one-half that amount. The lower doses still cause serum uric acid to increase, but the increments are small, 0.5 to 1.0 mg/dl. The nondiuretic antihypertensive agents have little or no effect on serum uric acid. It has been reported that those vasodilators that increase renal blood flow (i.e., the dihydropyridine calcium channel entry blockers) may actually reduce serum uric acid concentration by about 0.5 mg/dl. However, this small effect has no known clinical significance.

Clinical gout, expressed as acute urate crystal arthritis, is associated with hyperuricemia, yet its occurrence is not well related to the degree of serum uric acid elevation, per se. Acute gout is often treated with a short course of nonsteroidal anti-inflammatory agents (NSAIDs). Such agents may increase blood pressure or diminish the effect of antihypertensive drugs due to their inhibition of prostaglandin synthase and loss of the vasodilator prostaglandins. However, if given for only a few days to patients with normal renal function, NSAIDs seem to have no significant effect on long-term control of blood pressure. It has been suggested that some NSAIDs, notably sulindac, may have less effect on renal cyclo-oxygenase and thereby be less likely to cause decreased renal blood flow or hypertension. Colchicine, the ancient remedy for acute gout, is still effective and safe when given in proper doses. As prophylactic treatment for prevention of recurrent gout, daily colchicine and/or allopurinol, a xanthine oxidase inhibitor, are well established. The latter significantly decreases serum uric acid concentration and prevents or reverses chronic tophaceous gout, now a rarely seen phenomenon.

In hypertensive patients, there is no longer a rationale for uricosuric agents, such as probenecid. These drugs increase uric acid excretion and the risk of uric acid renal calculi. They have also been linked to interstitial nephritis. The one uricosuric diuretic agent to be approved for hypertension, ticrynafen, was withdrawn from the market after less than 1 year of use due to its severe and fatal adverse effects of hepatic necrosis and acute renal insufficiency.

Chronic prophylactic therapy to prevent gout is reserved for those with clearly documented acute uric acid-induced arthritis. In general, colchicine (0.6 mg/day) is used for those with minimal hyperuricemia. This dose of colchicine is well below that which causes diarrhea. Allopurinol (100 to 300 mg/day) is reserved for patients with gout and persistent hyperuricemia or those with hyperuricuria and uric acid renal calculi. Patients given allopurinol must be instructed to discontinue it if a rash appears; severe, and even fatal, Stevens-Johnston syndrome has been linked to this drug. It is clear that the progressive reduction in the average diuretic dose has reduced the number of treated patients with serum uric acid levels above 10 mg/dl. It is likely that there has been a parallel decrease in the prescribing of either uricosuric agents or allopurinol, to my mind a beneficial side effect of current trends in antihypertensive drug treatment.

DEPRESSION AND OTHER PSYCHIATRIC DISORDERS

As hypertension is so often found in the adult and especially the older population, it is not surprising that other highly prevalent diseases coexist with elevated blood pressure. The depressive disorders are among those that often require consideration in treating hypertensive patients. This is particularly so in older patients with elevated blood pressure in which symptoms suggesting cardiac disease or an adverse drug disorder may be difficult to distinguish from a depressive disorder. Those with established depressive syndromes pose several management problems. Their pathophysiology may alter diagnostic tests for secondary hypertension. For example, plasma catecholamines are slightly elevated in those with depression; a false-positive test result for pheochromocytoma may occur. There is less suppression of plasma cortisol by dexamethasone in depressed patients compared with normal persons[20]; Cushing syndrome may be suggested by a false-positive result.

Several antihypertensive drugs that have actions within the central nervous system have been associated with depressive reactions or depression-like symptoms. Reserpine, methyldopa, the α_2-agonists (e.g., clonidine), and the β-receptor blockers, particularly those that are lipophilic and thus more likely to cross the blood-brain barrier, have received attention for their depression-like adverse effects. A review of adverse effects related to propranolol that occurred during the therapeutic trials of antihypertensive therapy clearly implicates this β-blocker for induction of depression-like symptoms.[21] A retrospective review of β-blocker treatment in hypertension, however, suggests that once confounding influences, such as use of other drugs, particularly benzodiazepines, is adjusted for by multivariate analysis, the relationship between β-blockers and depression is less certain.[22] For those hypertensive persons with clear-cut depression, it is my conclusion that β-blockers should be avoided, particularly those that are lipophilic (propranolol, timolol, and metoprolol). Alternatives are available; verapamil may often be a useful choice because its cardiac actions are similar to those of β-blockade.

During the treatment of severe depression, electroshock therapy (ECT) may be necessary for relief of symptoms. Successful ECT may be associated with a subsequent fall in blood pressure, as has also been observed during treatment of depression with tricyclic antidepressants.[23] The abrupt transient increase in blood pressure during ECT has been considered a risk of this treatment, limiting its use in those with cardiovascular disease. Pretreatment with the α/β-receptor blocker labetalol can prevent the increases in arterial pressure, heart rate, and occurrence of cardiac arrhythmias during ECT and thus may increase the safety of this intervention.[24] Sublingual nifedipine has also been used to prevent ECT-induced elevations in arterial pressure, but this agent has no effect on the increase in heart rate.[25]

The physician who treats hypertensive patients must be aware of the effects of antidepressant or psychotropic drugs on the cardiovascular system and the many drug interactions between antidepressants and other drugs. Table 23-4 summarizes the most important effects of the various classes of the antidepressants and other agents used in the treatment of psychiatric illness on blood pressure or the treatment of hypertension. It is imperative that the treating physician know which drugs are being prescribed and taken by their patients during the course of antihypertensive therapy. If the patient is not certain about the treatment then communication with the psychiatrist to sort out this problem becomes necessary. Well-educated patients will, in general, keep careful records of their therapy for review by each doctor, since it is not unusual that regulation of medication is a joint project.

Many depressed patients are treated with the tricyclic agents in which orthostatic reduction in pressure is often found, if looked for. Measurement of seated and standing pressures at each visit is advisable for these patients, even if they do not express symptoms of orthostatic hypotension. The tricyclics block the adrenergic neuronal pump by which guanethidine and its analogs gain access to the neuron and deplete norepinephrine. This accounts for the diminished effectiveness of these peripheral neuron depletors in depressed patients during their treatment with the tricyclics. However, since the peripheral neuron depletors are now rarely used, this problem of drug interaction has virtually ceased. Tricyclics also cause conduction delays, even heart block, in those with cardiac disease or pre-existing conduction abnormalities.

Monoamine oxidase inhibitors (MAOIs) have a well-established record of causing hypertensive reactions if patients ingest tyramine-containing foods. Normally tyramine is metabolized by monoamine oxidase in the intestine and liver. When the intestinal and hepatic enzyme is blocked, ingested tyramine can gain access to the circulation and release norepinephrine from adrenergic nerve terminals, causing the hypertensive reaction. This is an α-receptor–mediated hypertension and can be reversed by α-receptor antagonists. The accompanying tachycardia is due to cardiac β-receptor stimulation and can be corrected by β-receptor blockade. As a result, the drug of choice for hypertensive/tachycardia crises due to the MAOI/tyramine syndrome is labetalol. Use of MAOIs alone may reduce blood pressure and/or cause orthostatic hypotension. At one time, an MAOI, pargyline, was approved and used for treatment of hypertension. The mechanisms by which MAOIs reduce blood pressure may have included (1) reduced release of norepinephrine to α_1-postsynaptic receptors as a direct effect or (2) accumulation of a false transmitter, octopamine, in neurons diluting the amount of norepinephrine available for neurosecretion. Occasionally, patients taking an MAOI have been noted to have abrupt increases in pressure without documentation of tyramine ingestion; the precise mechanism for such events is unknown.[26] It has been suggested that patients taking MAOIs are more sus-

Table 23-4. Effects of the Antidepressant and Psychotropic Drugs on Blood Pressure and Antihypertensive Drug Treatment

Drug Class or Drug	Effect
Tricyclic antidepressants	Orthostatic hypotension; reduce effect of some antihypertensive drugs, especially neuron depletors (i.e., guanethidine); overdose may cause hyper- or hypotension and cardiac conduction disturbances
Monoamine oxidase inhibitors (MAOIs)	Hypertensive reactions to tyramine-containing foods or wines, other drugs, and over-the-counter sympathomimetics; occasional spontaneous blood pressure elevations
Selective serotonin re-uptake inhibitors (fluoxetine, paroxetine, sertraline)	Hypertensive reactions with MAOIs, the "serotonin syndrome" of confusion, myoclonus, hypomania, diarrhea, and hypertension
Benzodiazepines	No significant effect on blood pressure
Lithium	Excretion may be reduced by diuretic agents and dehydration leading to toxic plasma levels
Phenothiazines, similar psychotropic drugs	Orthostatic hypotension, malignant neuroleptic syndrome (tachycardia, myocardial ischemia)
Bupropion	Occasional increase in pressure, orthostatic hypotension is rare

ceptible to blood pressure raising effects of the over-the-counter sympathomimetics, such as phenylpropanolamine, contained in decongestants and diet pills.[27] However, it is also likely that some of these patients may take overdoses of the over-the-counter drugs, resulting in hyperadrenergic hypertensive crises.

There is generally less information about the effect of the newer antidepressant agents. A study of buproprion in patients with pre-existing cardiac disease found that a small, but significant, increase in supine blood pressure was caused by 3 weeks treatment with this agent. Two hypertensive patients had clinically significant increases in blood pressure that were reduced when buproprion was discontinued.[28] It has been suggested that the selective serotonin re-uptake inhibitiors, such as fluoxetine, have fewer adverse effects than the older agents. This may be the case when these are used as monotherapy. The only recent drug interaction to be reported with relevance to blood pressure is the occurrence of hypertensive episodes when MAOIs are combined with fluoxetine.[29]

There is far less literature available to assess some of the other psychiatric disorders and treatment for their interaction with either blood pressure or antihypertensive therapy when compared with the depressive disorders. The usual anxiety syndromes that are treated with benzodiazepines pose no particular problem. However, the specific panic disorder syndrome is associated with hypertension as a diagnosis[30] and hypertensive episodes as a manifestation.[31] A study of the effect of benzodiazepine therapy on long-term patterns of blood pressure in this disorder would be of interest and relevance. Mania and hypomanic disorders are often treated with lithium, which has little or no effect on blood pressure, itself. However, lithium levels must be kept rigidly controlled during treatment to avoid the toxicity of high plasma concentrations. Dehydration is to be avoided; thus those patients taking lithium who are given diuretic agents should be carefully monitored to avoid lithium toxicity.

As a general rule for treatment of hypertensive patients with psychiatric disorders, I try to eliminate any drug that might alter their mental status or have an interaction with the agents prescribed for their disorder. More careful monitoring of standing blood pressure and the electrocardiogram (for conduction disturbances) is needed for patients taking tricyclic antidepressants. β-Blockers and verapamil are to be avoided in these patients whenever possible. On theoretical grounds, it appears that the ACE inhibitors and the dihydropyridine calcium channel entry blockers would be preferable for treatment of depressed hypertensive persons. These drug classes have good track records for quality of life indices, generally tend not to cause orthostatic hypotension, and also do not alter cardiac conduction. The same principle applies to patients with other severe psychiatric disorders, such as the psychoses. Often these patients are treated with large doses of psychotropic drugs and atropine-like agents (to reduce extrapyramidal manifestations). Thirst and water balance may be altered; diuretics are to be avoided.

For those with the panic disorder syndrome and intermittent hypertensive episodes not fully controlled on benzodiazepine treatment, the combination of α/β-blockers in the form of labetalol, as monotherapy, or as β- and α_1-receptor blockers (e.g., atenolol and doxazosin) might be effective. More studies are needed in this area.

REFERENCES

1. Radack K, Deck C: Beta-adrenergic blocker therapy does not worsen intermittent claudication in subjects with peripheral arterial disease: a meta-analysis of randomized controlled trials. Arch Intern Med 151:1769, 1991

2. Roberts DH, Tsao Y, Linge K et al: Double-blind comparison of captopril with nifedipine in hypertension complicated by intermittent claudication. Angiology 43:748, 1992

3. Svendsen TL, Jelnes R, Tonnesen KH: The effects of acebutolol and metoprolol on walking distances and distal blood pressure in hypertensive patients with intermittent claudication. J Intern Med 219:161, 1986

4. Lepantalo M Beta blockade and intermittent claudication. J Intern Med, suppl. 700:1, 1985

5. Solomon SA, Ramsay LE, Yeo WW et al: Beta blockade and intermittent claudication: placebo controlled trial of atenolol and nifedipine and their combination. BMJ 303:1100, 1991

6. Lewis P, Psaila JV, Davies WT et al: Nifedipine in patients with peripheral vascular disease. Eur J Vasc Surg 3:159, 1989

7. Catalano M, Libretti A: A multicenter study of doxazosin in the treatment of patients with mild or moderate essential hypertension and concomitant intermittent claudication. Am Heart J 121:367, 1991

8. Roberts DH, Tsao Y, McLoughlin GA, Breckenridge A: Placebo-controlled comparison of captopril, atenolol, labetalol, and pindolol in hypertension complicated by intermittent claudication. Lancet 2:650, 1987

9. Libretti A, Catalano M: Captopril in the treatment of hypertension associated with claudication. Postgrad Med J, suppl. 1. 62:34, 1986

10. Villanove X, Marthan R, Tunon de Lara JM et al: Sensitization decreases relaxation in human isolated airways. Am Rev Respir Dis 148:107, 1993

11. Ben Harari RR, Stenner M, Sutin KM: Clinical potency of calcium channel blockers in asthma may be related to their receptor-mediated phasic responses in vitro. Life Sci 51:2049, 1992

12. Imhof E, Elsasser S, Rosmus B et al: Verapamil in the prophylaxis of bronchial asthma. Is the bronchoprotective effect related to the plasma level? Eur J Clin Pharmacol 41:317, 1991

13. Riska H, Sovijarvi AR, Ahonen A et al: Effects of captopril on blood pressure and respiratory function compared to verapamil in patients with hypertension and asthma. J Cardiovasc Pharmacol 15:57, 1990

14. McTavish D, Sorkin EM: Verapamil. An updated review of its pharmacodynamic and pharmacokinetic properties, and therapeutic use in hypertension. Drugs 38:19, 1989

15. Kaufman J, Schmitt S, Barnard J, Busse W: Angiotensin-converting enzyme inhibitors in patients with bronchial responsiveness and asthma. Chest 101:922, 1992

16. Sanders BP, Portman RJ, Ramey RA et al: Hypertension during reduction of long-term steroid therapy in young subjects with asthma. J Allergy Clin Immunol 89:816, 1992

17. Pool JL, Shear CL, Downton M et al: Lovastatin and coadministered antihypertensive/cardiovascular agents. Hypertension 19:242, 1992

18. D'Agostino RB, Kannel WB, Stepanians MN, D'Agostino LC: Efficacy and tolerability of lovastatin in hypercholesterolemia in patients with systemic hypertension. Am J Cardiol 71:82, 1993

19. Os I, Bratland B, Dahlof B et al: Effect and tolerability of combining lovastatin witlh nifedipine or lisinopril. Am J Hypertens 6:688, 1993

20. Pfohl B, Rederer M, Coryell W, Stangl D: Association between post-dexamethasone cortisol level and blood pressure in depressed inpatients. J Nerv Ment Dis 179:44, 1991

21. Patten SB: Propranolol and depression: evidence from the antihypertensive trials. Can J Psychiatry 35:257, 1990

22. Bright RA, Everitt DE: Beta blockers and depression: evidence against an association. JAMA 267:1783, 1992

23. Swartz CM, Inglis AE: Blood pressure reduction with ECT response. J Clin Psychiatry 51:414, 1990

24. Stoudemire A, Knos G, Gladson M et al: Labetalol in the control of cardiovascular responses to electroconvulsive therapy in high-risk depressed medical patients. J Clin Psychiatry 51:508, 1990

25. Wells DG, Davies GG, Rosewarne F: Attenuation of electroconvulsive therapy induced hypertension with sublingual nifedipine. Anaesth Intensive Care 17:31, 1989

26. Keck PEJ, Pope HGJ, Nierenberg AA: Autoinduction of hypertensive reactions by tranylcypromine? J Clin Psychopharmacol 9:48, 1989

27. Harrison WM, McGrath PJ, Stewart JW, Quitkin F: MAOIs and hypertensive crises: the role of OTC drugs. J Clin Psychiatry 50:64, 1989

28. Roose SP, Dalack GW, Glassman AH et al: Cardiovascular effects of bupropion in depressed patients with heart disease. Am J Psychiatry 148:512, 1991

29. Feighner JP, Boyer WF, Tyler DL, Neborsky RJ: Adverse consequences of fluoxetine-MAOI combination therapy. J Clin Psychiatry 51:222, 1990

30. Noyes RJ, Woodman C, Garvey MJ et al: Generalized anxiety disorder vs. panic disorder. Distinguishing characteristics and patterns of comorbidity. J Nerv Ment Dis 180:369, 1992

31. White WB, Baker LH: Ambulatory blood pressure monitoring in patients with panic disorder. Arch Intern Med 147:1973, 1987

Appendix 1

LIST OF ANTIHYPERTENSIVE DRUGS

Table A1-1. Thiazide-Type Diuretic Agents[a]

Generic Name	Trade Name	Dose Range (mg/day)	Comments
Hydrochlorothiazide (HCTZ)	Hydrodiuril, Esidrix, Oretic	12.5–50	Protypical thiazide-type diuretic
Chlorthalidone	Hygroton	12.5–50	Long duration of action (≥24 hours)
Indapamide	Lozol	2.5–5	Very similar to chlorthalidone
Metolazone	Zaroxolyn	2.5–5	Similar to chlorthalidone
Metolazone	Mikrox	0.5–1.0	Much more bioavailable formulation than Zaroxolyn
Hydroflumethiazide	Diucardin	25–50	Similar to HCTZ
Chlorothiazide	Diuril	250–500	Identical action to HCTZ
Methyclothiazide	Enduron	2.5–5.0	Similar to HCTZ
Benzthiazide	Exna	25–50	Similar to HCTZ
Quinethazone	Hydromox	25–50	Similar to HCTZ

[a]All these drugs have a similar effect. When given (usually as once-a-day monotherapy) they reduce blood pressure in some patients. They are well known to be effective in combination with β-blockers, centrally acting agents, or ACE inhibitors. Adverse effects are similar for all: hypokalemia, hyperuricemia (occasional gout), hyponatremia, occasional impairment of glucose tolerance. Less frequent are hypercalcemia and thrombocytopenia. Modest increases in serum total and low-density lipoprotein cholesterol are well documented.

Table A1-2. Loop-Active and Potassium-Sparing Diuretic Agents

Generic Name	Proprietary Name	Dose Range	Comments
Loop-active diuretics			
Bumetanide	Bumex	Oral 0.5–2 mg/day Intravenous 0.5–1.0 mg	Like furosemide, useful for renal insufficiency and congestive heart failure
Furosemide	Lasix	Oral 20–80 mg bid Intravenous 20–100 mg	Most often used loop active diuretic in renal insufficiency and congestive heart failure
Ethacrynic acid	Edecrin	Oral 25–100 mg bid Intravenous 50–100 mg slow infusion	Gastrointestinal reactions reported; ototoxicity reported from intravenous use
Potassium-sparing diuretics			
Amiloride[a]	Midamor	5–10 mg/day	Well-tolerated sodium channel blocker; useful in combination with potassium-losing agents
Triamterene[a]	Dyrenium	50–100 mg bid	Sodium channel blocker; rare megaloblastic anemia reported
Spironolactone[a]	Aldactone	25–100 mg bid	Mineralocorticoid receptor antagonist; gynecomastia, menstrual disturbances limit use

[a]Can be given in combination with either thiazide-type agents or loop-active diuretics to reduce urinary potassium loss.

Table A1-3. Centrally Acting Agents

Generic Name	Proprietary Name	Dose Range	Comments
Clonidine	Catapres	0.1–0.3 mg bid (transdermal delivery [TTS] patches are available for use 1×/wk)	α_2-Agonist; overshoot hypertension reported Adverse effects: drowsiness, dry mouth, constipation
Guanabenz	Wytensin	4–16 mg bid	Very similar to clonidine, longer duration of action
Guanfacine	Tenex	1–3 mg/day	Longer duration of action than other α_2-agonists; may have less overshoot hypertension; no other differences
Methyldopa	Aldomet	250–1000 mg bid	Complex action as dopa decarboxylase inhibitor, false transmitter, and α_2-agonist Adverse effects: drowsiness, fatigue, positive Coombs test, hepatitis
Reserpine	Serpasil	0.1–0.5 mg/day	Central and peripheral neuron depletor; prolonged action Adverse effects: depression, hyperacidity

Table A1-4. Peripheral Antiadrenergic Drugs

Generic Name	Proprietary Name	Dose Range	Comments
			Adrenergic neuron depletors

Guanethidine	Ismelin	10–50 mg/day	Long acting
			Adverse effects:
			  orthostatic hypotension,
			  diarrhea, bradycardia

Guanadrel	Hylorel	10–40 mg bid	Shorter-acting agent than
			  guanethidine; less likely to
			  cause diarrhea

		α_1-Receptor antagonists[a]	

Prazosin	Minipress	1–5 mg tid	Short-acting agent
			Adverse effects: first dose and
			  orthostatic hypotension
			Can reduced low-density
			  lipoprotein and increase
			  high-density lipoprotein
			  cholesterol

Terazosin	Hytrin	1–5 mg/day or bid	Slightly longer duration of action than prazosin
Doxazosin	Cardura	1–10 mg/day	Longer duration of action suitable for once-a-day dosing
		Special drugs for pheochromocytoma	

Phenoxy-
  benzamine
	Dibenzyline	10–40 mg bid	Nonselective α-receptor blocker
			For prevention of hypertensive
			  episodes

Phentolamine	Regitine	1–5 mg IV bolus
		or infusion
			Nonselective α-receptor blocker
			For control of pressure in
			  patients with
			  pheochromocytoma

α-Methyl-
  meta-tyrosine
	Demser	250–1000 mg tid	Catecholamine synthesis
			  blocker
			Used in pheochromocytoma;
			  causes pseudoparkinsonian
			  state and crystalluria

		Combined α/β-blocker[b]	
Labetalol	Normodyne, Trandate	100–400 mg bid or tid 50-mg IV bolus	Fixed ratio receptor blocker; hepatotoxicity reported

[a]The α_1-receptor antagonists may combined with β-blockers for combined α/β-blockade. α_1-Receptor blockers may alleviate symptoms of prostatism, which may be useful in some hypertensive men.

[b]This is the only combined α/β-blocker available in the United States. The intravenous form may be used for hypertensive crises, especially if they are due to hyperadrenergic states (pheochromocytoma, amphetamine or diet pill overdose, MAOI/tyramine syndrome, or perhaps cocaine intoxication).

Table A1-5. β-Blockers[a]

Generic Name	Proprietary Name	Dose Range	Comments
Propranolol	Inderal, Inderal-LA	40–80 mg bid; the LA slow release form is given as 40–160 mg/day	Nonselective with short duration of action; lipid soluble; most widely used β-blocker
Timolol	Blocadren	10–20 mg bid	Very similar to propranolol in all important respects
Nadolol	Corgard	20–80 mg/day	Actions like propranolol; very long duration of action
Metoprolol	Lopressor	25–100 mg bid	β_1-Selective; also available in intravenous form
Metoprolol	Toprol XL	50–200 mg/day	Once-a-day formulation
Atenolol	Tenormin	25–100 mg/day	Longer acting, but similar to metoprolol
Pindolol	Visken	10–30 mg bid	Nonselective with ISA
Betaxolol	Kerlone	10–40 mg/day	Similar to atenolol, but long duration of action
Carteolol	Cartrol	2.5–10 mg/day	Nonselective with ISA
Penbutolol	Levatol	10–40 mg/day	Nonselective with slight ISA
Bisoprolol	Zebeta	5–10 mg/day	β_1-Selective without ISA; most recently approved in United States (1933); similar to atenolol
Acebutolol	Sectral	200–800 mg/day	β_1-Selective with mild ISA
Esmolol	Breviblock	Intravenous load 0.5 mg/kg/min, reduce as needed	Rapid action on and off; only for intravenous use

[a]There are differences in the β-blockers with regard to pharmacokinetics, selectivity for β_1- or β_2-receptors, and intrinsic sympathomimetic activity (ISA). Receptor selectivity diminishes at higher doses. ISA may occasionally be useful for those with bradycardia and limited tolerance for other β-blockers. Side effects profiles for β-blockers are remarkably similar despite theoretical differences.

Table A1-6. Angiotensin Converting Enzyme (ACE) Inhibitors[a]

Generic Name	Proprietary Name	Dose Range	Comments
Captopril	Capoten	12.5–100 mg bid	SH group; half-life 3–6 hours; can be given sublingually; very low doses may be effective in congestive heart failure
Enalapril	Vasotec	2.5–20 mg bid or daily IV 1.25–5 mg bolus	Prodrug; available in intravenous formulation as enalaprilat
Lisinopril	Prinivil, Zestril	5–40 mg/day	Less absorbtion, but longer duration of action than enalapril
Fosinopril	Monopril	10–40 mg/day	PO$_2$ group and prodrug; hepatic and renal elimination; half-life 11–12 hours
Quinapril	Accupril	10–80 mg/day	Prodrug; long duration of action; renal elimination
Benazepril	Lotensin	10–40 mg/day	Prodrug, similar to enalapril
Ramipril	Altace	2.5–20 mg/day	Prodrug; little difference from others

[a]ACE inhibitors differ from each other in their structure and pharmacokinetics. However, their actions as antihypertensive agents are remarkably similar. Except for captopril, they can be given once or twice daily. Cough is the most common adverse effect for all. Angioneurotic edema, within a few weeks of initiation, is rare, but seems to be a class effect. When added to diuretic therapy or α-blockers, low doses should be started to avoid hypotension. Potassium-sparing diuretics should not be given in combination with ACE inhibitors.

Table A1-7. Calcium Channel Entry Blockers[a]

Generic Name	Proprietary Name	Dose Range	Comments
Nondihydropyridines[b]			
Verapamil	Calan, Isoptin	40–120 tid	Short acting form; negative inotropic and chronotropic efffects; heart block, conduction defects may occur; constipation is common
Verapamil	Calan SR, Isoptin SR, Verelan	120–360 mg/ day	Long-acting, once-a-day formulations
Diltiazem	Cardizem	30–90 mg tid	Short-acting dose form; less myocardial effect than verapamil; occasional gastrointestinal disturbance, rash
Diltiazem	Cardizem SR	90–120 mg bid	Slow-release form for bid dosing
Diltiazem	Cardizem CD, Dilacor	180–360 mg/ day	Once-a-day formulations
Dihydropyridine calcium entry blockers[c]			
Nifedipine	Adalat, Procardia	10–30 mg tid	Short-acting dose form; frequent vasodilator adverse effects and edema
Nifedipine	Procardia XL, Adalat CC	30–90 mg/day	Once-a-day formulations; fewer vasodilator symptoms; edema most frequent side effect
Isradipine	Dynacirc	5–20 mg bid	Similar actions to nifedipine
Nicardipine	Cardine	20–40 mg tid	Pharmacologically more vasoselective than nifedipine; similar clinical effects
Nicardipine	Cardine SR	30–60 mg bid	Longer acting formulation
Felodipine	Plendil	10–40 mg/day	Highly vasoselective
Amlodipine	Norvasc	10–40 mg/day	Also vasoselective; long duration of action (>24 hr)

[a]As a class, the calcium channel blockers are vasodilators with or without effects on cardiac function. They are equally effective in various ethnic groups. As a group, they may be more effective, at lower doses, in patients >65 years, as monotherapy. All calcium blockers work well with ACE inhibitors, but to a varying extent with diuretics. The major symptomatic adverse effect is peripheral edema, which is not due to fluid retention.

[b]The nondihydropyridine calcium channel blockers impair cardiac conduction and ventricular contractility. They (especially verapamil) should not be given in combination with β-blockers.

[c]Dihydropyridine calcium channel blockers are almost pure vasodilators. Reflex tachycardia may occur and can be well controlled by β-blockers.

Table A1-8. Older Vasodilator Agents

Generic Name	Proprietary Name	Dose Range	Comments
Hydralazine	Apresoline	25–100 mg tid	Reactive tachycardia, fluid retention; useful in pregnancy due to safety record; frequent adverse effects: angina, systemic lupus erythematosus syndrome, neuropathy
Minoxidil	Loniten	5–20 mg bid	Very potent vasodilator; causes reflex tachycardia, fluid retention, hair growth; almost always given with diuretic and β-blocker
Diazoxide	Hyperstat	150–300 mg IV bolus	Only for hypertensive crises; reflex tachycardia, fluid retention, hyperglycemia

Table A1-9. Antihypertensive Drugs Not Approved by the Food and Drug Administration for Use as Antihypertensive Agents in the United States as of April 1, 1994

Agent	Comment
Bunazosin, Indoramin	α_1-Antagonists, similar to prazosin
Bethanidine, Deprisoquine	Neuron depletors, similar to guanadrel
Oxprenolol	β-Blocker, similar to metoprolol
Sotalol	β-Blocker, *approved in the United States only for refractory angina; associated with fatal arrhythmias*
Perindopril and others	Angiotensin converting enzyme inhibitors available outside the United States
Ketanserin	Serotonin receptor antagonist with central action, may also have α-receptor antagonism
Pinacidil	Vasodilator, similar to minoxidil—opens potassium ion channels
Nitrendipine, nisoldipine	Dihydropyridine calcium channel entry blockers, similar to nifedipine

Appendix 2

DIAGNOSTIC TESTS

The tests described in this section are those that can be performed in a clinic or office and can help, when combined with other assessments, to solve several of the diagnostic problems that often or occasionally emerge in the evaluation of hypertensive patients. I have included those tests that can now be undertaken using currently available technologies in many clinical reference laboratories. Normal ranges are given based on standard assays used in the Mount Sinai Hospital clinical laboratories and in agreement with those of other facilities. There remain a number of specialized assessments that are best conducted in research centers by clinical scientists with expertise in those areas.

SUPPLEMENTAL BLOOD PRESSURE MEASUREMENT

Ambulatory Blood Pressure Monitoring

Usual Indications

The indications for ambulatory blood pressure monitoring include (1) suspicion that the clinic pressure over- or underestimates average pressure, (2) determination of diurnal pattern of pressure, and (3) unexplained syncope-like symptoms where hypotension is suspected.

Method

Patients arrive at the test area in the morning, 8 to 10 AM. After the patient is comfortably seated, the procedure is explained by the nurse or technician. An appropriately sized cuff is snugly placed on the nondominant (less used) arm. Three separate pressures are taken by the monitor connected to a mercury manometer for comparison. The *average* monitor and manual pressures should agree within 5 mmHg. The monitor is then set to record pressures every 15 to 20 minutes during awake periods (usually 7:00 AM to 11:00 PM) and every 30 minutes during usual sleep hours. The patients are instructed to record their activity, especially hours of work, home, bedtime, awakening, and unusual activity or stress. Most monitors are not accurate with the arm in motion; patients are told to rest the arm or keep it still and at heart level during pressure recording.

Editing and Interpretation

Monitor recordings are now processed by software to give the following information: systolic pressure, diastolic pressure, mean arterial pressure, and heart rate. Standard deviations for pressures and heart rate are calculated. These are averaged for (1) 24 hours, (2) estimated awake time, and (3) estimated sleep time. Some programs also provide (1) hourly pressure and heart rate averages and (2) graphic display of the 24-hour pattern or histograms of frequency of pressure during various intervals. Usually a list of "error" readings is given. The opportunity to hand edit presumed outlier readings is often available.

Our group has chosen to omit hand editing of outlier readings and accept those permitted by the software restrictions. We rely primarily on the following for interpretation: average awake pressures, average sleep pressures, and the ratio of awake/sleep pressures. Ordinarily we consider as normal an awake average pressure of less than 135/85 mmHg and an awake/sleep ratio of more than 1.05. Definite hypertension is present if the daytime average is 140/90 mmHg or higher. See Chapter 6 for further information on these issues.

Home Blood Pressure Determination

Indications

The indications for determination of home blood pressure include borderline office or clinic pressures and the inability to use ambulatory blood pressure monitoring.

Method

Many patients buy sphygmomanometers and, with varying degrees of enthusiasm and obsessiveness, take their own blood pressure or have a companion take it. The devices range from mercury manometers and stethoscopes to semiautomatic, battery-powered units that print the results. The devices should be tested for accuracy concurrently with a mercury manometer by a well-trained individual. Patients need counseling and instruction if they are going to take their pressures at home. They are then trained to use the device and record, in an orderly fashion, the date and time of each measurement and their systolic pressure, diastolic pressure, and heart rate. A printed form is useful. We explain the need for *enough recordings to establish a meaningful average* for interpretation. Usually two recordings in the morning and evening for 5 separate days over a 2-week period is adequate, giving a total of 20 recordings for calculation of average pressures and standard deviations. Calculations are easily made using spreadsheet software (e.g., *Lotus 1-2-3* or *Excel*).

Interpretation

In general, average home pressures are compared using the same standards as clinic pressure; for the diagnosis of hypertension, the dividing points are 140 mmHg for systolic and 90 mmHg for diastolic pressure. Some patients can guide their own therapy using home pressures. If a new treatment has no effect on home pressures, drug titration can be made over the phone. I prefer an *average* of at least 10 home readings to compare with a baseline before adjustment of medication. Finally, one or two elevated readings at home usually means little. Some patients call in because a single reading is elevated, having been taken after a stressful event or minor medical illness (e.g., tension headache). Some education and counseling may be needed, but such patients are often among the "worried well," and rarely is there a significant change in their medical status.

CLINICAL ASSESSMENT OF THE RENIN-ALDOSTERONE SYSTEM

Renin Profiling

Still somewhat controversial, the renin profile with concurrent measurement of plasma aldosterone provides a screening assessment that includes a prognosis, pathogenetic basis for hypertension with implications for treatment, and a beginning in the detection of secondary hypertension. It is best performed early in the evaluation of patients, before starting drug treatment.

Method

Patients are advised to avoid excess dietary salt (salt shaker and salty foods) for 1 week before the profile. They are to collect a 24-hour urine specimen in a washed, water-rinsed bottle, starting the day before coming to the clinic and concluding on the day of the visit. The visit is scheduled from morning to midday. A venous blood sample is obtained for plasma renin activity and aldosterone concentration determinations; serum electrolytes are repeated if necessary.

The blood samples for renin activity and aldosterone are immediately sent to the testing laboratory with a fraction of the urine collection. Measurements of plasma renin activity and aldosterone concentration are interpreted by comparison to normal values as related to 24-hour sodium excretion. Other fractions of the urine collection can be used for other tests, if indicated, such as metanephrine excretion, free cortisol, microalbumin excretion, total protein excretion, or creatinine clearance.

Interpretation

When the urine sodium excretion is between 100 and 150 mmol/24 hr, interpretation of the renin-aldosterone profile is most accurate. The relationship between renin and aldosterone is necessary, rather than use of either one separately. Table A2-1 provides a basis for classification into nine potential groups based on low, normal, or high for either plasma renin activity or aldosterone.

Table A2-1. Interpretation of Renin-Aldosterone Profile Studies[a]

Aldosterone Level	PRA Low (<0.8 ng/ml/hr)	PRA Normal (0.9–5.0 ng/ml/hr)	PRA High (≥5.0 ng/ml/hr)
Low (<10 ng/dl)	Nonaldosterone mineralocorticoid excess	Unresponsive aldosterone? nonmodulator	Aldosterone deficiency; possible enzyme defect or adrenal insufficiency
Normal (10–30 ng/dl)	Low renin essential hypertension	Normal renin hypertension	Some high renin hypertension
High (≥30 ng/dl)	Primary aldosteronism	Rarely found, may indicate prolonged adrenal stimulation by angiotensin	High-renin state with secondary aldosteronism, rule out renal artery stenosis

[a]Ranges for plasma renin activity (PRA) and plasma aldosterone concentration are given for 24-hour urine sodium of 100–150 mmol.

Captopril or Angiotensin Converting Enzyme Inhibitor Tests for Secondary Hypertension

A more detailed analysis of the role of the renin-aldosterone system for blood pressure control and diagnosis of possible secondary hypertension can be provided by assessing the blood pressure and renin and aldosterone responses to angiotensin converting enzyme (ACE) inhibition by either oral captopril or intravenous enalapril. The test described in the following paragraphs is designed to be used for detection of either renal artery stenosis or primary aldosteronism.

Method

Patients should be withdrawn from antihypertensive medication for 1 week and allowed a moderate salt intake (100 to 150 mmol/day of sodium). A 24-hour urine collection, starting the day before the test, should be brought to the laboratory or clinic (see previous section). A light fluid breakfast is allowed, without caffeinated beverages. Tests are usually performed between 8:00 and 10:00 AM. Patients are placed in a comfortable, semiupright position. Preparation is made for noninvasive blood pressure measurements every 10 minutes and repeated venous blood samples (placement of an indwelling intravenous catheter). After a 60-minute baseline period, blood samples for plasma renin activity and aldosterone determinations are obtained (a blood sample for plasma 18-OH corticosterone should be included if primary aldosterone is under consideration). The patient is given captopril, 25 to 50 mg by mouth (as an option, 2.5 mg enalaprilat may be given intravenously). The tablet may be briefly dissolved in water a few minutes before swallowing to speed absorption. Repeat blood samples are obtained 1 hour after captopril or enalapril. Blood pressure measurements continue for the postcaptopril period for another hour.

Caution: The captopril test may lead to excessive hypotension in high renin elderly patients with impaired cardiovascular reflexes or in those who are hypovolemic due to excessive diuresis or taking α_1-receptor blockers.

Interpretation

Most patients will have a decrease in blood pressure of 10 to 20 percent, with the nadir at about 60 minutes after a single dose of captopril by mouth or enalapril intravenously. Those with high baseline renin states (e.g., unilateral renal artery stenosis) tend to have greater reductions in pressure to 30 percent; patients with very low renin levels, such as in primary aldosteronism, will have little change in pressure. The blood pressure response should be related to both the baseline and post-ACE inhibitor plasma renin activity and aldosterone concentration. In general, high renin states (baseline plasma renin activity 3 ng/ml/hr or higher) are characterized by (1) a greater fall in blood pressure, (2) higher baseline plasma renin activity, (3) a two- to fivefold increase in plasma renin activity, and (4) a 25 to 50 percent fall in plasma aldosterone. The low renin states have (1) little change in pressure (less than 10 percent/decrease), (2) low baseline plasma renin activity (less than 0.8 ng/ml/hr), (3) little increase in plasma renin activity after ACE inhibition, and (4) little change in plasma aldosterone concentration. In primary aldosteronism due to a functioning adrenal adenoma, there is either no change in plasma aldosteronce concentration or a small reduction. Patients with no change in aldosterone are thought to have adenomas responsive to adrenocorticotropic hormone but not to angiotensin II.

As described in Chapters 6 and 10, the accuracy of the captopril test, using the post-captopril renin level and the percentage of increase in plasma renin to detect renal artery stenosis, is variable from series to series (sensitivity, 70 to 90-plus percent; specificity, 70 to 90 percent overall). Of patients with high renin essential hypertension, about 30 to 40 percent will have positive captopril tests, based on renin criteria.[1] It is clear that additional tests are needed to confirm or exclude renal artery stenosis as a cause of reversible hypertension.

In primary aldosteronism due to a functioning adrenal adenoma, either there is no change in plasma aldosterone concentration or a small reduction. Patients with no change in aldosterone are thought to have adenomas responsive to adrenocorticotropic hormone but not responsive to angiotensin II.

The integrated responses of arterial pressure, plasma renin activity, and plasma aldosterone after ACE inhibition provide a dynamic view of the renin system's participation in control of arterial pressure rather than a specific diagnosis. The results, taken together with all relevant clinical information, should provide guidance to the next diagnostic or therapeutic steps.

Postural Responses of the Renin-Aldosterone System

Postural responses of the renin-aldosterone system may also be used for characterization of the system and has been used as an alternative to the captopril test.

Method

Patients are best studied off of antihypertensive medication and with a salt intake of 100 to 150 mmol/day. the patient should arrive at the study area between 7:30 and 8:00 AM and is placed in a supine position; an indwelling venous catheter is placed for blood samples. After the patient has been supine for 60 minutes, a blood sample is obtained for plasma renin activity and plasma aldosterone determinations. The patient is then allowed to be upright—seated, standing, or walking—for 3 hours, and then must return to the clinic for the second blood sample. If primary aldosterone is being considered, supine and upright blood samples for plasma cortisol and 18-OH corticosterone should be included.

Interpretation

Normally plasma renin activity and plasma aldosterone increase about twofold from the supine to upright position. The increase from a high baseline level (3.0 ng/ml/hr or higher) is often three- to fourfold in high-renin states (e.g., renal artery stenosis). In low-renin states, there is little change with the upright position. In most, but not all, patients with aldosterone-producing adenomas, plasma aldosterone falls in parallel with cortisol, after the 3 hours of upright posture, suggesting that the adenoma is mainly responsive to adrenocorticotropic hormone. Furthermore, the baseline plasma aldosterone level is usually 30 ng/dl or more and the plasma 18-OH corticosterone level is 50 ng/dl or more. Perhaps 20 percent of patients with aldosterone-producing adenomas have no change or an increase in plasma aldosterone with standing, possibly reflecting a persistant responsiveness to angiotensin II.

CLINICAL ASSESSMENT OF ADRENERGIC FUNCTION

Plasma Catecholamine Reponses to Posture

Occasionally, it is necessary to determine whether the function of the sympathetic nervous system, as reflected by its neurotransmitter norepinephrine and its adrenomedullary hormone epinephrine, is abnormal. Measurement of supine and upright plasma catecholamine levels is the usual approach to this issue.

Method

Patients are prepared as for the posture studies of the renin-aldosterone system. Antihypertensive medications are discontinued, as are other drugs that might alter adrenergic function. The patient should arrive at the study area between 7:30 and 8:00 AM and is placed in a supine position; an indwelling venous catheter is placed for blood samples. After the patient has been supine for 60 minutes, a blood sample is obtained for plasma catecholamine (norepinephrine and epinephrine) determination. The patients then stands upright for 10 minutes, and a second blood sample is obtained.

Table A2-2. Normal Plasma Catecholamine Concentrations

Plasma Catecholamines (pg/ml)	Supine	Standing
Norepinephrine	150–600	300–1200
Epinephrine	0–50	10–80

Interpretation

The normal ranges for the plasma catecholamines are given in Table A2-2. With standing, there is a twofold increase in plasma norepinephrine level and a 50-percent increase in plasma epinephrine level. Excessive increases in these hormones usually reflect hypovolemia. High baseline plasma norepinephrine levels (600 to 1500 pg/ml) may be observed in some hypertensive persons, those with excessive anxiety, or those in cardiac failure. Baseline plasma norepinephrine levels above 2000 pg/ml strongly suggest pheochromocytoma. By contrast, low plasma norepinephrine (less than 150 ng/ml) with little or no response to standing suggests peripheral autonomic failure.

Clonidine Suppression Test

The clonidine suppression test is used primarily for diagnosis of pheochromocytoma. It is most useful when supine plasma catecholamine concentrations are between 600 and 2000 pg/ml (i.e., the upper limit of normal and below the level usually found in pheochromocytomas.

Method

Ideally the patient should be withdrawn from antihypertensive drugs, but may continue α-blockers if necessary for prevention of hypertensive episodes. The patient is prepared as for postural studies by placement in the supine position with an indwelling intravenous catheter placed for blood samples. We routinely monitor blood pressure and heart rate every 10 minutes throughout the study. After the patient has been supine for 60 minutes, two baseline blood samples, 10 minutes apart are obtained. Then the patient swallows 0.3 mg clonidine with 30 to 60 ml water. The patient is kept supine. Blood samples are taken 2 and 3 hours after the clonidine. All samples are analyzed for plasma norepinephrine and epinephrine.

Caution: It is not unusual for patients to fall asleep for 30 to 60 minutes after clonidine. Blood pressure usually falls 10 to 20 percent with a lesser decrease in heart rate. At the end of the study, patients may have orthostatic dizzyness, feel unusually fatigued, and notice a dry mouth. These symptoms cease within another 30 to 60 minutes.

Interpretation

Patients with a normal sympathetic nervous system have a greater than 40 percent decrease in plasma norepinephrine 2 to 3 hours after clonidine. Normal suppression is observed in persons with essential hypertension and high baseline plasma catecholamine levels and in patients with the panic disorder syndrome. A reduction of less than 20 percent in the plasma norepinephrine level strongly suggests defective suppression most likely due to autonomous production of catecholamines by a chromaffin tumor (i.e., pheochromocytoma).

Glucagon Stimulation Test

Administration of glucagon to normal subjects and to patients with essential hypertension has little effect on plasma norepinephrine concentration, but plasma epinephrine may double. By contrast, patients with pheochromocytoma may have a substantial increase in plasma norepinephrine concentration. The glucagon stimulation test is the most useful test for detection of pheochromocytoma when this tumor is suspected but neither urinary catecholamine metabolites nor plasma catecholamine concentrations are elevated. This is most likely to occur in two situations: (1) asymptomatic family members of patients with either multiple endocrine neoplasia type II or one of the "birthmark" syndromes[2] or (2) incidentally found adrenal tumors in which other endocrine disorders have been excluded.

Method

We recommend reserving the glucagon stimulation test for patients suspected of pheochromocytoma with nondiagnostic urinary excretion of metanephrine or VMA and normal or borderline high levels of plasma norephinephrine. Antihypertensive drugs, except for α-blockers, are withheld on the test day. Phentolamine (Regitine) should be available for intravenous injection (5 mg in a syringe) in case a hypertensive crisis occurs after glucagon administration.

Patients should be in a comfortable supine position. An intravenous catheter is placed in a forearm vein and the blood pressure is measured in the opposite arm. During a control period of 30 minutes, the blood pressure and heart rate are taken every 10 minutes. Two blood samples for plasma catecholamine concentration (norepinephrine and epinephrine) are obtained 15 minutes and 5 minutes before glucagon is given. At the end of the baseline period, 1 mg of glucagon is given by rapid intravenous bolus. Repeat blood samples are obtained 1 and 2 minutes after the glucagon injection, with concurrent measurement of blood pressure and heart rate. If the blood pressure increases significantly (to greater than 180 mmHg systolic or to greater than 120 mmHg diastolic pressure), phentolamine should be injected to reverse the hypertensive crisis. The clonidine suppression test described above may be performed on the same day, at least 1 hour after the glucagon test. A repeat baseline period is necessary before giving the clonidine.

Interpretation

A recent large series from the National Institutes of Health describes a positive glucagon test as the combination of a post-glucagon plasma norepinephrine concentration that is greater than 2,000 pg/ml *and* an increase in plasma norepinephrine that is greater than 200 percent.[3] This occurred in 77 percent of patients with pheochromocytoma and in only 1.4 percent of those without the tumor. The value of the test was greatest in patients with a baseline plasma norepinephrine concentration of 500 to 1,500 pg/ml.

REFERENCES

1. Gerber LM, Mann SJ, Muller FB et al: Response to the captopril test is dependent on baseline renin profile. J Hypertens 12:173, 1994

2. Aprill BS, Drake AJ III, Lasseter DH, Shakir KM: Silent adrenal nodules in von Hippel-Lindau disease suggest pheochromocytoma. Ann Intern Med 120:485, 1994

3. Grossman E, Goldstein DS, Hoffman A, Keiser HR: Glucagon and clonidine testing in the diagnosis of pheochromocytoma. Hypertension 17:733, 1991

INDEX

Page numbers followed by *f* indicate figures; those followed by *t* indicate tables.